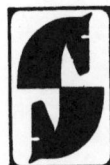

Shinji Takahashi

An Atlas of Axial Transverse Tomography and its Clinical Application

With 576 Figures

Springer-Verlag Berlin Heidelberg GmbH 1969

SHINJI TAKAHASHI, M. D.
Professor of Radiology, Nagoya University School of Medicine,
Showaku, Nagoya, Japan

ISBN 978-3-642-85565-8   ISBN 978-3-642-85563-4 (eBook)
DOI 10.1007/978-3-642-85563-4

Preface

In spring this year it will be 23 years since I began to study rotation technique as applied to radiology. In applying this technique to roentgenography the name Rotation Radiography was adopted publicly in 1946. Since then this study has revealed that the technique is valuable not only in diagnosis but also in radiotherapy, and the name Conformation Radiotherapy was publicly announced in 1960.

Through these studies it became clear that it is possible to show the axial transverse cross section of the human body roentgenographically, which could be of great value medically, but it was realized that no detailed roentgenograms of the axial transverse cross section covering the whole of the normal human adult have been published so far. To prepare an atlas was therefore considered basic for the practical application of this method, since without it further developments of this type of roentgenography cannot be expected. Consequently it was decided first to prepare the atlas. In addition, the clinical application of this method to the diagnostic and therapeutic field was described with brief notes on the essential features of the method.

This work was planned a few years ago, but actual work commenced in September 1966. A further year was spent in the preparation of the manuscript, and its publication was made possible by the help of numerous coworkers. The preparation of the axial transverse tomograms has been our direct responsibility, but the revision of the anatomical diagrams drawn by us was made by courtesy of Dr. *Seiho Nishi*, Professor Emeritus of Anatomy, Tokyo University. The preparation of this book was made possible by the help of members of our Department staffs, especially of Drs. *T. Sasaki*, *S. Sakuma* and *A. Takeuchi*. In addition, Drs. *F. Hayashi*, *K. Ban*, *K. Hiramatsu*, *Y. Ayakawa*, *T. Fujita*, *T. Kato*, *S. Koga*, *Y. Tanaka* and others cooperated in the preparation of the respective figures, Mr. *K. Ito* in the conduct of the radiography, Mr. *R. Ando* in the preparation of the photographs, Mr. *H. Maekoshi* in the drawing of the anatomical figures and Miss *T. Nishikawa* in the arrangement and printing of the original manuscripts. Dr. *K. Morita* of the Czerny Krankenhaus, Heidelberg, kept in close contact with the publisher to expedite the printing. Dr. *T. Oyama* undertook the labors of translating one part of the manuscript from Japanese to English.

For the final decision of publication by Springer-Verlag, Professor *O. Olsson*, Lund, kindly gave recommendations and advice to me and the publisher.

I wish to take this opportunity to express my deep appreciation to all these persons.

Nagoya, May 1969 *Shinji Takahashi*

Contents

Introduction

Knowledge of roentgenological anatomy is essential in roentgen diagnosis, as only when the normal state of the human body is known can abnormal, i.e. pathological findings be ascertained roentgenologically.

As for the axial transverse tomography, *de Abreau* (1), *Amisano* (4, 6), *Duhamel* et al. (19), *Frain* et al. (24—26, 28), *Gebauer* and *Wachsmann* (32), *Gebauer* (33), *Justztusz* (47), *de Maestri* (59), *Shimazaki* (117, 116), *Stevenson* (119,) *Takahashi* (121, 122, 126, 128), *Takahashi* et al. (123, 124, 129), *Vieten* (161), *Watson* (167) and especially *Vallebona* (147—158) have worked as pioneers in determining the fundamentals of this method of roentgenography or in applying this method to roentgen diagnosis.

In several European countries this roentgenographic method was developed from tomography, while in Japan it grew out of rotation radiography rather than the method of tomography.

The terms of this method thus differed individually, but in accordance with the recommendation of ICRU (1962) (p. 15, NBS Handbook 80) the term "axial transverse tomography" may perhaps be the most fitting.

This method is useful not only for diagnosis but also in undertaking treatment, especially in the field of radiotherapy, as it is necessary to know accurately and concretely the state of the lesion in the body, to set up an irradiation plan and to confirm whether or not the plan is being carried out properly. Such planning and confirmation are difficult to carry out by means of existing radiography methods alone. Axial transverse tomography can solve these problems, and thus it is believed that it should be used more widely in the fields of roentgen diagnosis and radiotherapy.

Monographs on axial transverse tomography, by *Bonte* et al. (169), *Farr* et al. (170), *Gebauer* et al. (171), *Gebauer* et al. (172), *Takahashi* (173—175), *Vallebona* et al. (176), *Vallebona* (177), total nine as far as I could collect, but these are mostly concerned with the diagnosis of chest diseases, though *Gebauer's* work contains good descriptions of almost all parts of the body.

In axial transverse tomography, despite the promise of wide clinical application, there is no monograph that explains systematically and clearly the roentgenological anatomy of every part of the body.

At present, when applying axial transverse tomography to all areas of the body for medical purposes, there is no other way but to refer to existing atlases illustrating anatomical cross sections of such regions prepared from cadavers. The books by *Doyen* et al. (178), *Hovelacque* et al. (179), *Nishi* et al. (180, 181), *Pernkopf* (182), *Roy-Camille* (183) and *Eycleshymer* (184) are listed in the bibliography. Distortion is sometimes seen in the figures due to their preparation post mortem. Further, some troubles arise because there is no way to refer the roentgen findings to the whole cadaver because the relevant roentgenogram is missing. In addition, an atlas containing cross-section figures of all parts of the human body in systematic order with thin layers of cross section is not usually obtainable even as an anatomical atlas.

These are the direct reasons for the publication of our monograph which takes as its subject the living standard adult.

To prepare the atlas of axial transverse tomograms, the level to be imaged should be determined as accurately as possible as, when the level in relation to the body axis at which the section is made moves even slightly, the appearance of the sectional figures will differ greatly. Again, unless the atlas of the axial transverse cross section is made systematically by one and the same author, there will be differences in the style of illustrating the axial transverse tomograms. One author will illustrate the figure of the axial transverse cross section right side left or left side right, and the other upside down or down side up, and this will cause confusion in the interpretation of tomograms based on such figures. It is hoped that the preparation of this atlas will contribute to the correction of such defects and drawbacks in existing books.

To avoid guesswork when giving anatomical interpretations of the cross sections, contrast medium was used as often as possible in order to obtain roentgen images of the various viscera and tissues. It was, of course, not possible to prepare roentgenograms of all body regions from the same individual. Needless to say, this was due to consideration of the roentgen dose to which the individual is exposed. The concentrated use of various contrast media was also avoided, as some of these media are not always harmless, and the administration of different contrast media can be a burden to the subject used. In other words, the study could fall into a study for its own sake. In view of the above, the subjects to be examined were made to vary in accordance with the several parts of the body and roentgen images of various organs of the same body region were prepared with or without the use of contrast medium and the diagrams of the anatomical figures were prepared by integration of these images.

Part 1

Axial Transverse Tomography
of the Normal Adult

I. Conduct of Axial Transverse Tomography

A description will be made of the apparatus and of the tomographic procedure used in the preparation of this Atlas.

1. Tomographic Apparatus

Axial transverse tomography has been developed over the last twenty years. After the clinical value of this technique was proved by the pioneers, roentgenographic units for taking axial transverse tomograms have been commercially manufactured in Italy, France and Germany, and soon after in Japan. Most of this apparatus was of the type for taking tomograms of sitting or standing patients, e.g. axial transverse tomograph of erect type. In addition to this type, a unit for taking tomograms of lying patients, axial transverse tomograph of horizontal type, was suggested as superior to the erect type by *Janker* (45) and *Takahashi* (121, 128, 175), and a unit of this type has been manufactured since 1950 and is widely used in Japan.

Roentgenography here was carried out by an axial transverse tomograph of horizontal type. The patient is made to lie still on the tomography table while the roentgen tube and film are rotated around the patient from 0° to 360°. This apparatus was originally designed and manufactured to work with the range of rotation from 0° to 210°. Although a perfect image is obtained with the range of rotation of 360° (*Oliva* (83), *Bonte* et al. (169), *Frik* (29)), the range of rotation of 210° also provides good tomograms, suitable for clinical practice, when the following technique is applied as described below (*Takahashi* (124, 129)).

A. Roentgenography of Every Part of the Body

The tomographic table is made of wood and is 30 cm wide, 5.4 cm thick and 354 cm long. The rotation axis of the unit is approximately 12 cm above the surface of the tomography table. The position of the plane g to be cross sectioned, i.e. to be tomographed, is specific to the apparatus and is about 142.5 cm from the end of the table to which the tomography unit is attached. The plane g is the place where the lights converge from projectors located on both walls and on the bar of the support of the roentgen tube (T_1) for tomography. Hence, the part of the subject to be tomographed is easily adjusted to this plane g by means of the light projectors (Figs. 1 and 2).

The tomography table is approximately 2 times the length of the human body, so it is possible to place any part of the body on plane g with ease. With a unit of the erect type, it is usually difficult to take an axial transverse tomogram of every part of the body, though there is a paper on examination of the extremities made by means of this type of tomograph (*Lacroix* (51)).

In axial transverse tomography a normal roentgenogram of the body part to be tomographed is also taken with the patient in the same posture. On this normal roentgenogram the axial transverse level of the body at which the tomography is made should be clearly indicated. The location of the plane g crosses the focus of the roentgen tube T_2 fixed to the ceiling, while the cassette holder B is placed horizontally below the table. On the front cover of the cassette, either right across or halfway across, a lead line is placed to meet or coincide with the plane g. Directly before or after the axial transverse tomography, a normal roentgenogram of the part of the body being tomographed is taken with roentgen tube T_2 and film B.

When the subject to be examined lies supine on the bare table, the X-ray absorption rates of the soft tissues of the body are approximately equal to those of the tomography table and cause the contours of the dorsal regions of the body to be indistinct, due to lack of contrast between them. Hence, a cotton mat 3 cm thick is placed on the tomography table. This procedure makes it possible to produce a roentgen image of the entire contour of the cross section of the body by axial transverse tomography.

B. Quality of Image on the Tomogram

In general, the nearer contour of the body imaged on the axial transverse tomogram is too dense and renders interpretation between that part and the ground density of the tomogram difficult. Hence, a moving filter (*Matsuda* (72, 73)) was attached to the radiation mouth of the tube housing. This made the density of the contour and the ground density reasonable and made interpretation easy (Fig. 3).

Next, a wedge grid whose grid ratio is high at one side and low at the opposite side was placed with the high grid ratio close to the body and the grid itself perpendicular to the central X-rays and covering the entire area of the film (*Matsuda* (75)). This helped to remove the fog induced by scattered rays increasing at the parts of the film close to the body, and generally to improve the contrast of the tomograms.

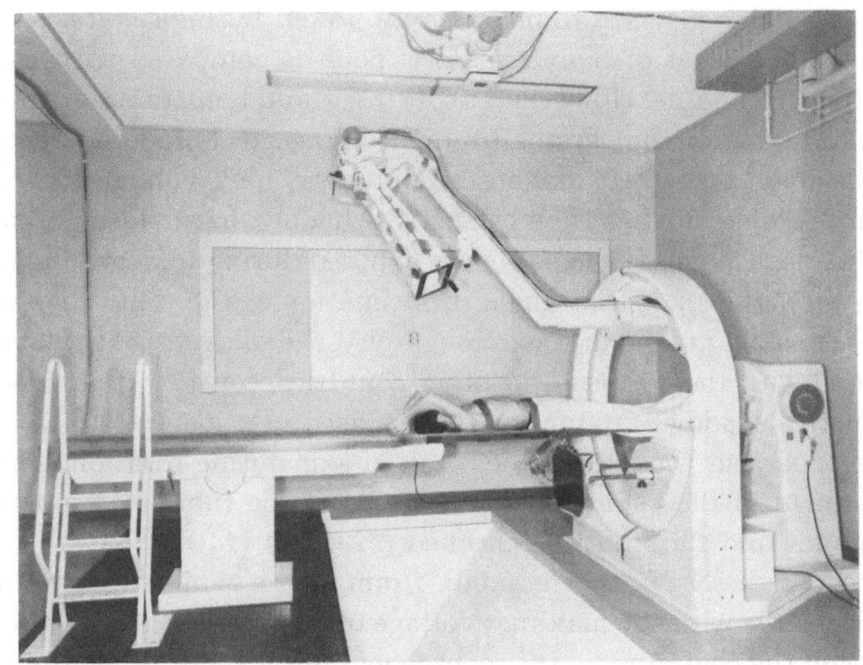

Fig. 1. Axial transverse tomograph of horizontal type (Toshiba) in action

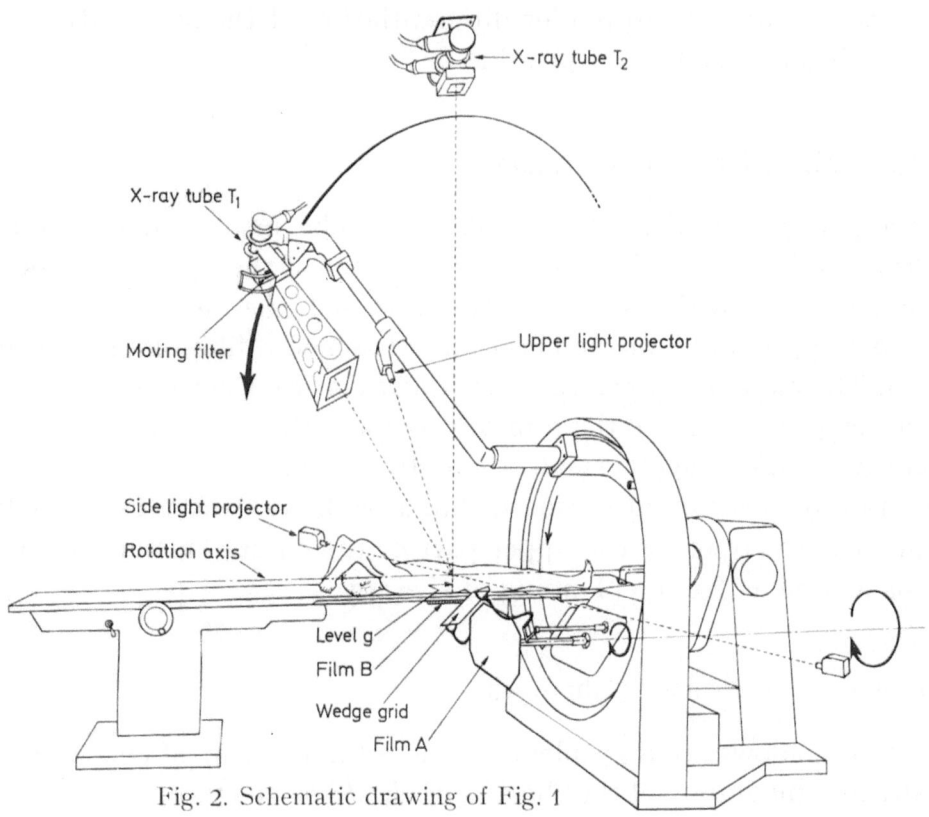

Fig. 2. Schematic drawing of Fig. 1

As these axial transverse tomograms are taken by high voltage technique (125 kVp), the contrast of bony tissues is poor as compared with that taken by low voltage technique. However, as soft tissue and bony tissue are reasonably distinct, the taking of tomograms by high voltage technique does not hinder the establishment of correct diagnoses. Moreover, high voltage technique has the advantage of removing the obstructive shadow, harmonising density and reducing the dose to which the patient is exposed during tomography (*Matsuda* (70), *Takahashi* (138)). As the angle of inclination of the central X-ray to the film is rather small, i.e. 20° in this tomography, the thickness of the layer is thin. As compared with the 30° usual in other countries, contrast of images is lower but obstructive shadows are markedly decreased (*Takahashi* (123)).

In this apparatus the play of the rotation axis during rotation is negligible. The adjustment of the alignment of the focus of the tube, rotation centers of the X-ray unit and the film was checked (*Matsuda* (74)).

The focus of the X-ray tube is small, 1 mm in size, while the capacity of the tube is fairly large with the maximal voltage of 150 kVp. 67 mA for 15 seconds.

As a result the penumbra of the roentgenograms is small, while the sharpness of the image is very good. Even with such a small bone as the lingual bone, the images were so sharp as to render differentiation of the substantia compacta from the substantia spongiosa possible.

C. Low Magnification Rate of Image

In this apparatus the distance between the tube focus and rotation axis is 212.5 cm, while that between the rotation center of the apparatus and that of the film is 62.5 cm, with a magnification rate of 1.24 times.

For roentgenography of the chest and abdomen a film of 14×17 inch size was used. The rectangular cassette is cut away at its 4 corners. The cassette is placed as near as possible to the rotation center of the apparatus. As the magnification rate of the image is small, the entire contours of the axial transverse cross section of the normal standard Japanese body can be contained within the film with exception of the upper part of the chest. This is convenient for diagnosis as well as for the planning of therapy.

D. Removal of Obstructive Shadows

Obstructive shadows are a problem for the establishment of correct diagnosis, especially in tomography of the chest (*Takahashi* et al. (130), *Takahashi* (134)).

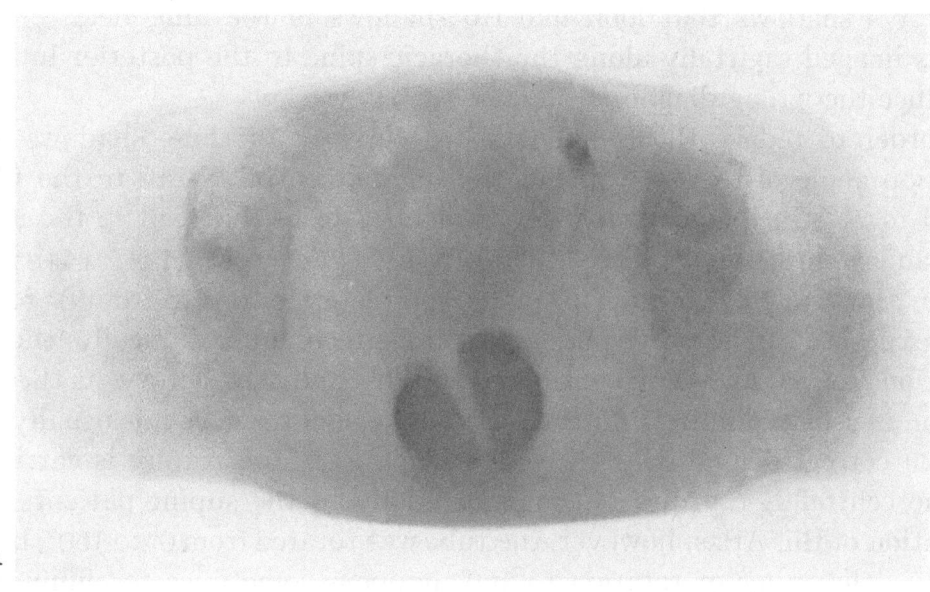

A

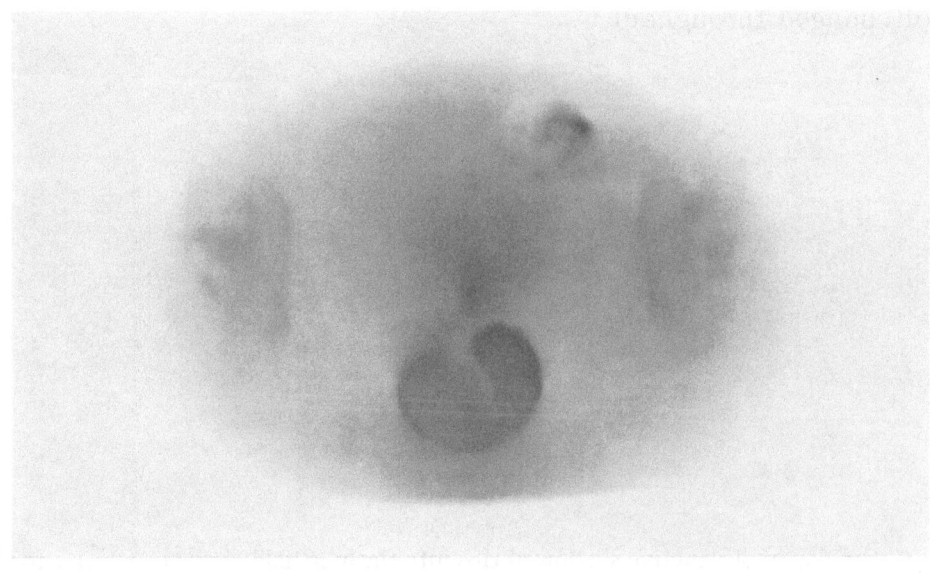

B

Fig. 3 A and B. Axial transverse tomograms of the pelvis at the same level in the same person. A with moving filter. B without moving filter. Entire contour of the body is seen perfectly on A, but imperfectly on B

Obstructive shadows that look like rib shadows in the lung field, or linear shadows imaged sagittally along the thoracic spine to the posterior lung field will induce the wrong diagnosis.

In order to reduce the frequency of occurrence of these shadows a) the inclination angle of the tube (inclination of the central X-ray to the film) is reduced to 20°; b) the central X-ray is inclined from the head to the feet i.e. craniocaudal direction of the central X-ray (*Takeuchi* (143, 144)); c) if possible, the range of rotation is made complete, i.e. rotate from 0° to 360°; and d) exposure is made with the high voltage technique. Clinically, the range of rotation from 0° to 220° is considered suitable and satisfactory, as the size of the room is usually limited and the obstructive shadow does not usually interfere with correct diagnosis, if the axial transverse tomography is carried out with the central X-ray directed craniocaudally to the supine patient. In the preparation of this Atlas, however, the tube was rotated from 0° to 360°, because increasing the range of rotation to 360° happens sometimes to eliminate the obstructive shadows found with 0° to 220° (Fig. 4). Obstructive shadows become practically negligible and it is thus possible to prepare standard illustrations of axial transverse cross sections of the body. In regions other than the chest these obstructive shadows do not usually appear and it is thus not necessary to rotate the tube from 0° to 360°. However, in order to maintain the standardized exposure conditions, the inclination angle of the tube and range of rotation were not changed throughout.

Fig. 4 A—C. Overlap of obstructive shadow of ribs into the lung field. Axial transverse tomograms of the chest at the same level in the same person. A rotation angle of 360°: negligible obstructive shadow (⁄). B rotation angle of 220°, with the craniocaudal direction of central X-ray: slight obstructive shadow (⁄). C rotation angle of 220°, with the caudalocranial direction of central X-ray: excessive obstructive shadow (⁄)

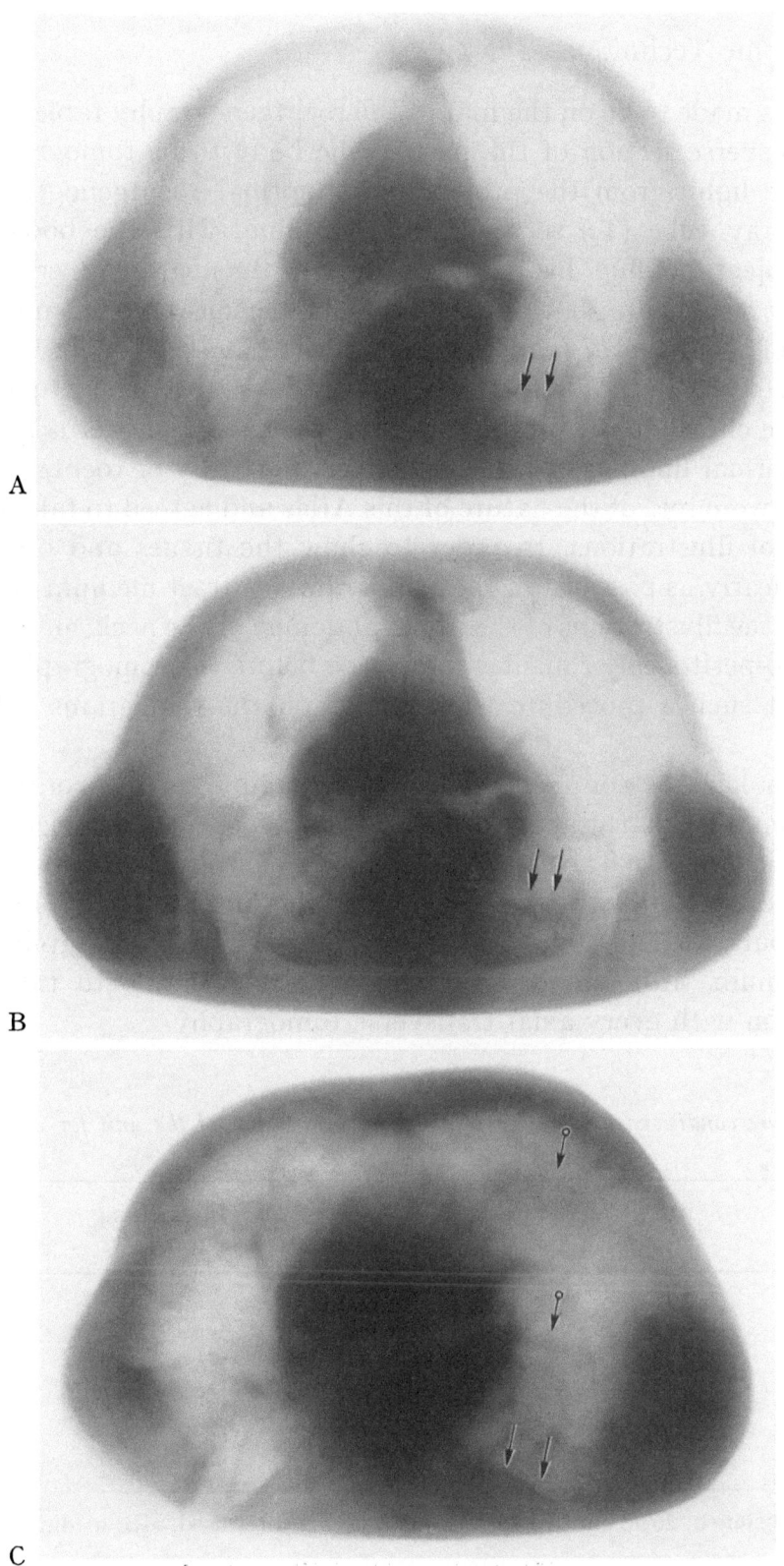

A

B

C

2. Tomographic Technique

The subject is made to lie on the mat of the roentgenography table on his back, and the transverse section of the part of the body to be tomographed is adjusted to the lights from the projectors. A normal roentgenogram is taken with the X-ray tube (T_2) secured to the ceiling, with the body kept still and the subject holding his breath. The roentgenographic conditions for various body regions are shown in Table 1. All persons used as subjects in the illustration of this Atlas are cancer patients who have passed the reproductive age. The parts selected to be tomographed are normal. For example, in tomography of the chest a patient suffering from the cancer of uterus is employed, with no abnormal findings in the chest, either clinically or roentgenologically. The patients were told of the nature of this Atlas and agreed to take part in the preparation of illustrations. In order to show the tissues and organs of the sections as clearly as possible on the tomogram, contrast medium is employed. In preparing the illustrations of the upper abdomen or the neck, air is insufflated into the retro-peritoneal or mediastinal space before the tomography is carried out. Without such a procedure the findings on the tomograms will be very poor.

Radiation hazards for technicians are negligible as the control room is separate from the tomography room. Exposure of patients per transverse tomography is shown in Table 1. In order to reduce the patient dose, the X-ray beams are prevented from protruding beyond the film by the diaphragm of the radiation mouth. Further, the amount of normal roentgenography was kept to the minimum, although it would have been desirable to take one a.p. roentgenogram with every axial transverse tomography.

Table 1. *Exposure conditions and air dose at the rotation center of the unit for one axial transverse tomography*

	kV	mA	sec	Intensifying screens	Air dose (mR)
Head	110	5	15	MS	150
Neck	95	5	15	MS	100
Chest	120	3	15	MS	110
Abdomen	125	10	15	MS	340
Arm	60—65	5	15	MS	35— 43
Leg	70—90	5	15	MS	50—100

Focus film distance: 262.8 cm. Wedge grid and moving filter used. MS: medium speed screen

II. Interpretation of Axial Transverse Tomogram

Up to the present research work on the individual parts of the body in the normal adult has appeared in several papers: axial transverse encephalotomography was studied by *di Chiro* (17), *Takahashi* et al. (131), the head by *Takahashi* et al. (132), the neck by *Takahashi* (133), the chest by *Duhamel* (20), *Gardella* (31), *Gebauer* (34), *Matsuda* (63), *Ono* (87), *Retzepis* (95), the gall bladder by *Imaoka* (44), the stomach and duodenum by *Matsuda* et al. (68), and *Sasaki* (110), the upper abdomen by the pneumoretroperitoneal technique by *de Albertis* (2), *Macarini* et al. (58), *Matsuda* et al. (66) or *Sasaki* (111) and by the pneumoperitoneal technique by *Sato* (113). The axial transverse tomography of the pelvis was reported by *Kubota* et al. (50).

In this Atlas, series of axial transverse tomograms taken for each level of every part of the human body will be illustrated, the illustrations extending across 2 pages for each level.

First, in order to know at what level and how the tomogram is taken, see the top of the right page, where at top left is shown a normal roentgenogram in the anteroposterior view of the subject taken at time of the transverse tomography; the horizontal line drawn through the roentgenogram represents the level at which the tomography is made. At the top right is a diagram, drawn from normal photographs taken in lateral view at time of tomography, which shows the level relative to the body at which the transverse tomography is carried out.

On the left page a tomogram is shown at the top. In the lower part of this page is a tomogram identical with that at the top but developed with less density and retouched, as it is sometimes difficult to reproduce all the details of the original tomogram. However, it should be emphasized here that *in this retouched illustration of the tomogram only the findings actually seen on the original tomogram are drawn.* In other words, there are no imaginary findings on the figure. The anatomical terms are attached to these roentgen findings to facilitate interpretation.

At the bottom of the right page is a diagram showing as faithfully as possible the topographical relation with the axial transverse tomogram. However, as muscles, tendons, nerves etc. do not produce roentgen images, reference was made to existing anatomical atlases (178—184) and these features were inserted, though compared with these anatomical section figures the muscles have been inserted as simply as possible, due to special stress on the practical utility of this Atlas and the desire to avoid as much as possible the insertion by mere conjecture of findings that did not actually appear. Illustrations and diagrams of the tomogram are reduced accurately to one third the size of the original tomogram.

As indicated in the figures, the transverse section figures were prepared as such for this Atlas (Fig. 5). After cutting the body in the supine position at the required levels of body axis, the lower part is removed and the sectional surface of the upper part observed from the horizontal direction.

This arrangement of the illustrations has been our practice since we developed rotation radiography in 1946 (*Takahashi* (174, 175)) for the following clinical reasons: when an interpretation of the axial transverse tomogram is made, the normal roentgenogram with the horizontal line is placed adjacent to the axial transverse tomogram in the viewing box and examined. For convenience of interpretation, the right of the axial transverse cross section view of the body is better placed to the left of the figure, so as to be similar to the normal roentgenogram taken posteroanteriorly.

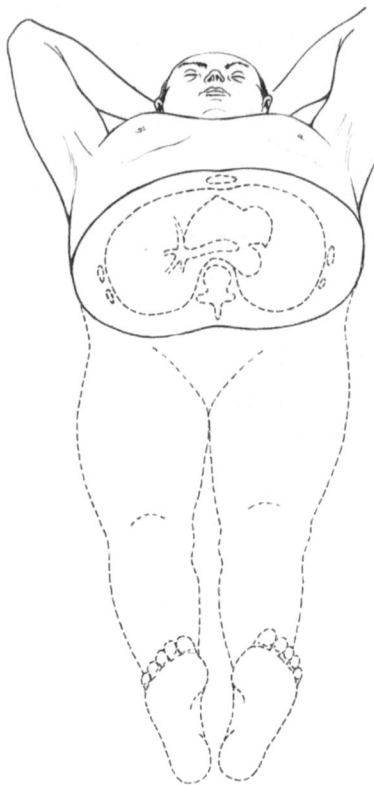

Fig. 5. Schematic drawing of our manner of viewing the axial transverse tomogram. An axial transverse cross section of the upper part of the body is inspected

This manner of viewing the illustration, that is, with the back of the body at the bottom of the illustration, is convenient for planning the positioning of the patient in radiation therapy.

On the following pages, the axial transverse tomograms are arranged in the order of the head, the neck, the chest, the upper abdomen, the female and male lower abdomen, and the arm and the leg.

Appendices are attached to each group of parts of the body in order to add the information which is difficult to include in the relevant illustrations.

Head

Eight axial transverse tomograms,
including encephalotomogram, taken
parallel to the orbitomeatal line

and

Ten axial transverse tomograms, including encephalotomogram, taken
parallel to the acanthiomeatal line.

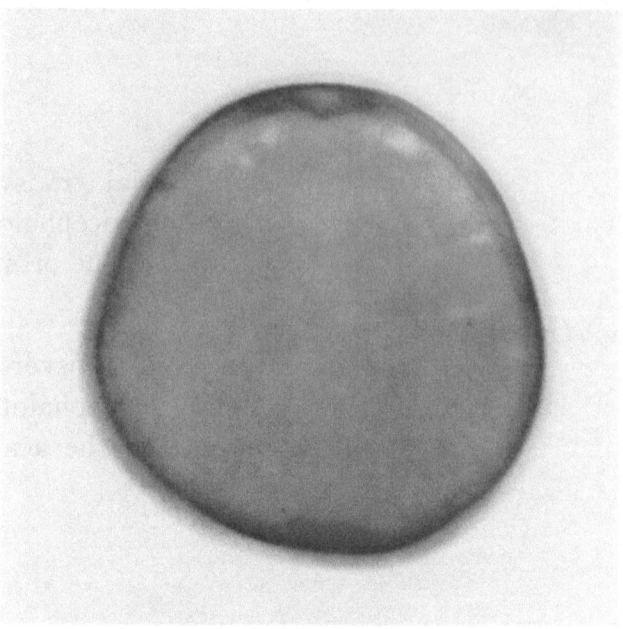

Fig. 6. Axial transverse tomogram

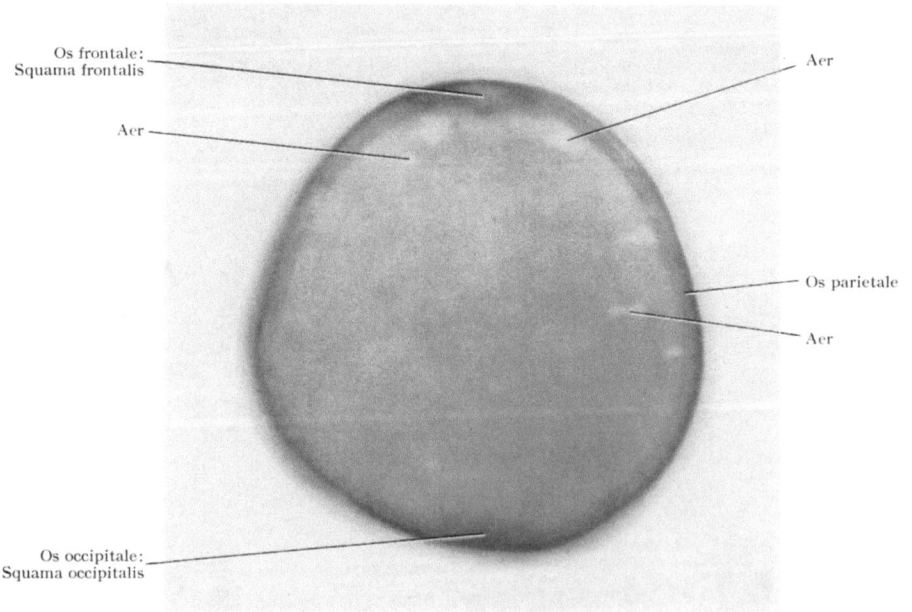

Fig. 7. Interpretation

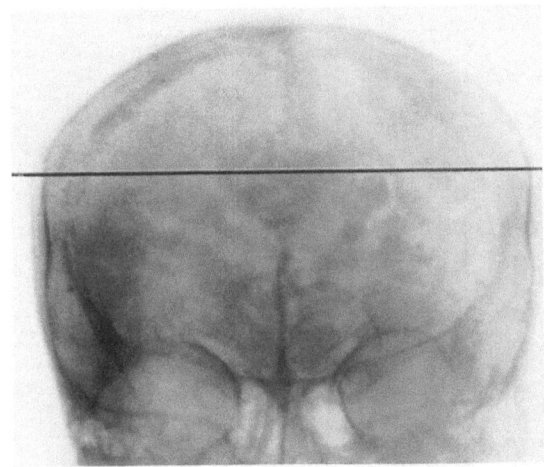

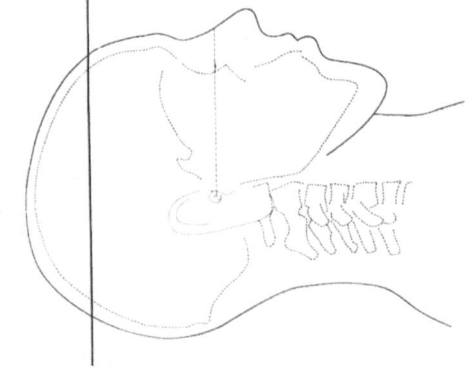

Fig. 8. Normal roentgenogram. Horizontal line showing the level tomographed

Fig. 9. Schema of tomographed level (solid line) 8 cm above the orbitomeatal line (dashed line)

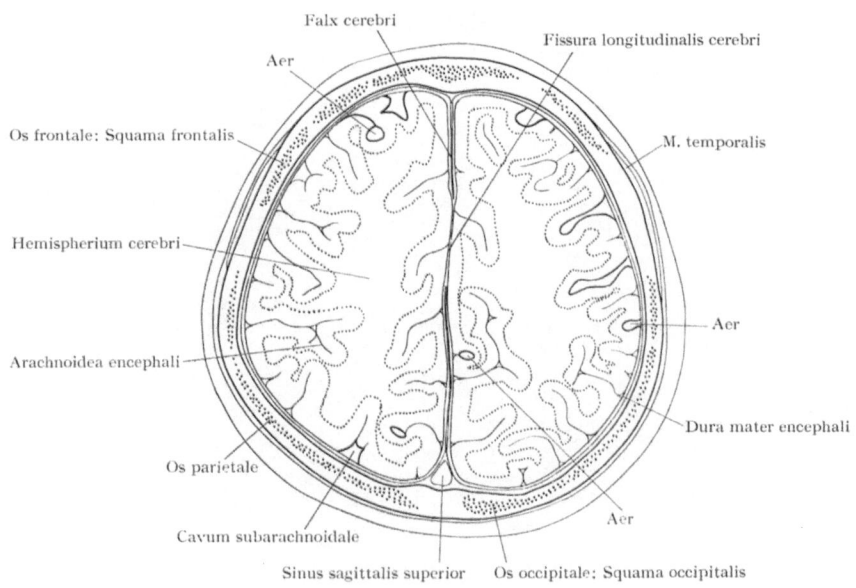

Fig. 10. Anatomical chart

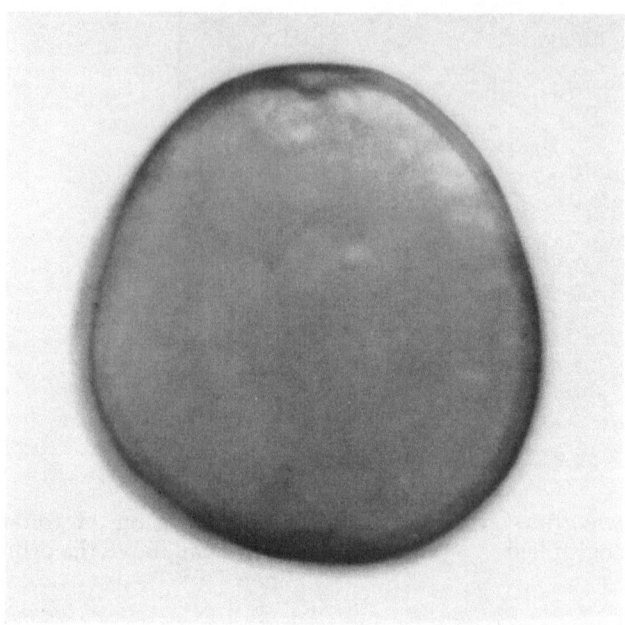

Fig. 11. Axial transverse tomogram

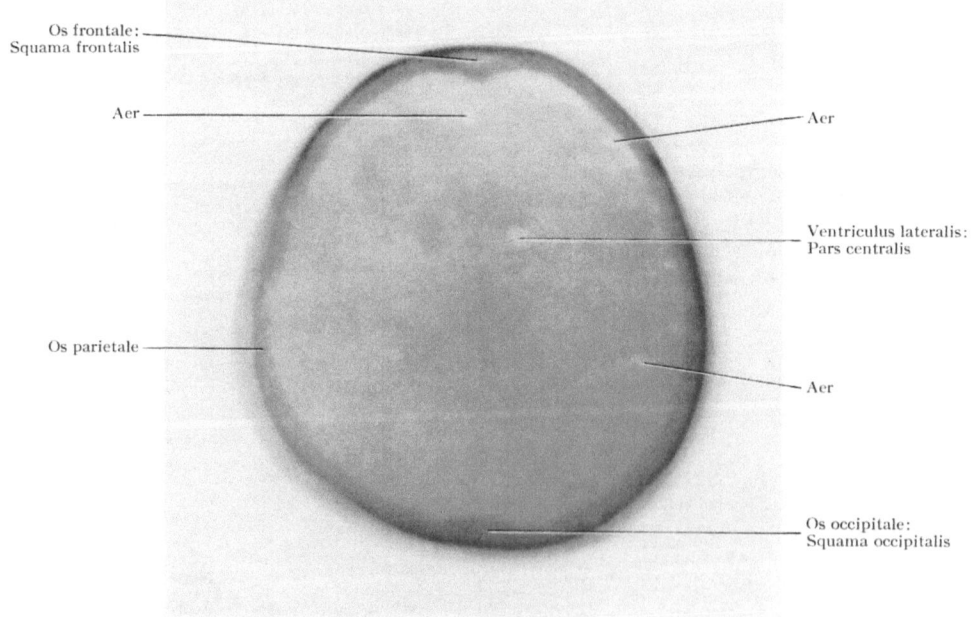

Fig. 12. Interpretation

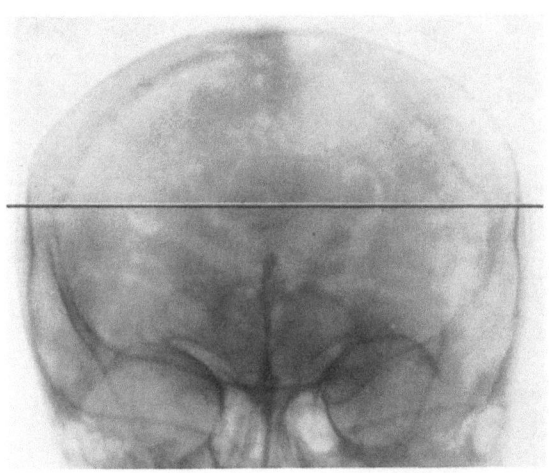

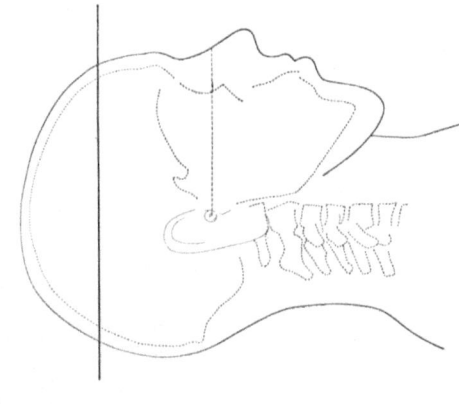

Fig. 13. Normal roentgenogram. Horizontal line showing the level tomographed

Fig. 14. Schema of tomographed level (solid line) 7 cm above the orbitomeatal line (dashed line)

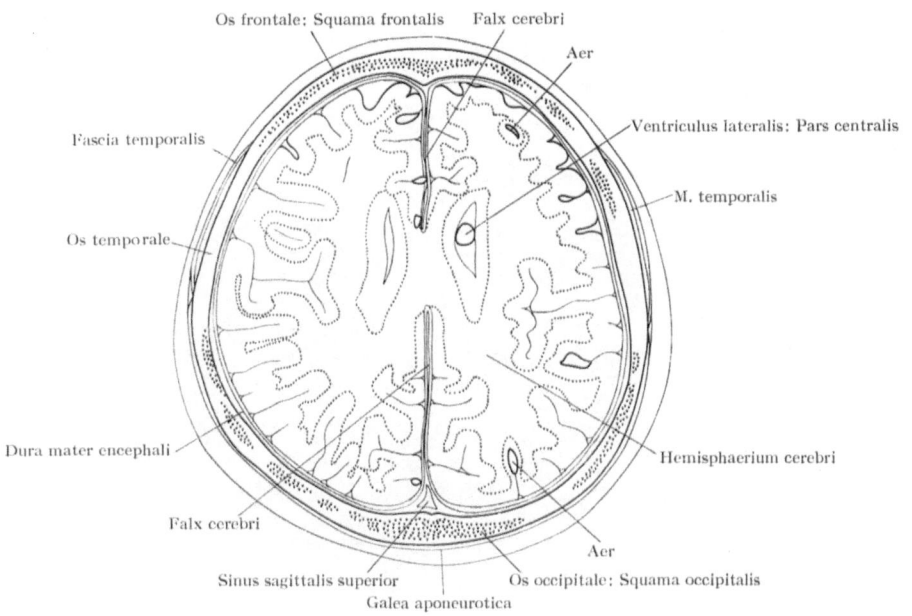

Fig. 15. Anatomical chart

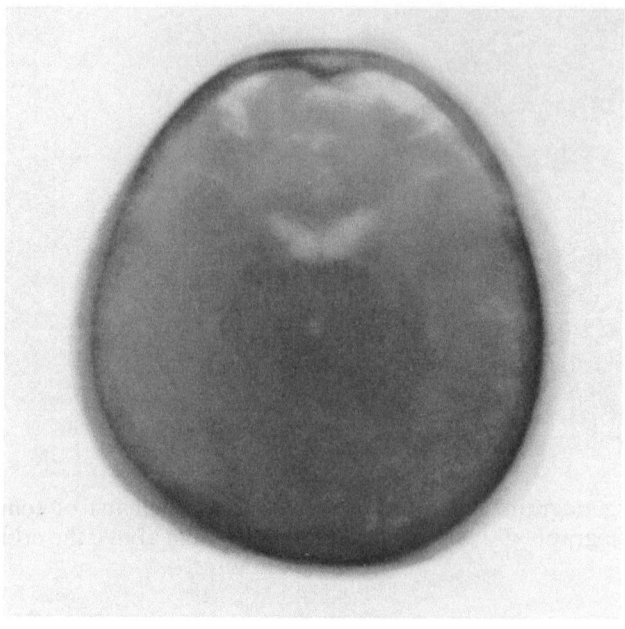

Fig. 16. Axial transverse tomogram

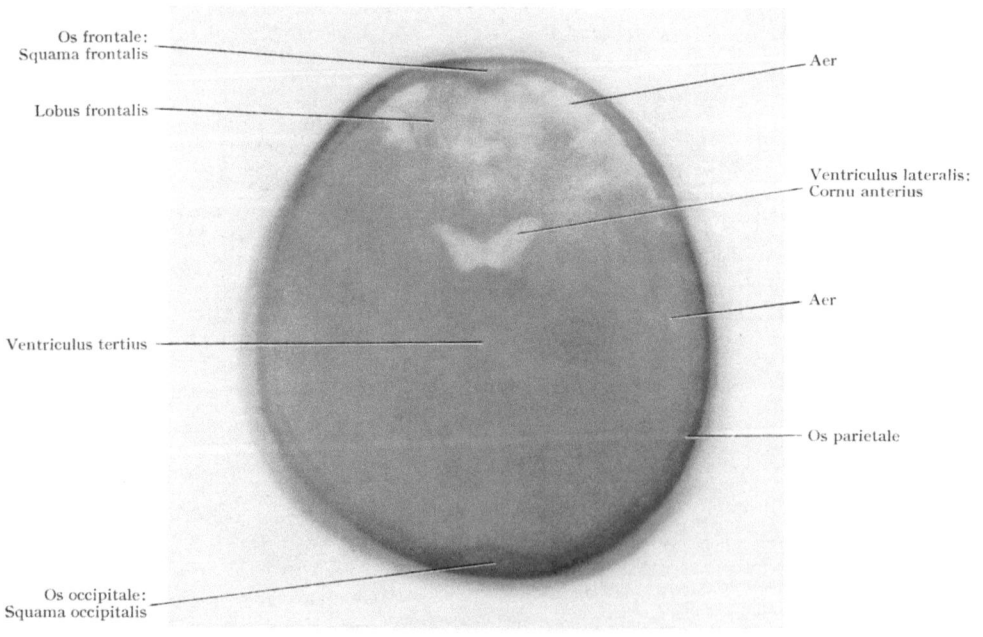

Os frontale:
Squama frontalis

Aer

Lobus frontalis

Ventriculus lateralis:
Cornu anterius

Ventriculus tertius

Aer

Os parietale

Os occipitale:
Squama occipitalis

Fig. 17. Interpretation

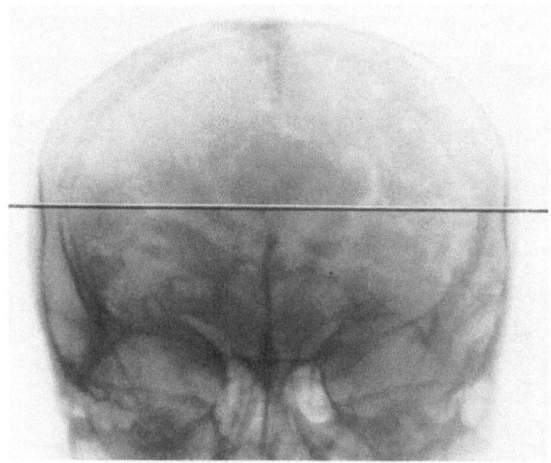
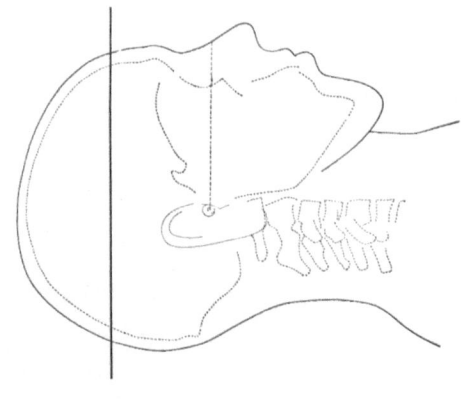

Fig. 18. Normal roentgenogram. Horizontal line showing the level tomographed

Fig. 19. Schema of tomographed level (solid line) 6 cm above the orbitomeatal line (dashed line)

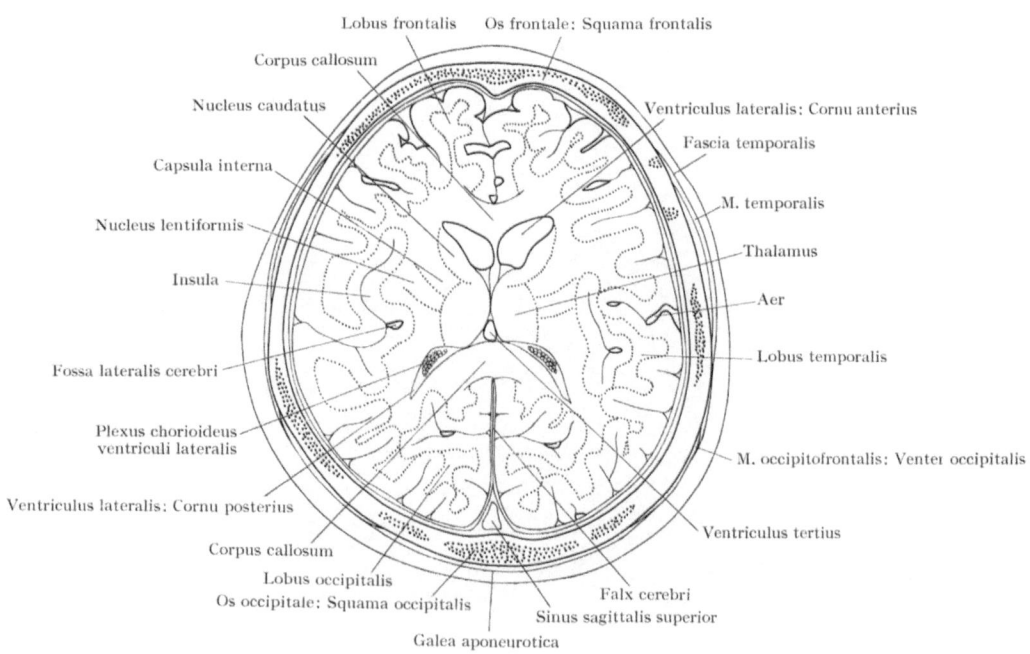

Fig. 20. Anatomical chart

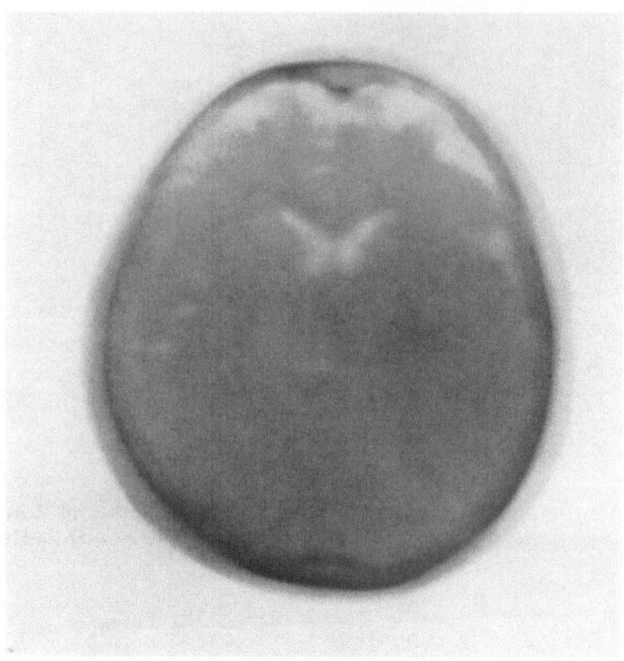

Fig. 21. Axial transverse tomogram

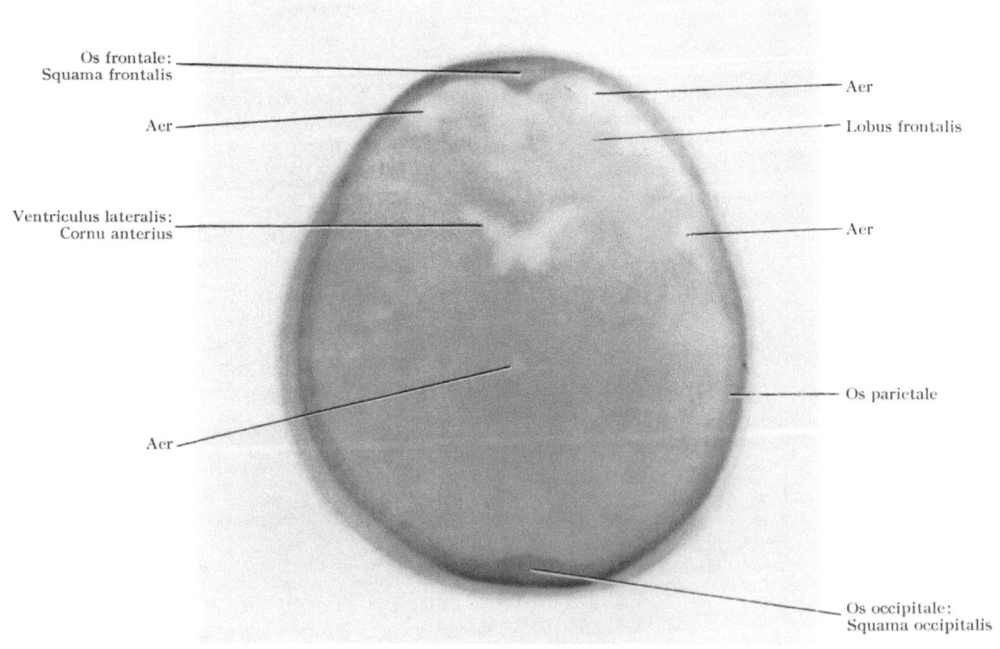

Os frontale: Squama frontalis

Aer

Ventriculus lateralis: Cornu anterius

Aer

Aer

Lobus frontalis

Aer

Os parietale

Os occipitale: Squama occipitalis

Fig. 22. Interpretation

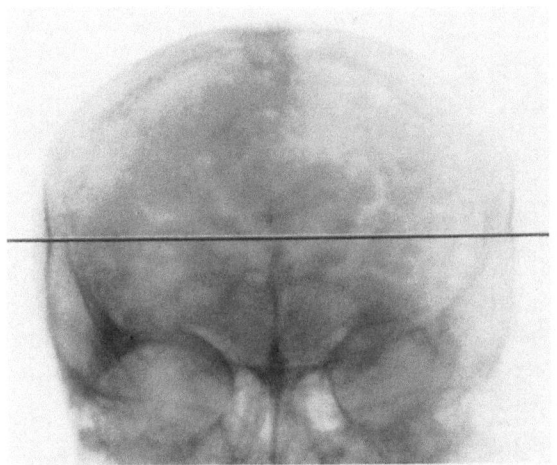

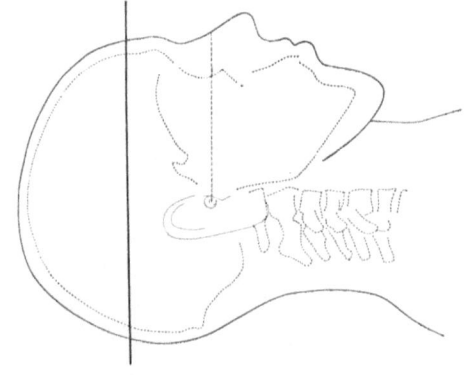

Fig. 23. Normal roentgenogram. Horizontal line showing the level tomographed

Fig. 24. Schema of tomographed level (solid line) 5 cm above the orbitomeatal line (dashed line)

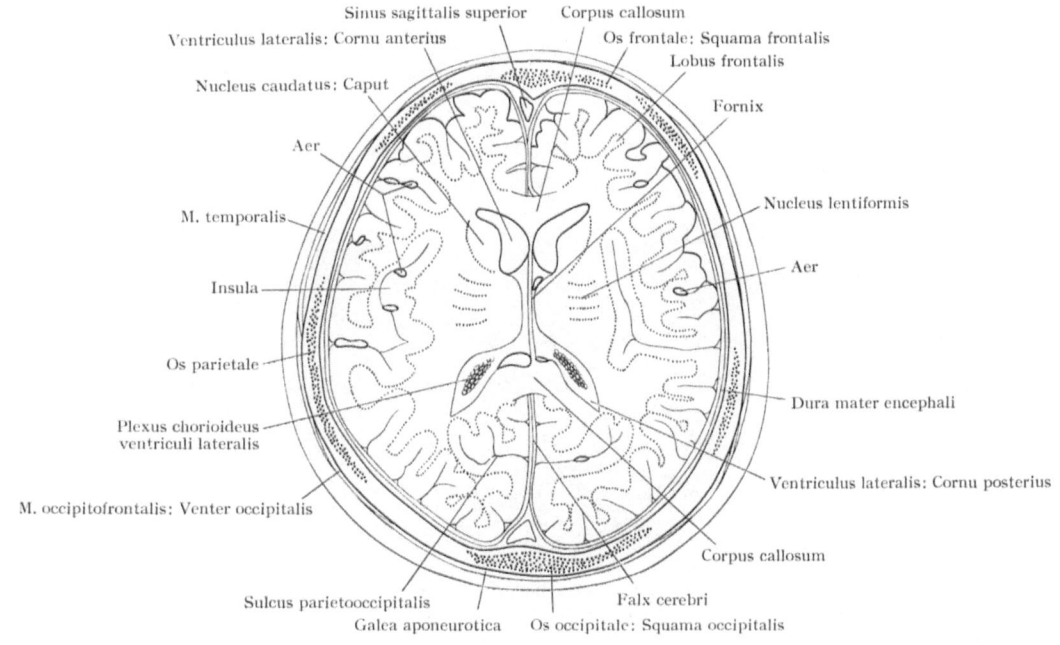

Fig. 25. Anatomical chart

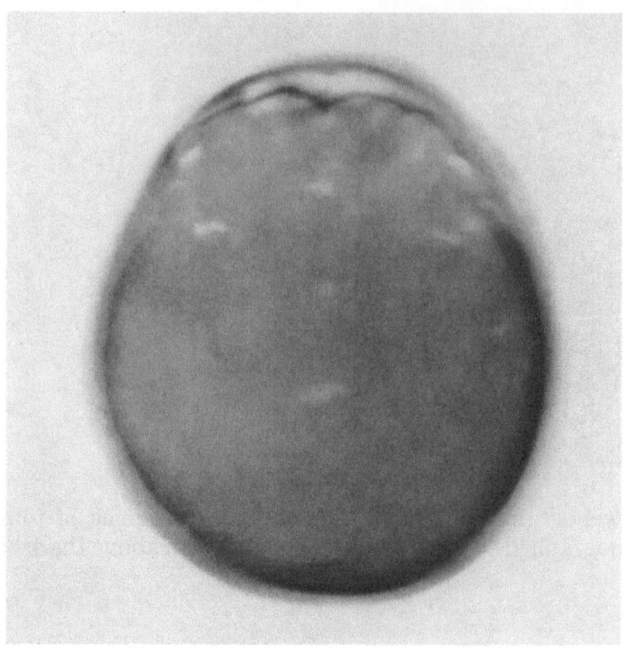

Fig. 26. Axial transverse tomogram

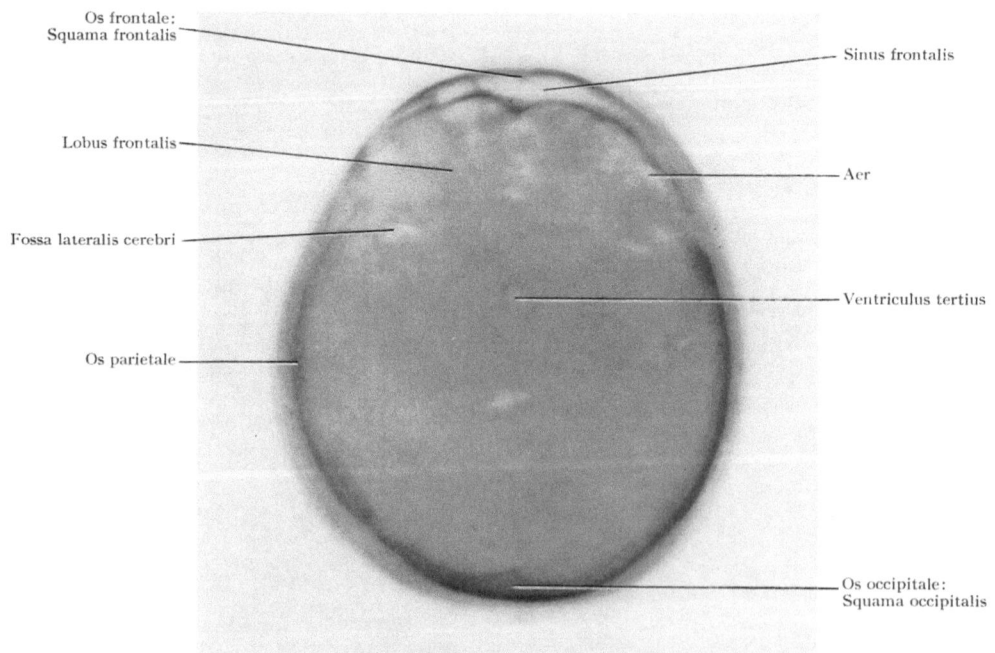

Fig. 27. Interpretation

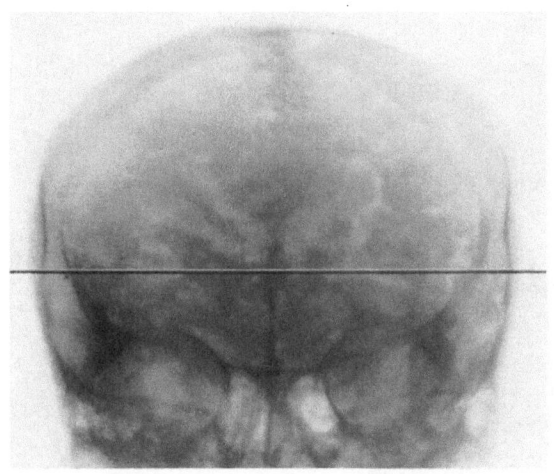
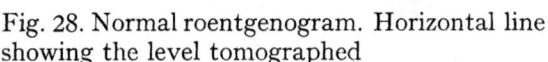

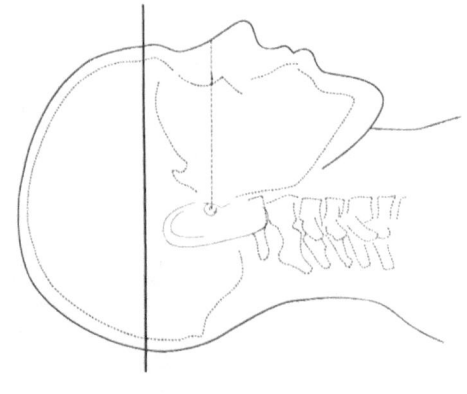

Fig. 28. Normal roentgenogram. Horizontal line showing the level tomographed

Fig. 29. Schema of tomographed level (solid line) 4 cm above the orbitomeatal line (dashed line)

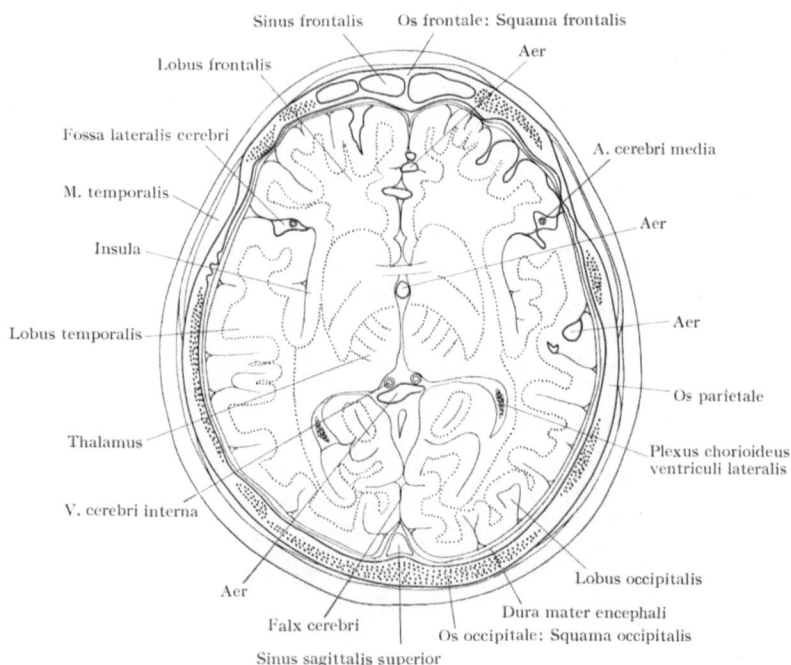

Fig. 30. Anatomical chart

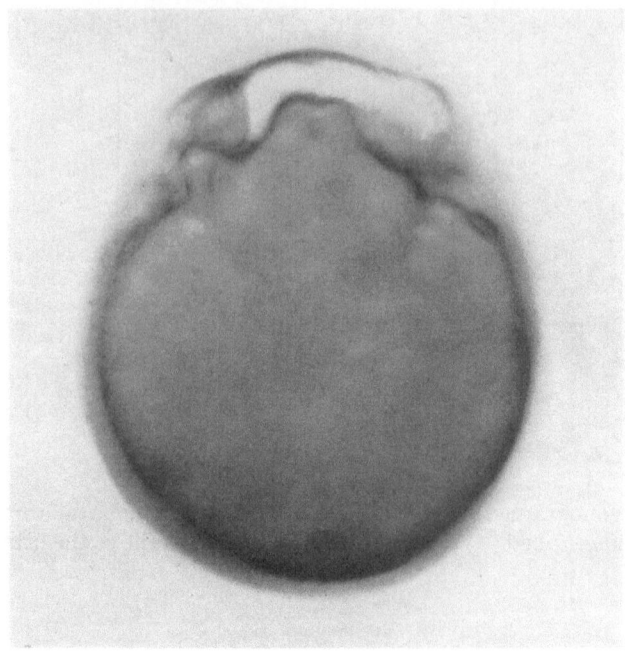

Fig. 31. Axial transverse tomogram

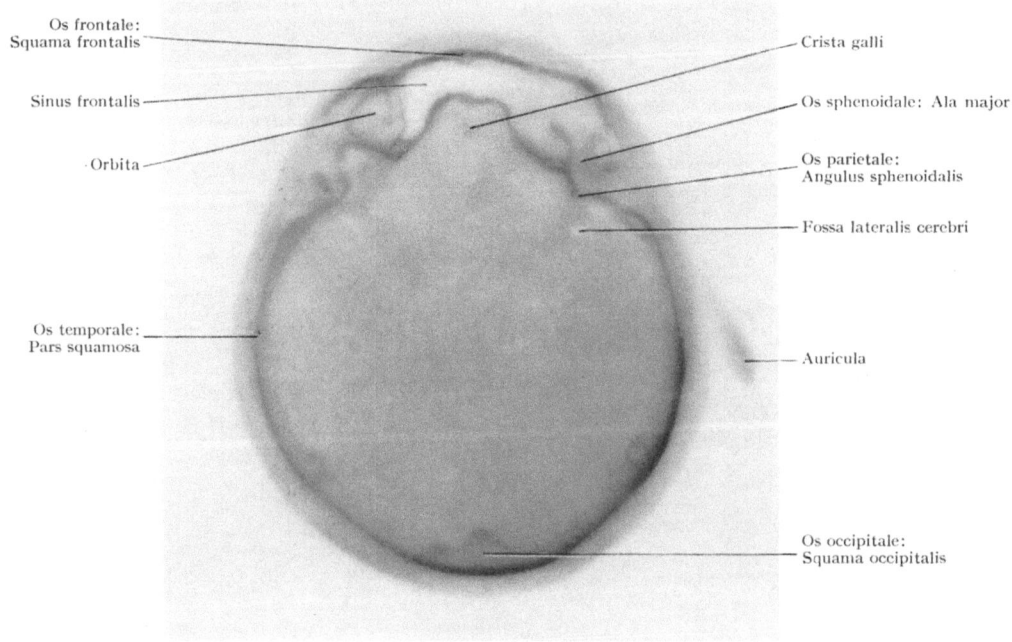

Os frontale:
Squama frontalis

Sinus frontalis

Orbita

Os temporale:
Pars squamosa

Crista galli

Os sphenoidale: Ala major

Os parietale:
Angulus sphenoidalis

Fossa lateralis cerebri

Auricula

Os occipitale:
Squama occipitalis

Fig. 32. Interpretation

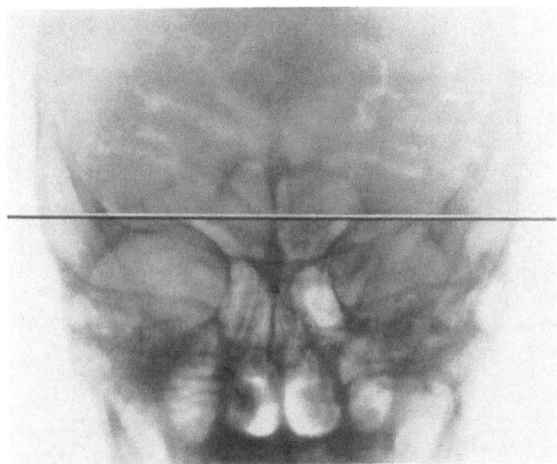

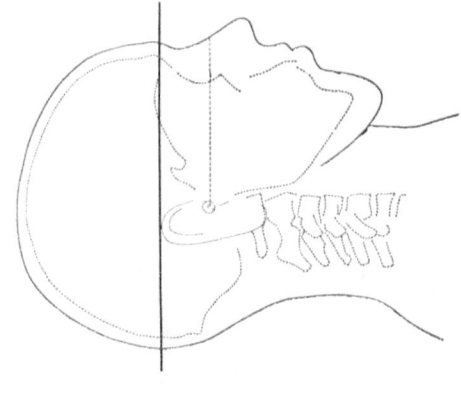

Fig. 33. Normal roentgenogram. Horizontal line showing the level tomographed

Fig. 34. Schema of tomographed level (solid line) 3 cm above the orbitomeatal line (dashed line)

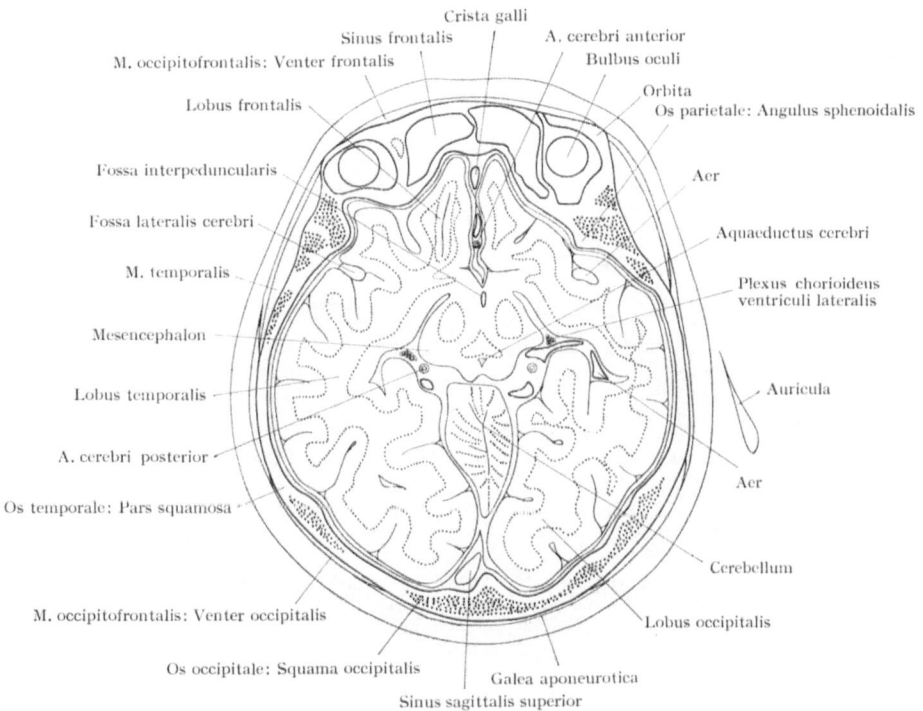

Fig. 35. Anatomical chart

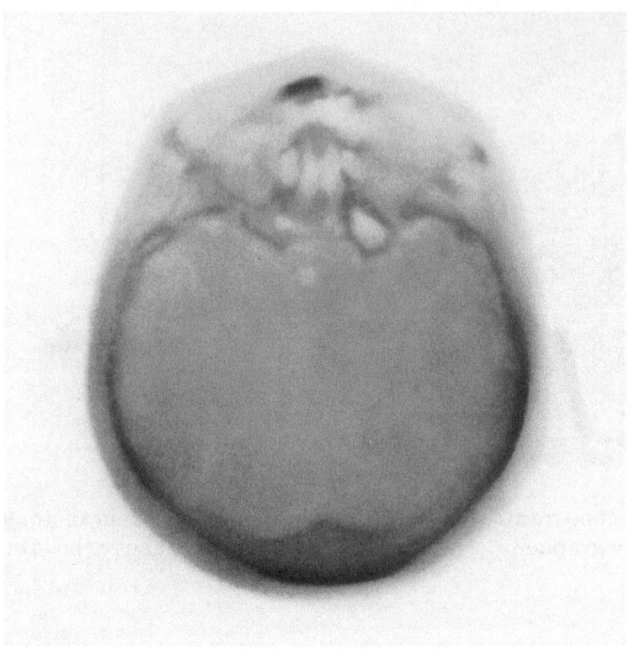

Fig. 36. Axial transverse tomogram

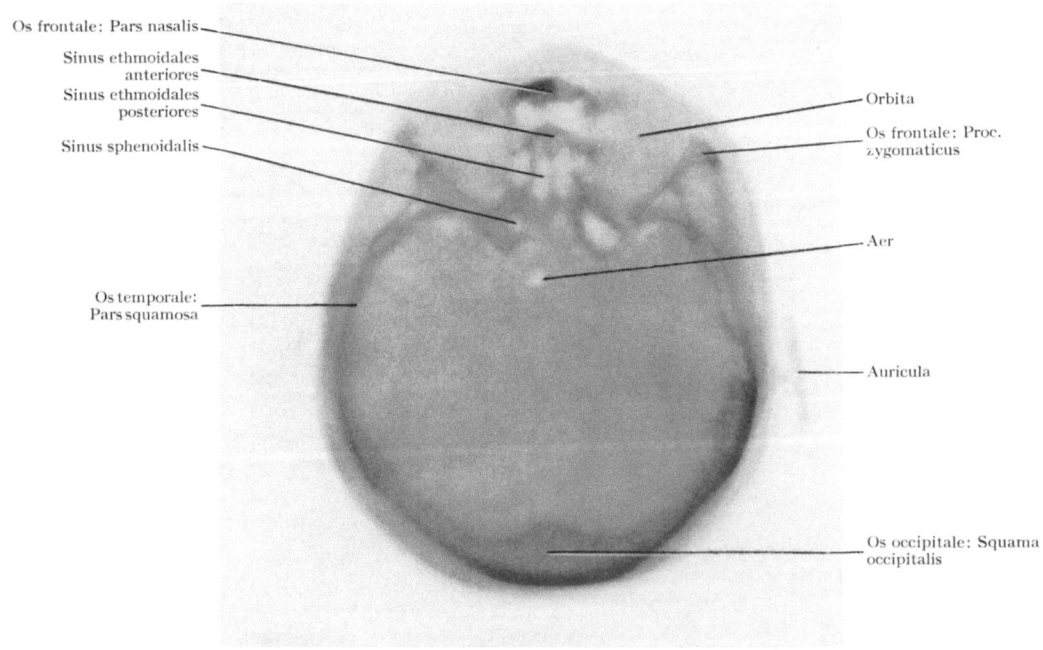

Os frontale: Pars nasalis

Sinus ethmoidales anteriores

Sinus ethmoidales posteriores

Sinus sphenoidalis

Os temporale: Pars squamosa

Orbita

Os frontale: Proc. zygomaticus

Aer

Auricula

Os occipitale: Squama occipitalis

Fig. 37. Interpretation

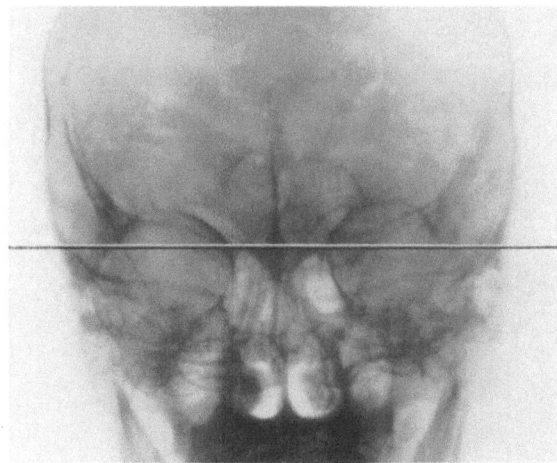

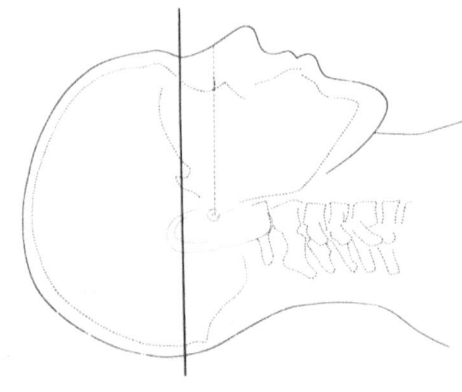

Fig. 38. Normal roentgenogram. Horizontal line showing the level tomographed

Fig. 39. Schema of tomographed level (solid line) 2 cm above the orbitomeatal line (dashed line)

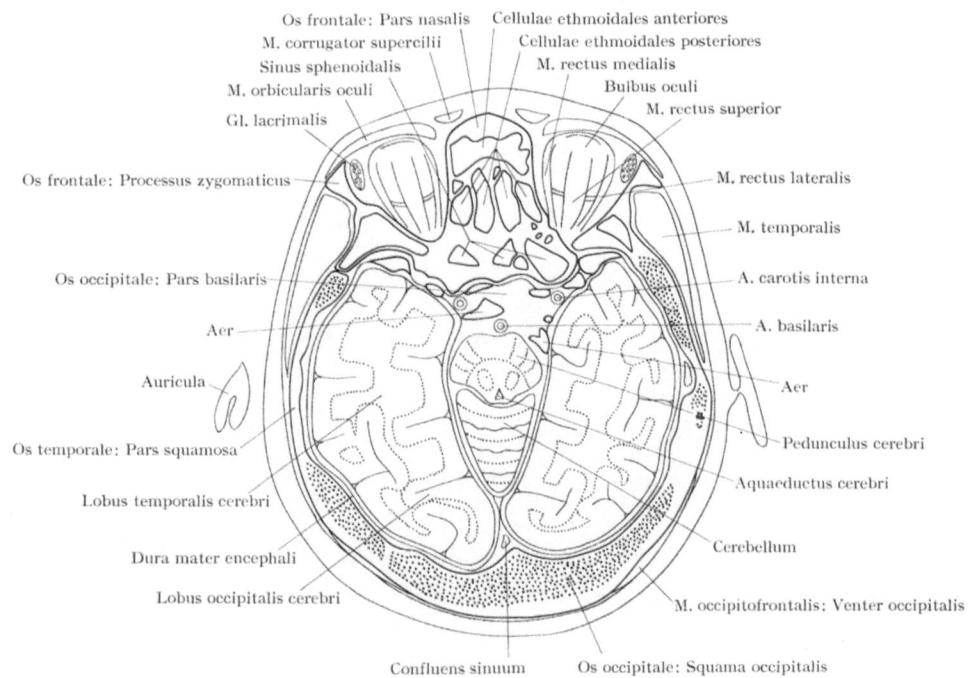

Os frontale: Pars nasalis
M. corrugator supercilii
Sinus sphenoidalis
M. orbicularis oculi
Gl. lacrimalis

Cellulae ethmoidales anteriores
Cellulae ethmoidales posteriores
M. rectus medialis
Bulbus oculi
M. rectus superior

Os frontale: Processus zygomaticus

M. rectus lateralis

M. temporalis

Os occipitale: Pars basilaris

A. carotis interna

Aer

A. basilaris

Auricula

Aer

Os temporale: Pars squamosa

Pedunculus cerebri

Lobus temporalis cerebri

Aquaeductus cerebri

Dura mater encephali

Cerebellum

Lobus occipitalis cerebri

M. occipitofrontalis: Venter occipitalis

Confluens sinuum

Os occipitale: Squama occipitalis

Fig. 40. Anatomical chart

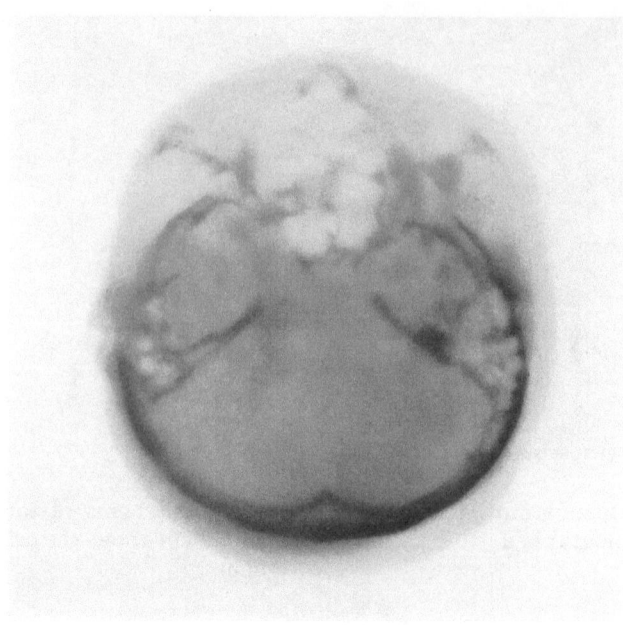

Fig. 41. Axial transverse tomogram

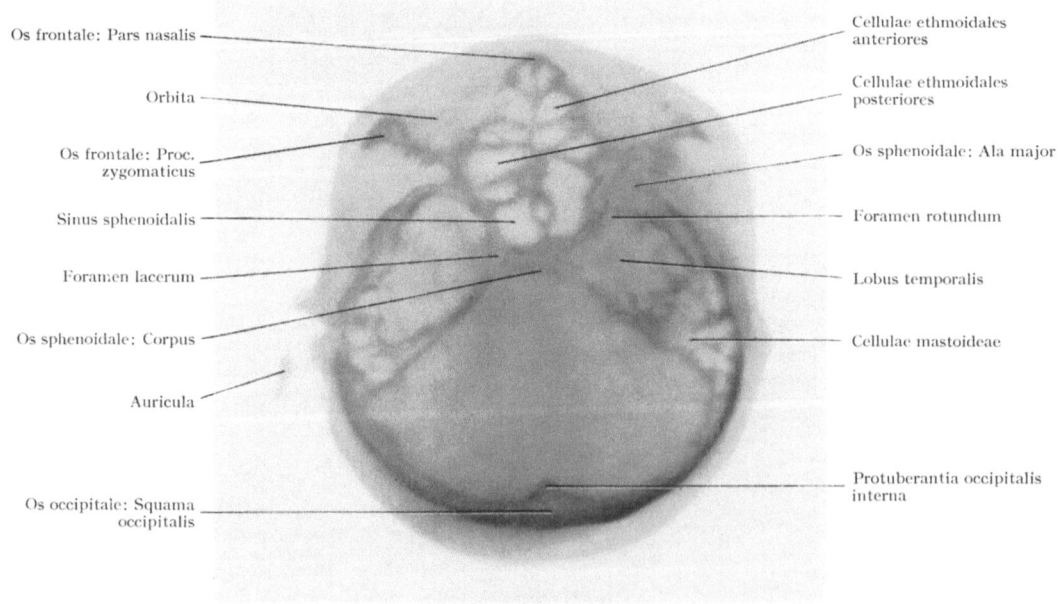

Os frontale: Pars nasalis

Orbita

Os frontale: Proc. zygomaticus

Sinus sphenoidalis

Foramen lacerum

Os sphenoidale: Corpus

Auricula

Os occipitale: Squama occipitalis

Cellulae ethmoidales anteriores

Cellulae ethmoidales posteriores

Os sphenoidale: Ala major

Foramen rotundum

Lobus temporalis

Cellulae mastoideae

Protuberantia occipitalis interna

Fig. 42. Interpretation

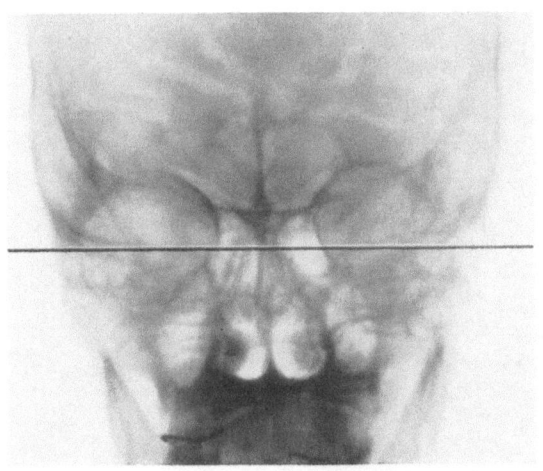

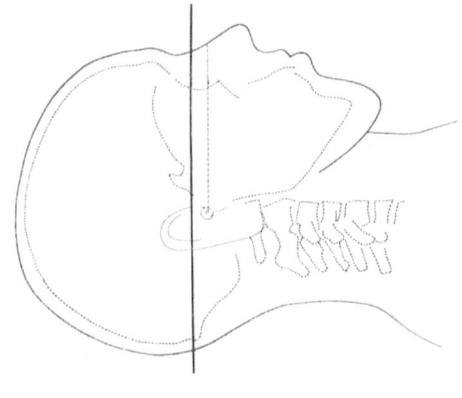

Fig. 43. Normal roentgenogram. Horizontal line showing the level tomographed

Fig. 44. Schema of tomographed level (solid line) 1 cm above the orbitomeatal line (dashed line)

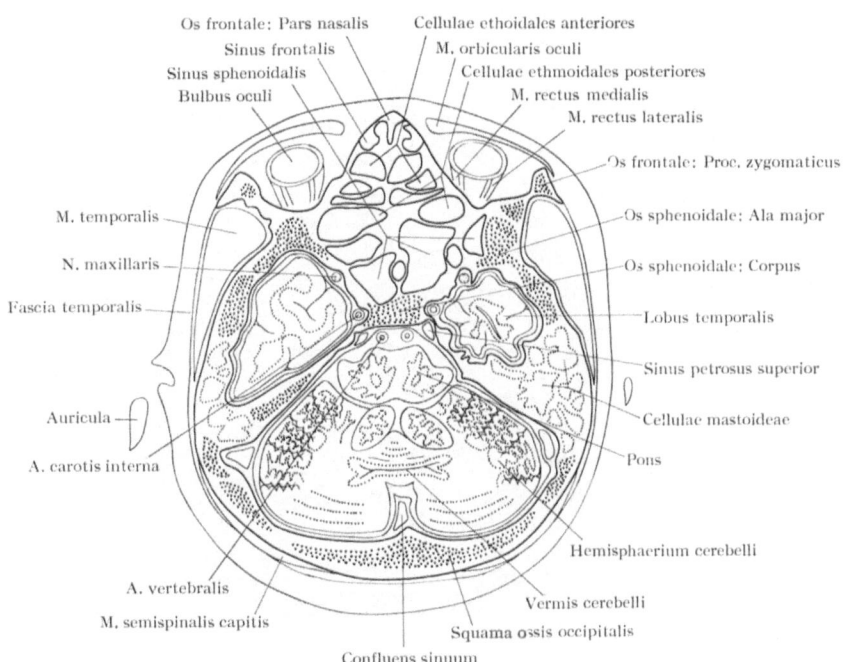

Os frontale: Pars nasalis
Sinus frontalis
Sinus sphenoidalis
Bulbus oculi
Cellulae ethoidales anteriores
M. orbicularis oculi
Cellulae ethmoidales posteriores
M. rectus medialis
M. rectus lateralis
M. temporalis
N. maxillaris
Fascia temporalis
Os frontale: Proc. zygomaticus
Os sphenoidale: Ala major
Os sphenoidale: Corpus
Lobus temporalis
Sinus petrosus superior
Cellulae mastoideae
Pons
Auricula
A. carotis interna
Hemisphaerium cerebelli
Vermis cerebelli
A. vertebralis
M. semispinalis capitis
Squama ossis occipitalis
Confluens sinuum

Fig. 45. Anatomical chart

31

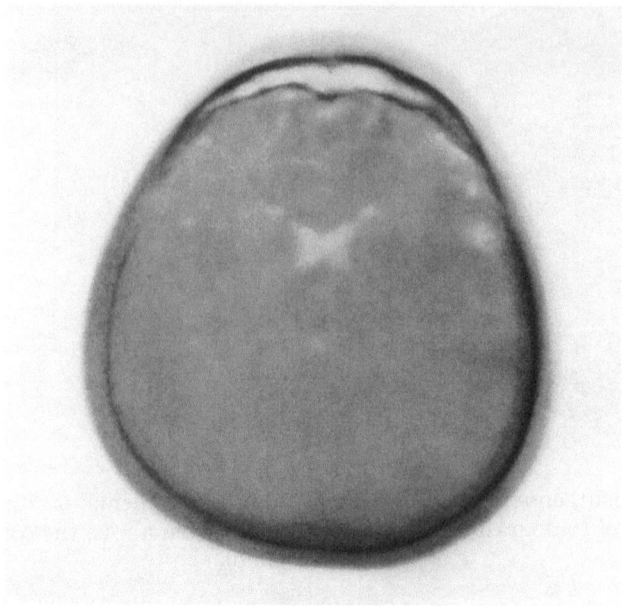

Fig. 46. Axial transverse tomogram

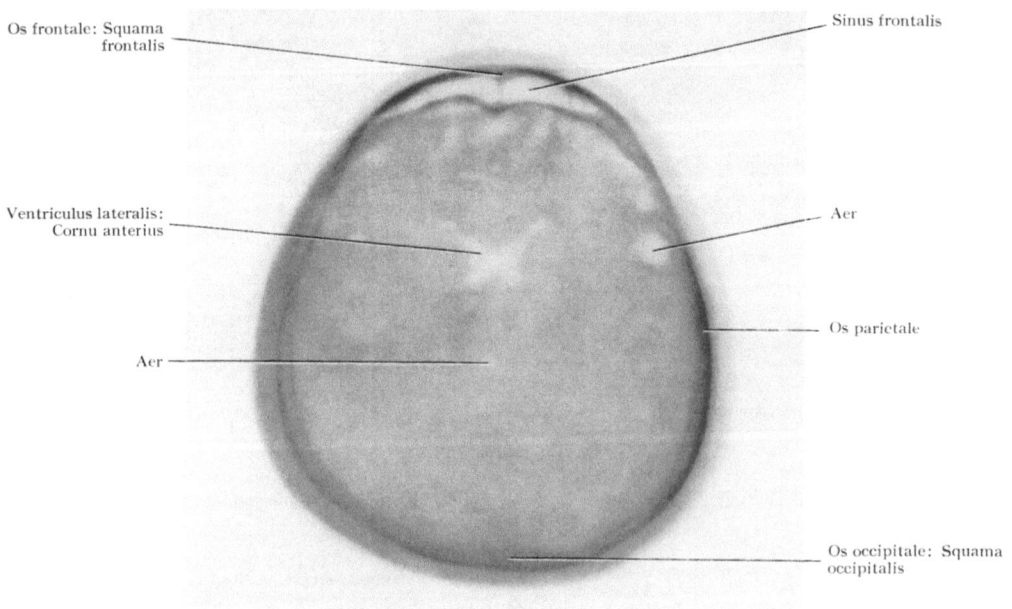

Fig. 47. Interpretation

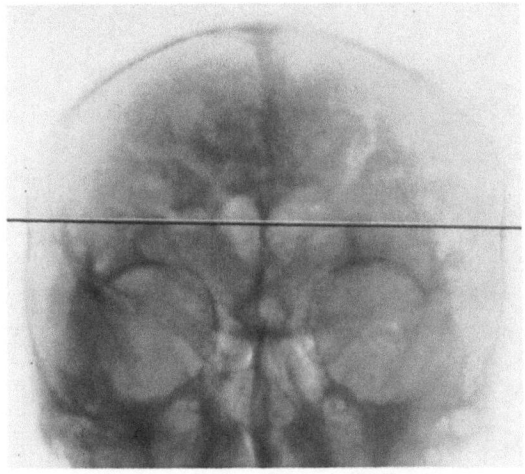

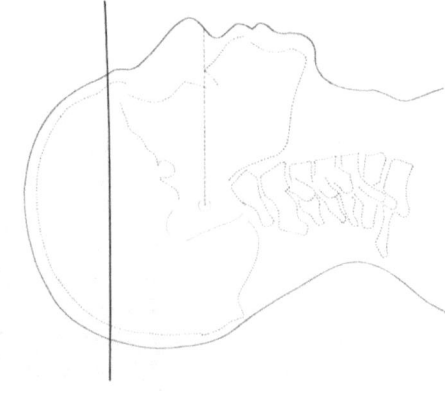

Fig. 48. Normal roentgenogram. Horizontal line showing the level tomographed

Fig. 49. Schema of tomographed level (solid line) 6 cm above the acanthiomeatal line (dashed line)

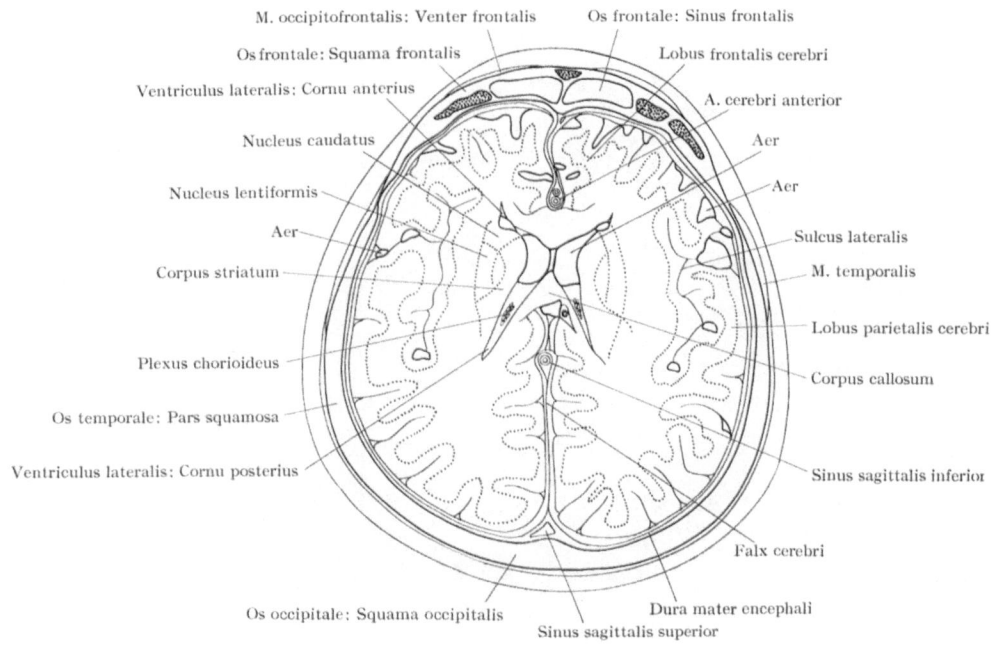

Fig. 50. Anatomical chart

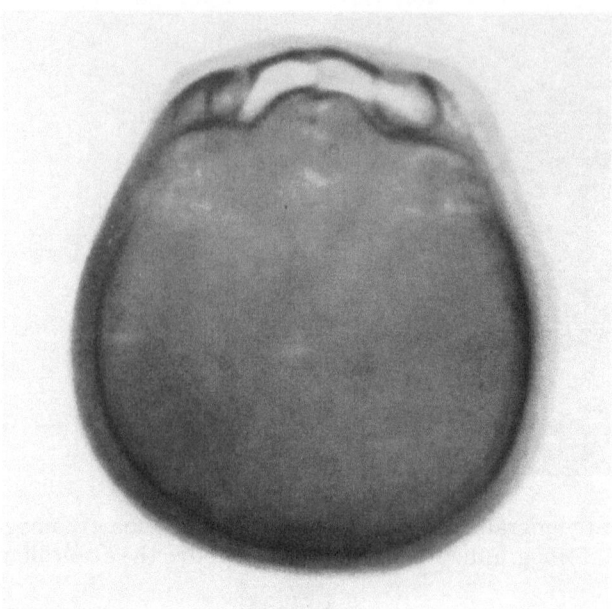

Fig. 51. Axial transverse tomogram

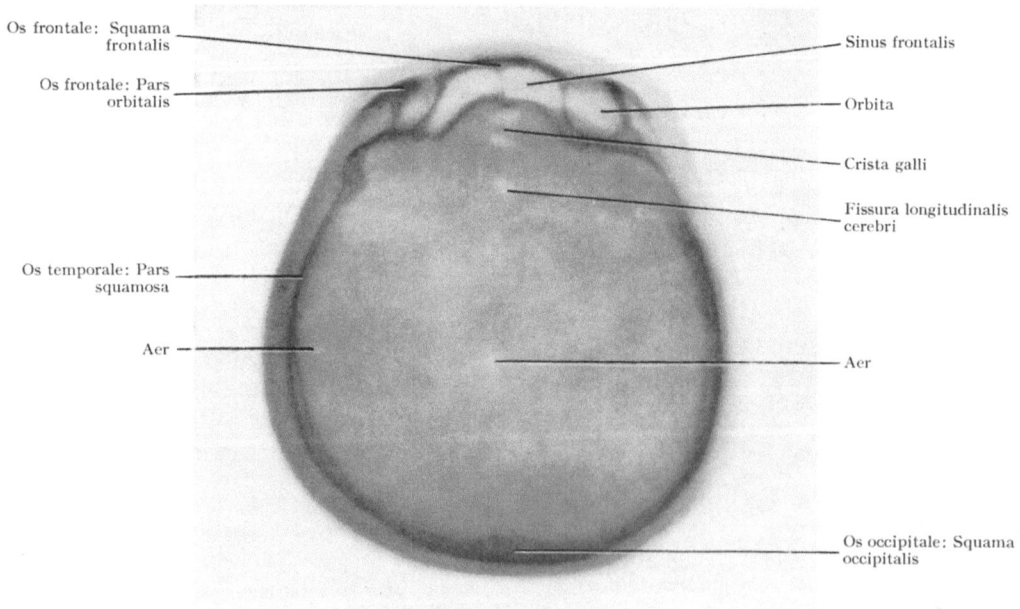

Os frontale: Squama frontalis

Os frontale: Pars orbitalis

Os temporale: Pars squamosa

Aer

Sinus frontalis

Orbita

Crista galli

Fissura longitudinalis cerebri

Aer

Os occipitale: Squama occipitalis

Fig. 52. Interpretation

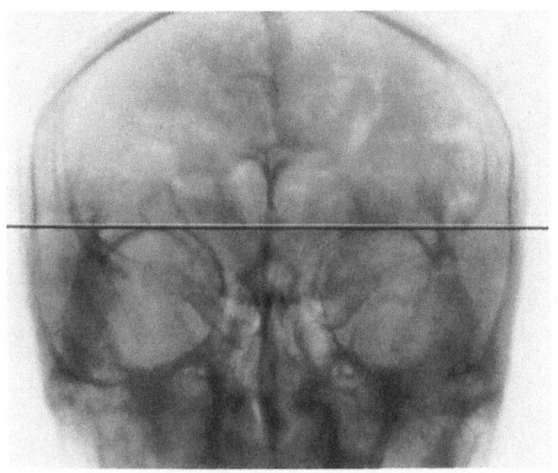

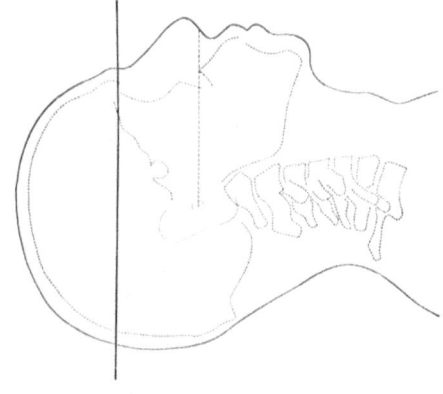

Fig. 53. Normal roentgenogram. Horizontal line showing the level tomographed

Fig. 54. Schema of tomographed level (solid line) 5 cm above the acanthiomeatal line (dashed line)

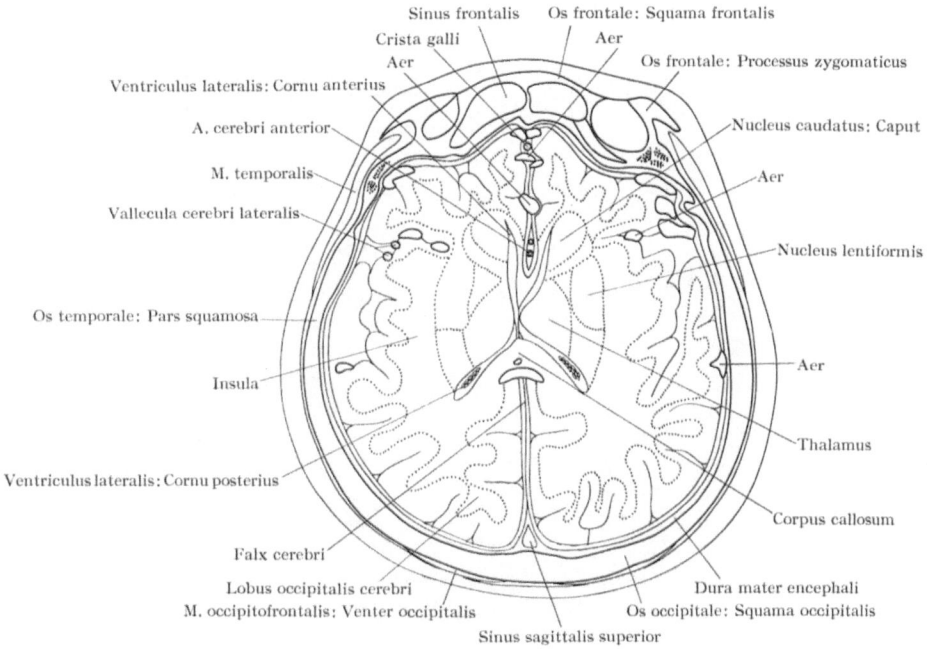

Fig. 55. Anatomical chart

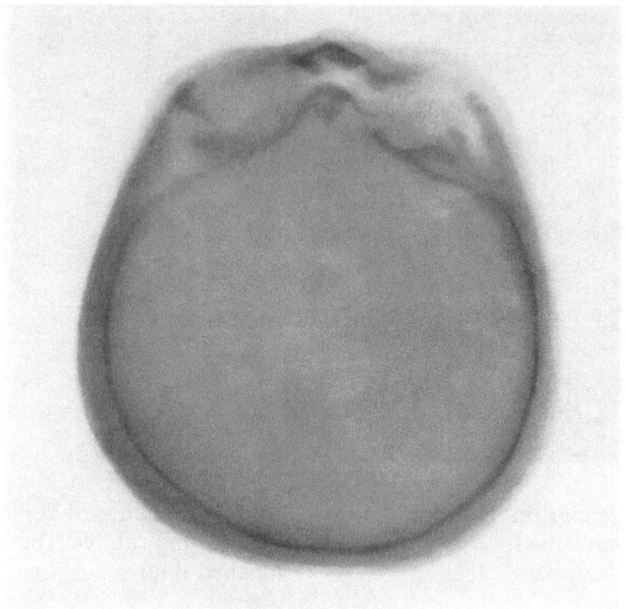

Fig. 56. Axial transverse tomogram

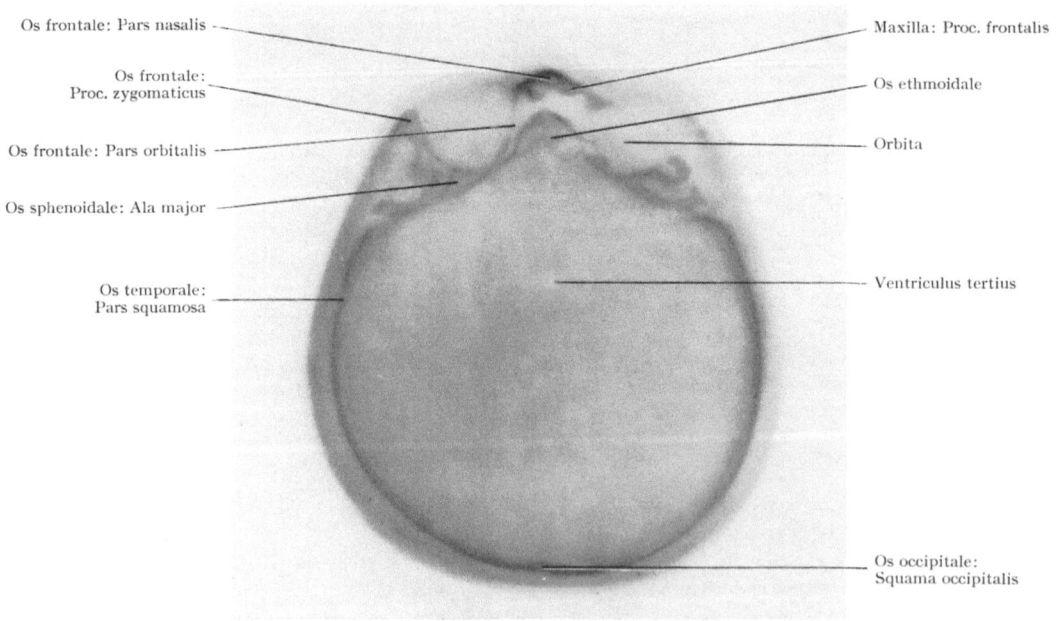

Os frontale: Pars nasalis

Os frontale:
Proc. zygomaticus

Os frontale: Pars orbitalis

Os sphenoidale: Ala major

Os temporale:
Pars squamosa

Maxilla: Proc. frontalis

Os ethmoidale

Orbita

Ventriculus tertius

Os occipitale:
Squama occipitalis

Fig. 57. Interpretation

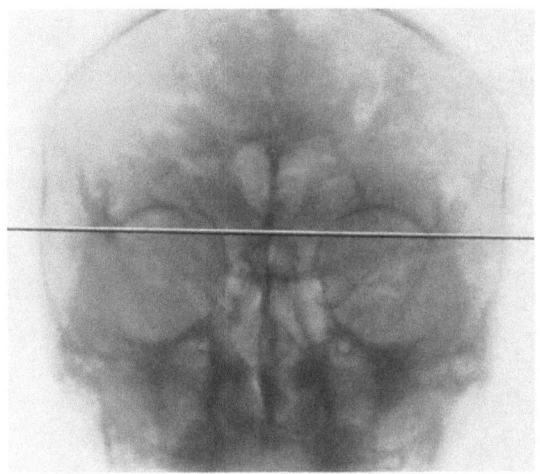

Fig. 58. Normal roentgenogram. Horizontal line showing the level tomographed

Fig. 59. Schema of tomographed level (solid line) 4 cm above the acanthiomeatal line (dashed line)

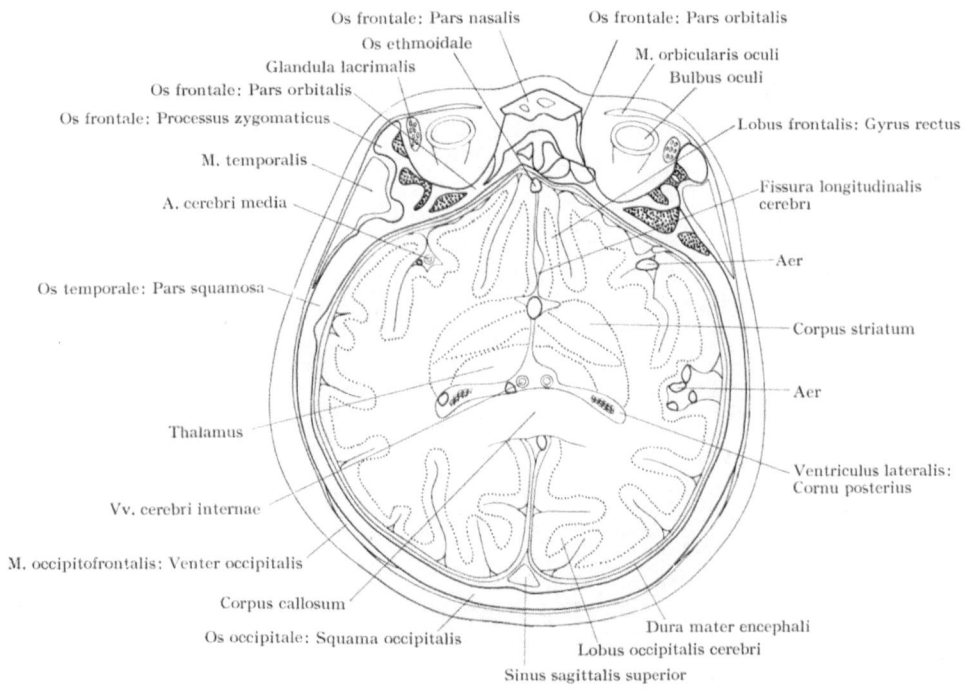

Os frontale: Pars nasalis
Os ethmoidale
Glandula lacrimalis
Os frontale: Pars orbitalis
Os frontale: Processus zygomaticus
M. temporalis
A. cerebri media
Os temporale: Pars squamosa
Thalamus
Vv. cerebri internae
M. occipitofrontalis: Venter occipitalis
Corpus callosum
Os occipitale: Squama occipitalis

Os frontale: Pars orbitalis
M. orbicularis oculi
Bulbus oculi
Lobus frontalis: Gyrus rectus
Fissura longitudinalis cerebri
Aer
Corpus striatum
Aer
Ventriculus lateralis: Cornu posterius
Dura mater encephali
Lobus occipitalis cerebri
Sinus sagittalis superior

Fig. 60. Anatomical chart

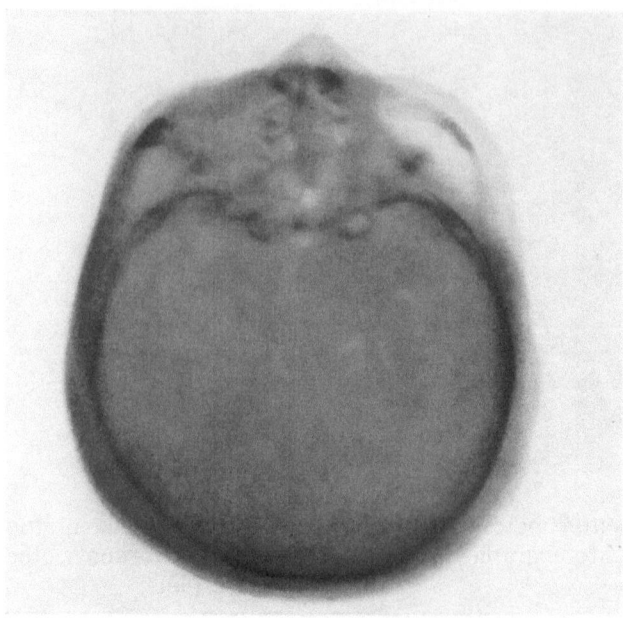

Fig. 61. Axial transverse tomogram

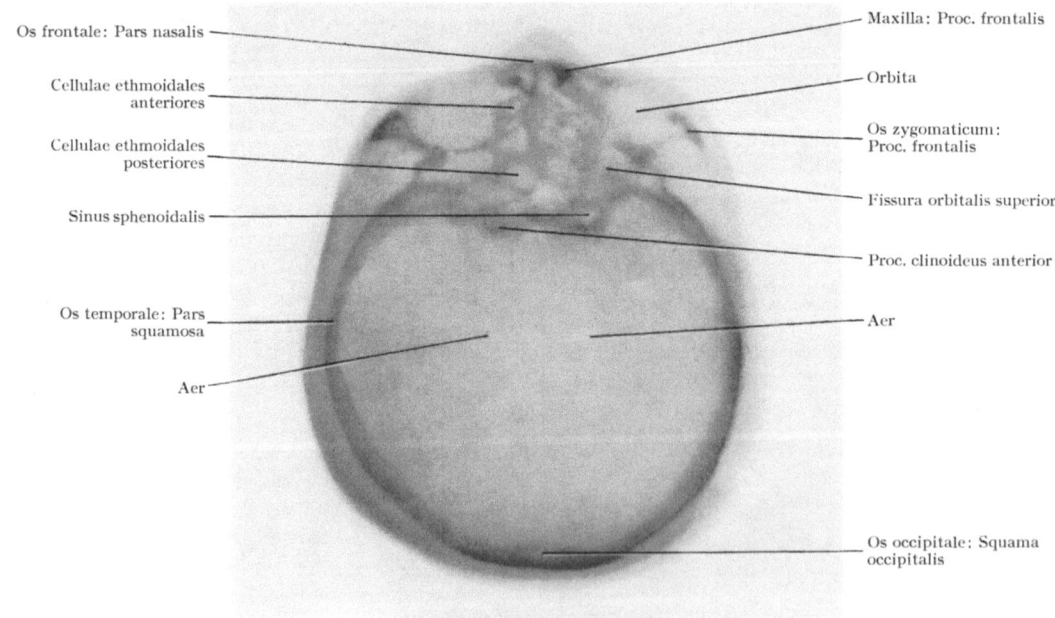

Os frontale: Pars nasalis

Cellulae ethmoidales anteriores

Cellulae ethmoidales posteriores

Sinus sphenoidalis

Os temporale: Pars squamosa

Aer

Maxilla: Proc. frontalis

Orbita

Os zygomaticum: Proc. frontalis

Fissura orbitalis superior

Proc. clinoideus anterior

Aer

Os occipitale: Squama occipitalis

Fig. 62. Interpretation

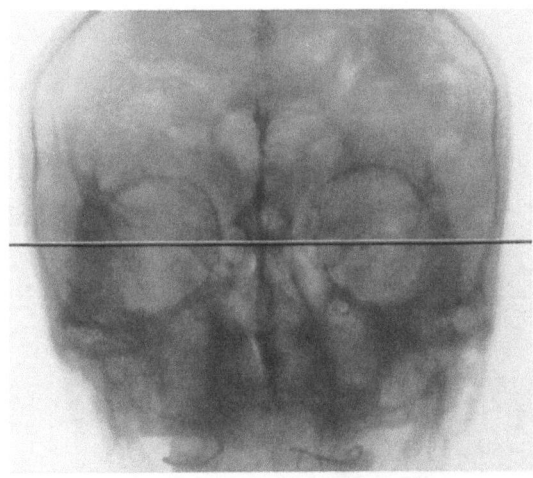

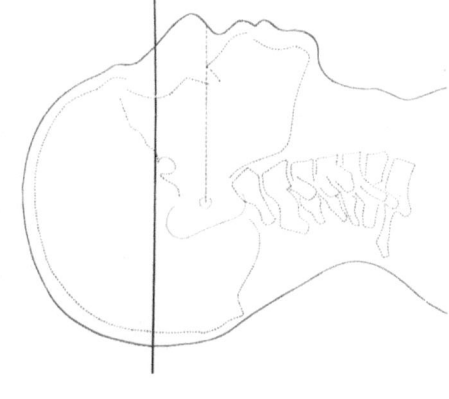

Fig. 63. Normal roentgenogram. Horizontal line showing the level tomographed

Fig. 64. Schema of tomographed level (solid line) 3 cm above the acanthiomeatal line (dashed line)

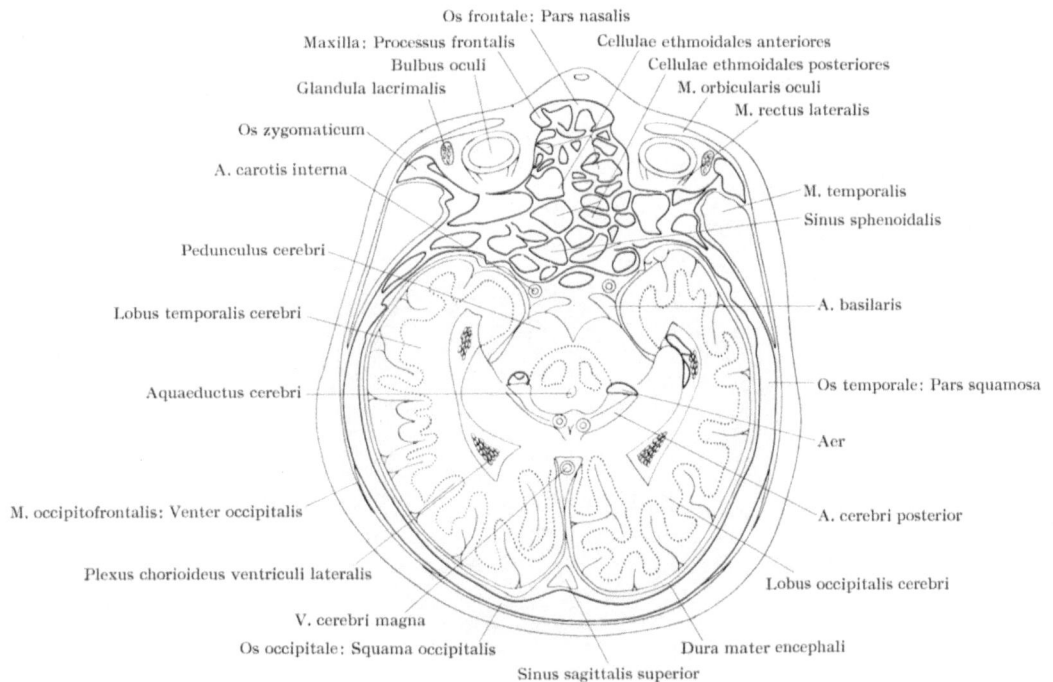

Os frontale: Pars nasalis
Maxilla: Processus frontalis
Bulbus oculi
Glandula lacrimalis
Os zygomaticum
A. carotis interna
Pedunculus cerebri
Lobus temporalis cerebri
Aquaeductus cerebri
M. occipitofrontalis: Venter occipitalis
Plexus chorioideus ventriculi lateralis
V. cerebri magna
Os occipitale: Squama occipitalis
Sinus sagittalis superior
Cellulae ethmoidales anteriores
Cellulae ethmoidales posteriores
M. orbicularis oculi
M. rectus lateralis
M. temporalis
Sinus sphenoidalis
A. basilaris
Os temporale: Pars squamosa
Aer
A. cerebri posterior
Lobus occipitalis cerebri
Dura mater encephali

Fig. 65. Anatomical chart

39

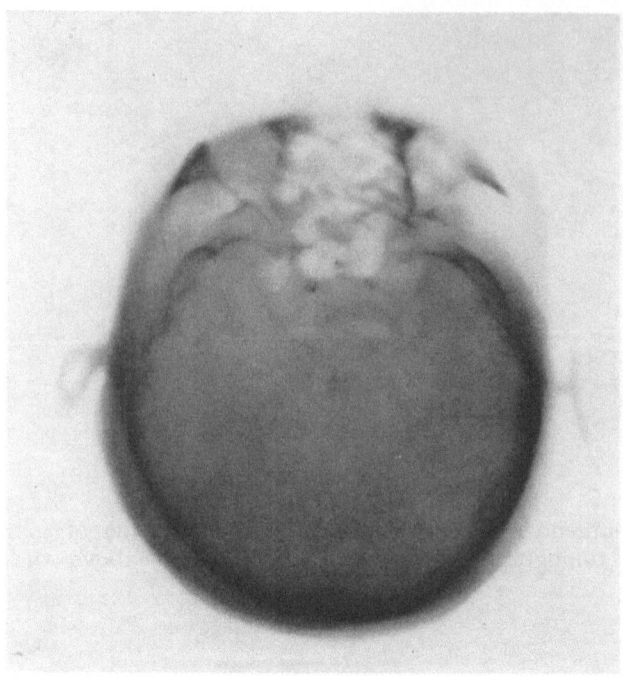

Fig. 66. Axial transverse tomogram

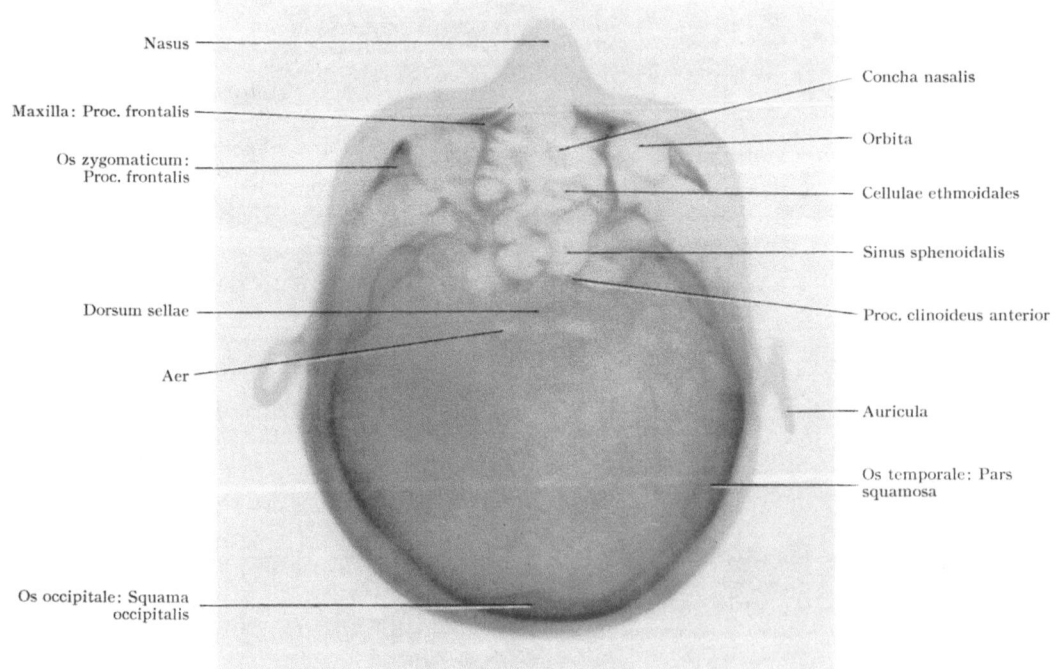

Nasus

Maxilla: Proc. frontalis

Os zygomaticum:
Proc. frontalis

Dorsum sellae

Aer

Os occipitale: Squama
occipitalis

Concha nasalis

Orbita

Cellulae ethmoidales

Sinus sphenoidalis

Proc. clinoideus anterior

Auricula

Os temporale: Pars
squamosa

Fig. 67. Interpretation

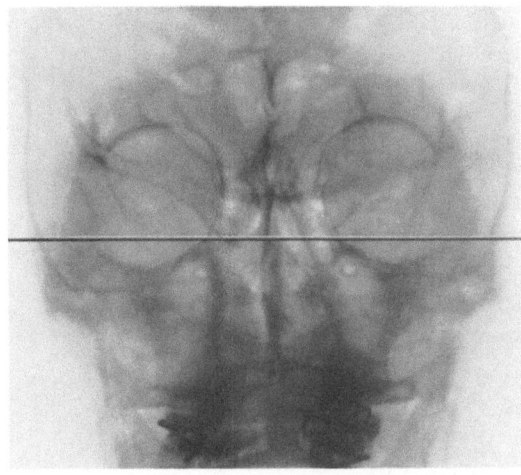

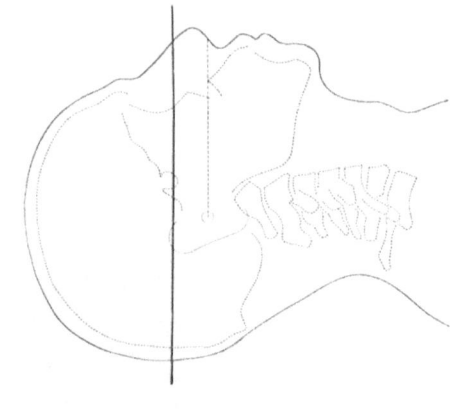

Fig. 68. Normal roentgenogram. Horizontal line showing the level tomographed

Fig. 69. Schema of tomographed level (solid line) 2 cm above the acanthiomeatal line (dashed line)

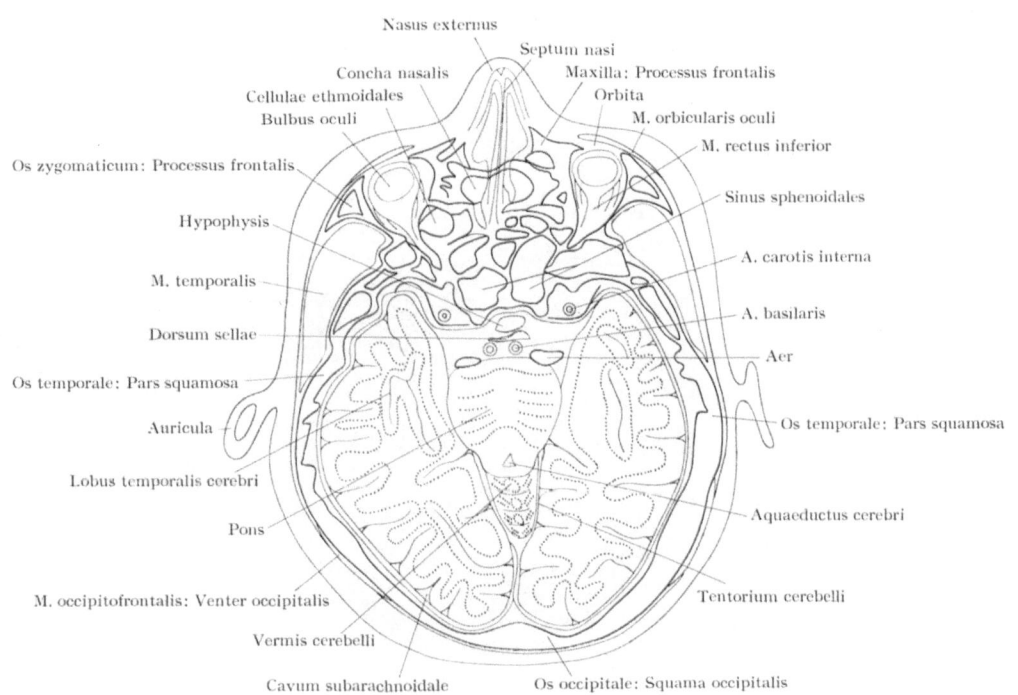

Fig. 70. Anatomical chart

Nasus externus
Septum nasi
Concha nasalis
Maxilla: Processus frontalis
Cellulae ethmoidales
Orbita
Bulbus oculi
M. orbicularis oculi
M. rectus inferior
Os zygomaticum: Processus frontalis
Sinus sphenoidales
Hypophysis
A. carotis interna
M. temporalis
A. basilaris
Dorsum sellae
Aer
Os temporale: Pars squamosa
Os temporale: Pars squamosa
Auricula
Lobus temporalis cerebri
Aquaeductus cerebri
Pons
M. occipitofrontalis: Venter occipitalis
Tentorium cerebelli
Vermis cerebelli
Cavum subarachnoidale
Os occipitale: Squama occipitalis

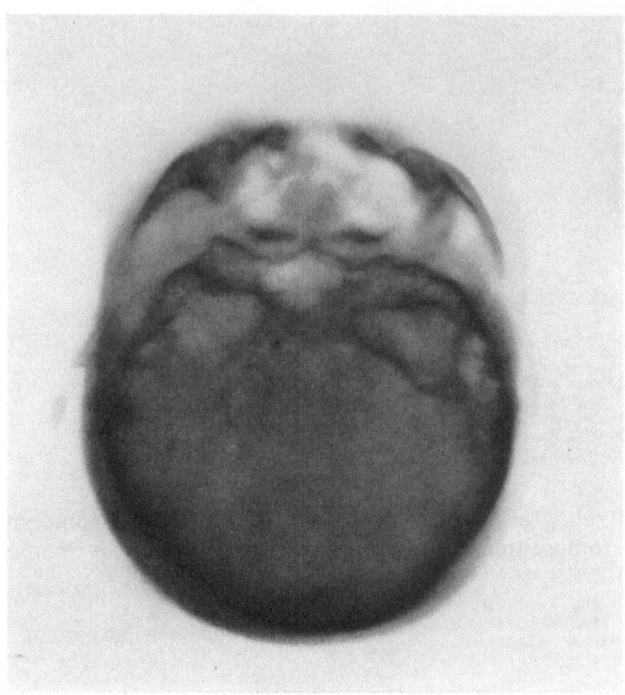

Fig. 71. Axial transverse tomogram

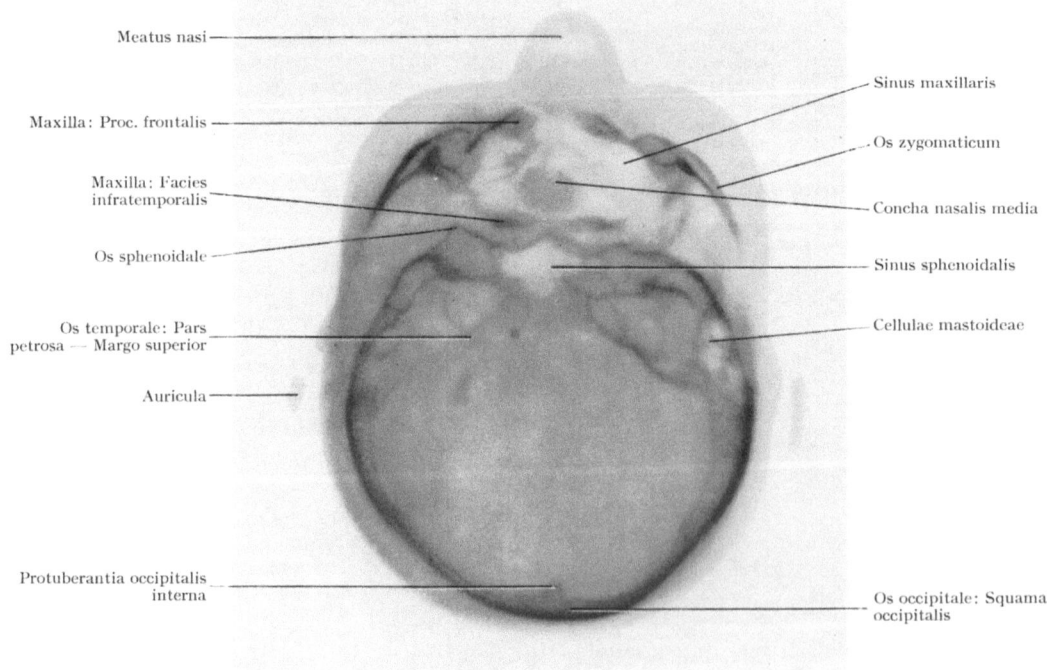

Meatus nasi

Maxilla: Proc. frontalis

Maxilla: Facies
infratemporalis

Os sphenoidale

Os temporale: Pars
petrosa — Margo superior

Auricula

Protuberantia occipitalis
interna

Sinus maxillaris

Os zygomaticum

Concha nasalis media

Sinus sphenoidalis

Cellulae mastoideae

Os occipitale: Squama
occipitalis

Fig. 72. Interpretation

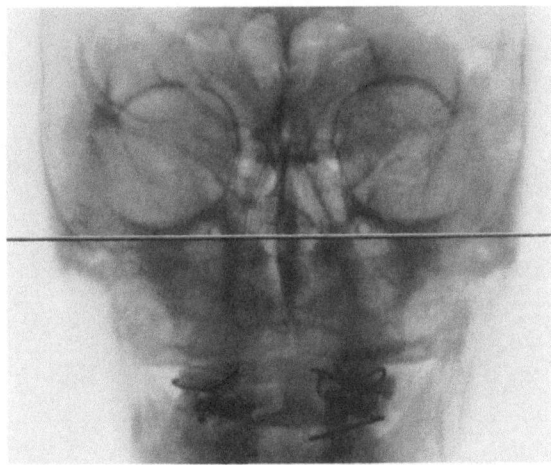

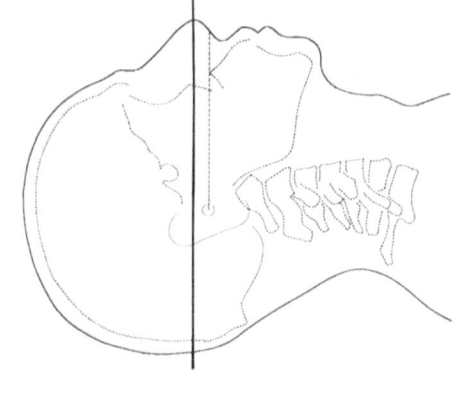

Fig. 73. Normal roentgenogram. Horizontal line showing the level tomographed

Fig. 74. Schema of tomographed level (solid line) 1 cm above the acanthiomeatal line (dashed line)

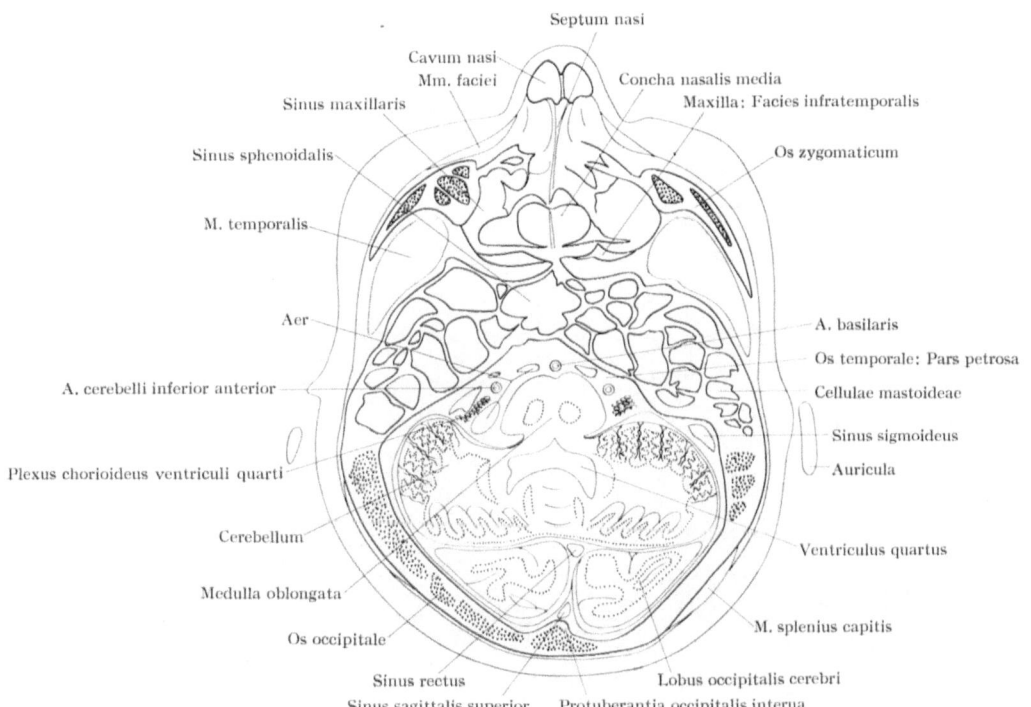

Fig. 75. Anatomical chart

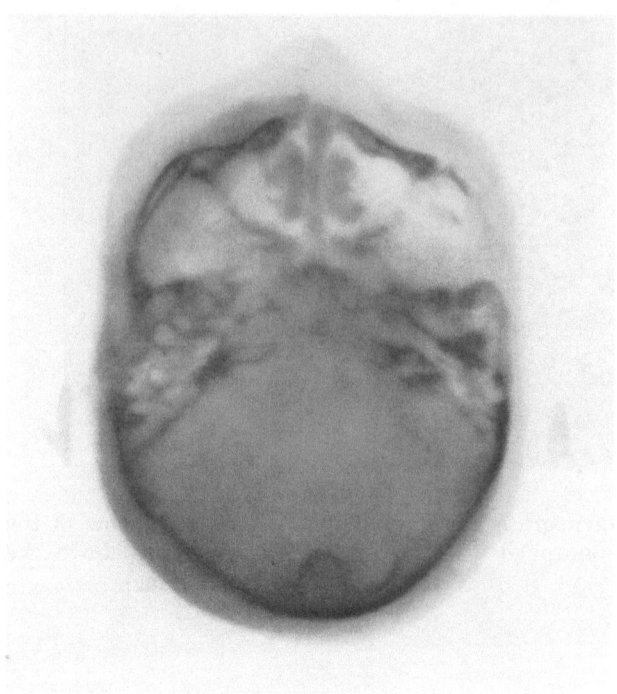

Fig. 76. Axial transverse tomogram

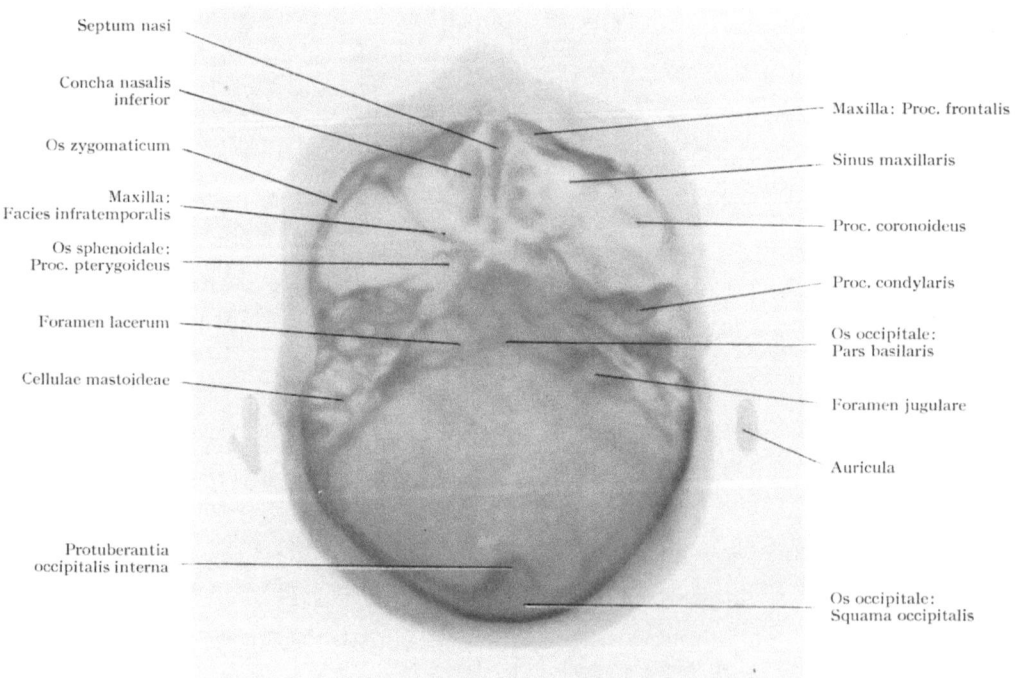

Septum nasi

Concha nasalis
inferior

Os zygomaticum

Maxilla:
Facies infratemporalis

Os sphenoidale:
Proc. pterygoideus

Foramen lacerum

Cellulae mastoideae

Protuberantia
occipitalis interna

Maxilla: Proc. frontalis

Sinus maxillaris

Proc. coronoideus

Proc. condylaris

Os occipitale:
Pars basilaris

Foramen jugulare

Auricula

Os occipitale:
Squama occipitalis

Fig. 77. Interpretation

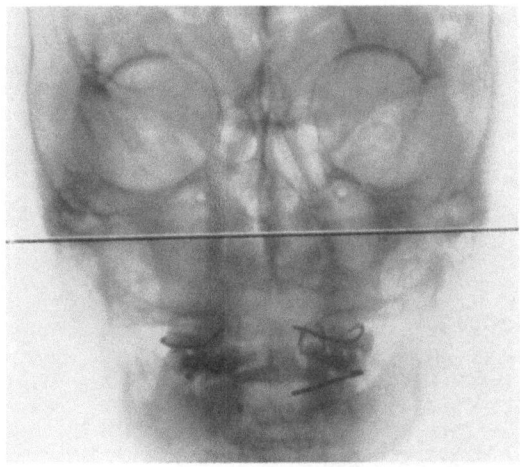

Fig. 78. Normal roentgenogram. Horizontal line showing the level tomographed

Fig. 79. Schema of tomographed level (solid line) along the acanthiomeatal line

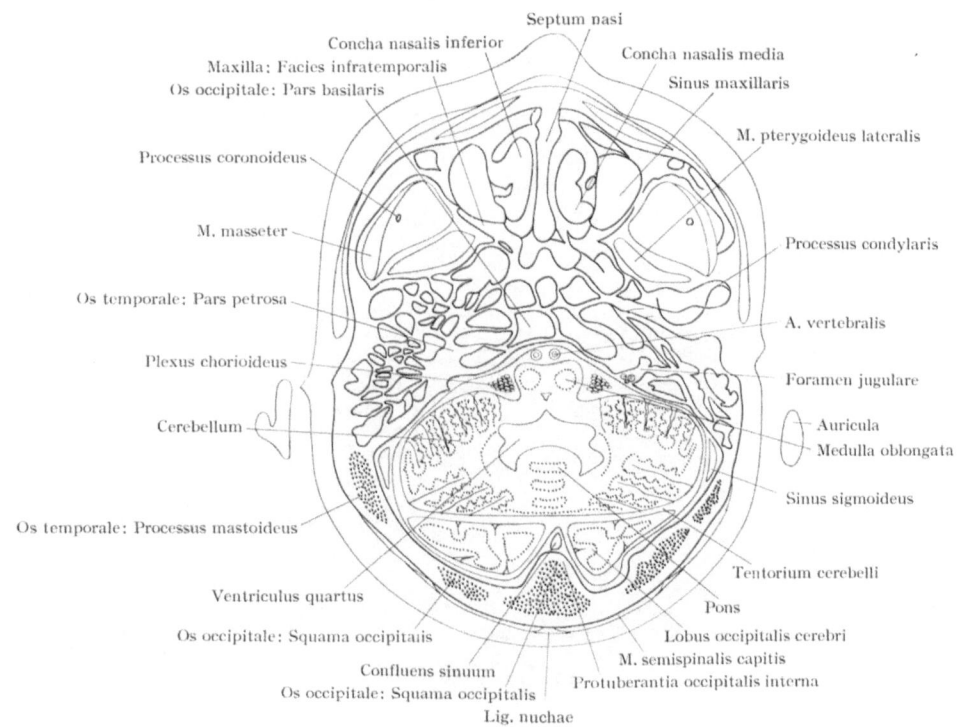

Septum nasi
Concha nasalis inferior
Maxilla: Facies infratemporalis
Os occipitale: Pars basilaris
Concha nasalis media
Sinus maxillaris
Processus coronoideus
M. pterygoideus lateralis
M. masseter
Processus condylaris
Os temporale: Pars petrosa
A. vertebralis
Plexus chorioideus
Foramen jugulare
Cerebellum
Auricula
Medulla oblongata
Os temporale: Processus mastoideus
Sinus sigmoideus
Tentorium cerebelli
Ventriculus quartus
Pons
Os occipitale: Squama occipitalis
Lobus occipitalis cerebri
M. semispinalis capitis
Confluens sinuum
Protuberantia occipitalis interna
Os occipitale: Squama occipitalis
Lig. nuchae

Fig. 80. Anatomical chart

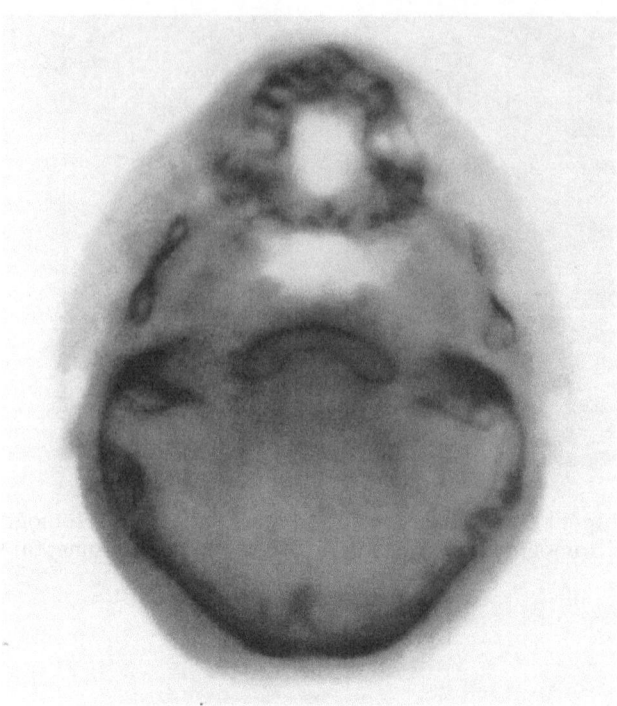

Fig. 81. Axial transverse tomogram

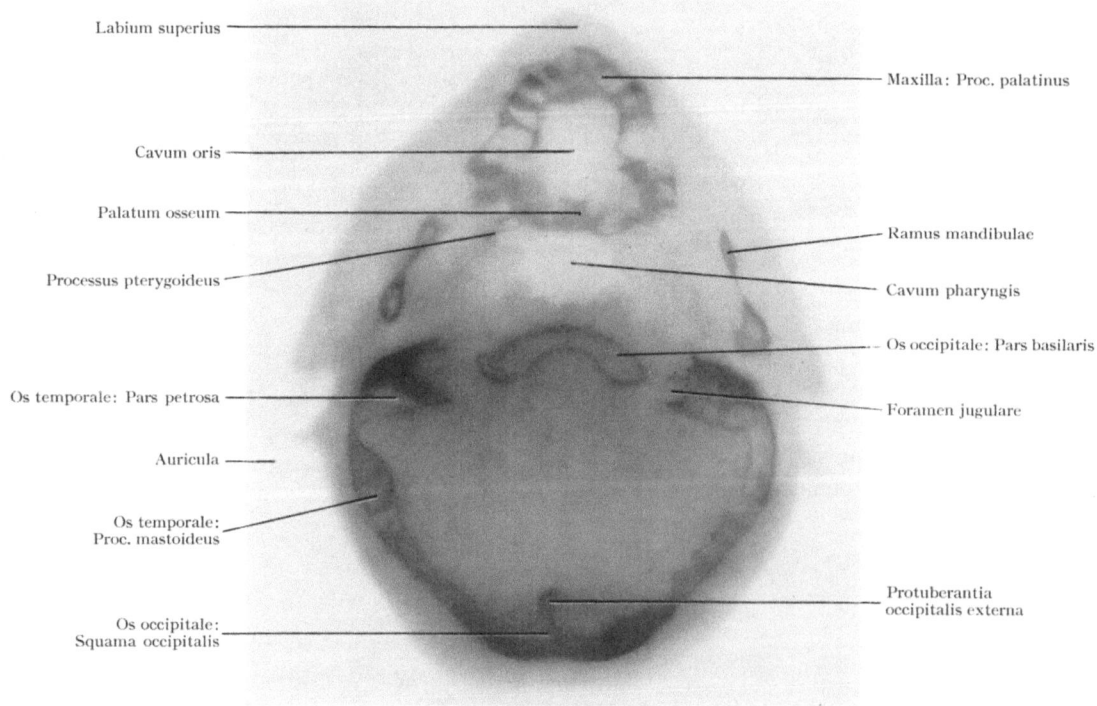

Labium superius

Cavum oris

Palatum osseum

Processus pterygoideus

Os temporale: Pars petrosa

Auricula

Os temporale:
Proc. mastoideus

Os occipitale:
Squama occipitalis

Maxilla: Proc. palatinus

Ramus mandibulae

Cavum pharyngis

Os occipitale: Pars basilaris

Foramen jugulare

Protuberantia
occipitalis externa

Fig. 82. Interpretation

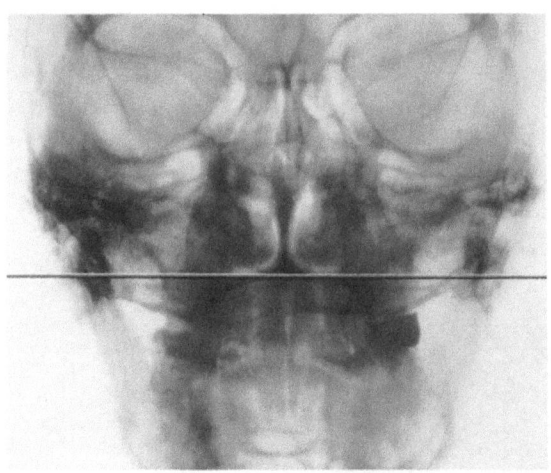

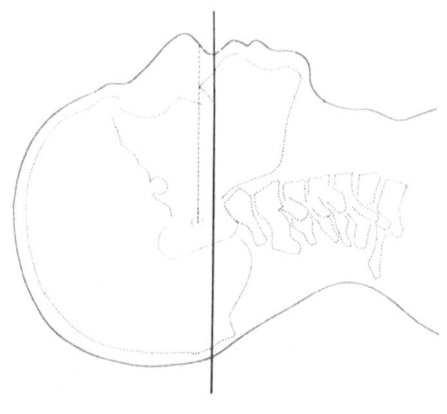

Fig. 83. Normal roentgenogram. Horizontal line showing the level tomographed

Fig. 84. Schema of tomographed level (solid line) 1 cm below the acanthiomeatal line (dashed line)

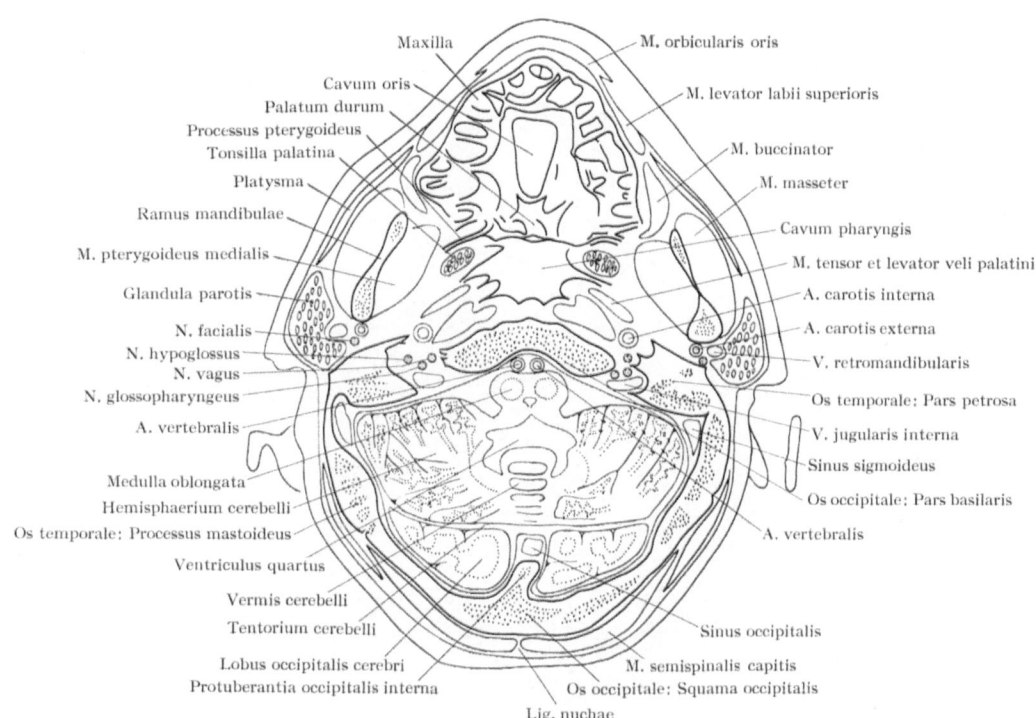

Fig. 85. Anatomical chart

47

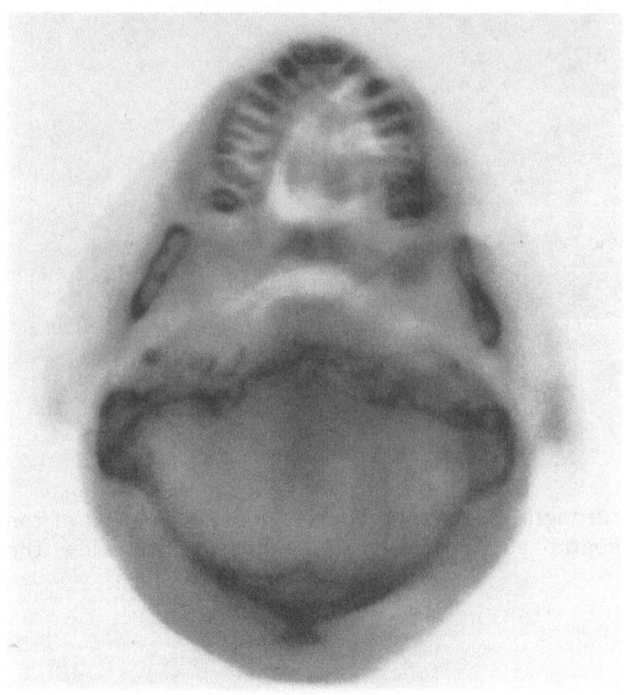

Fig. 86. Axial transverse tomogram

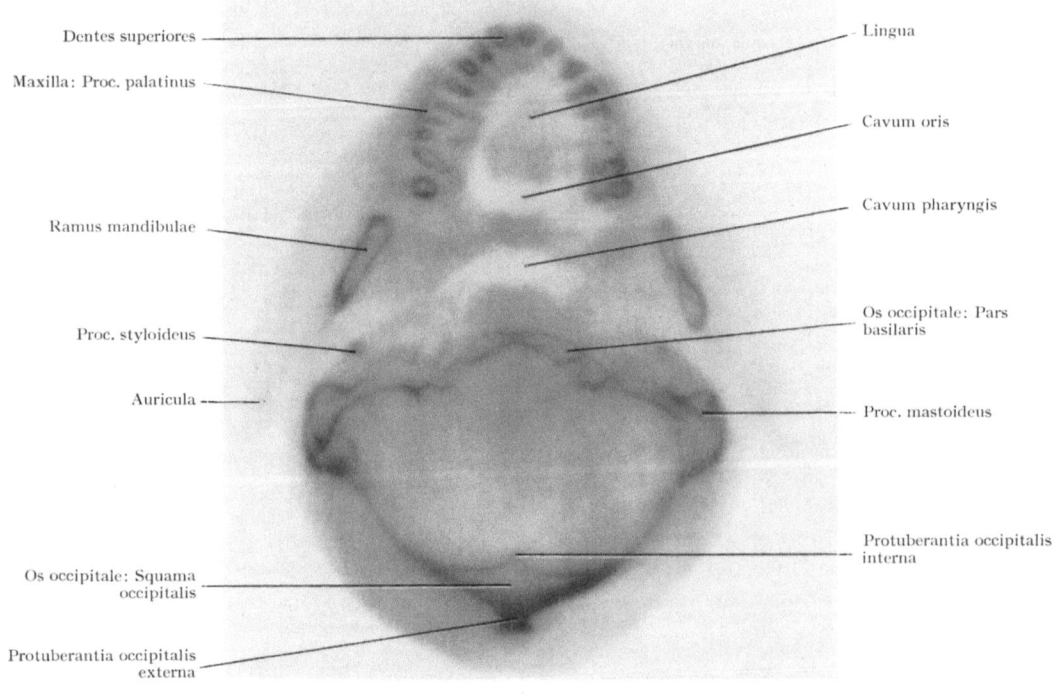

Dentes superiores

Maxilla: Proc. palatinus

Ramus mandibulae

Proc. styloideus

Auricula

Os occipitale: Squama occipitalis

Protuberantia occipitalis externa

Lingua

Cavum oris

Cavum pharyngis

Os occipitale: Pars basilaris

Proc. mastoideus

Protuberantia occipitalis interna

Fig. 87. Interpretation

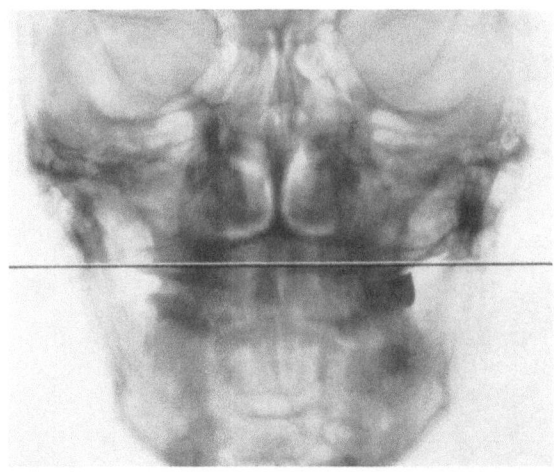

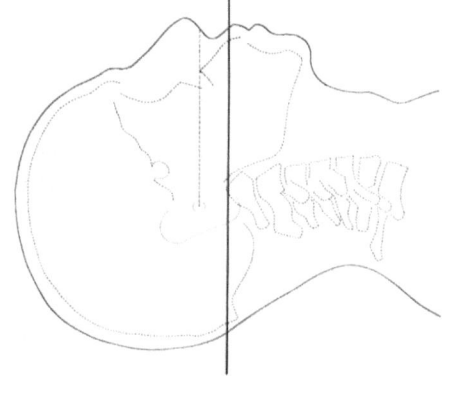

Fig. 88. Normal roentgenogram. Horizontal line showing the level tomographed

Fig. 89. Schema of tomographed level (solid line) 2 cm below the acanthiomeatal line (dashed line)

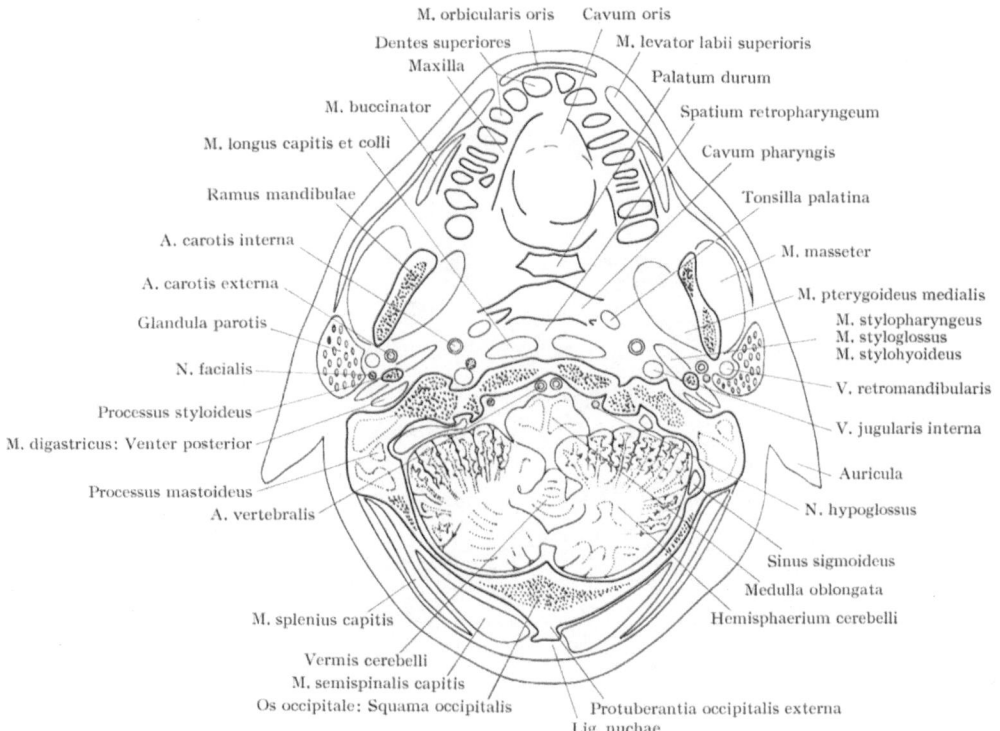

Fig. 90. Anatomical chart

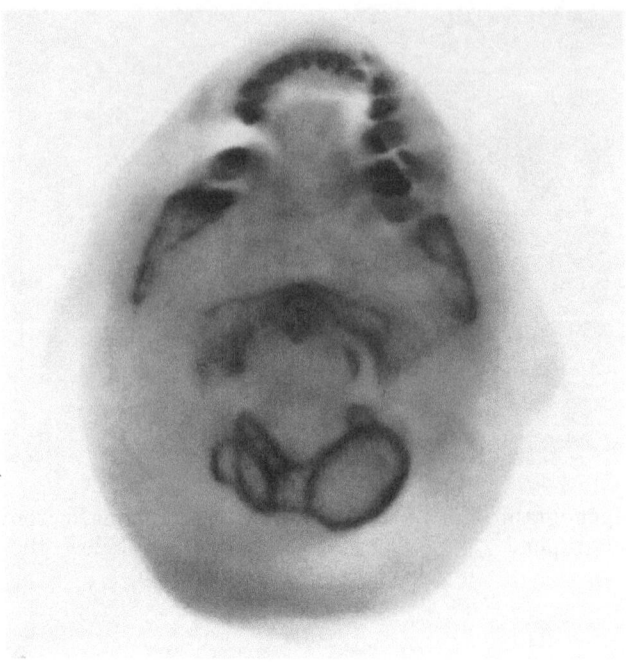

Fig. 91. Axial transverse tomogram

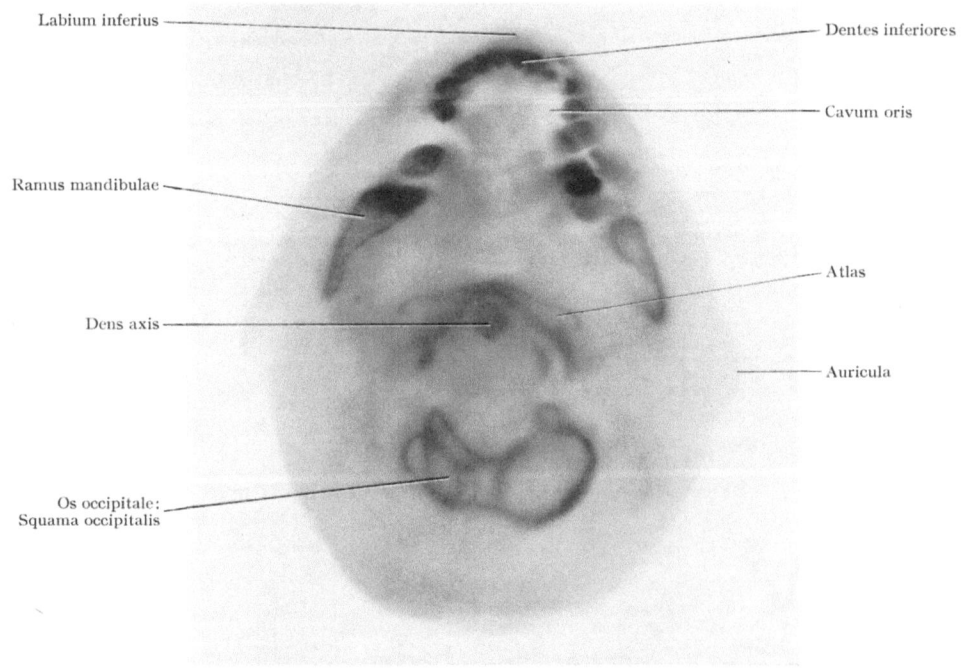

Labium inferius

Ramus mandibulae

Dens axis

Os occipitale:
Squama occipitalis

Dentes inferiores

Cavum oris

Atlas

Auricula

Fig. 92. Interpretation

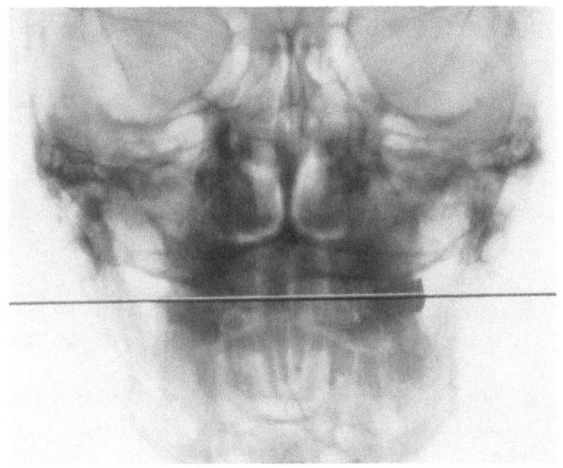

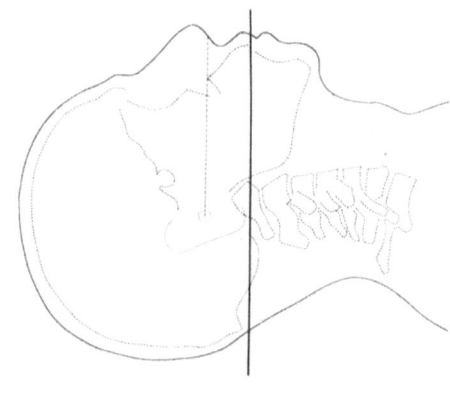

Fig. 93. Normal roentgenogram. Horizontal line showing the level tomographed

Fig. 94. Schema of tomographed level (solid line) 3 cm below the acanthiomeatal line (dashed line)

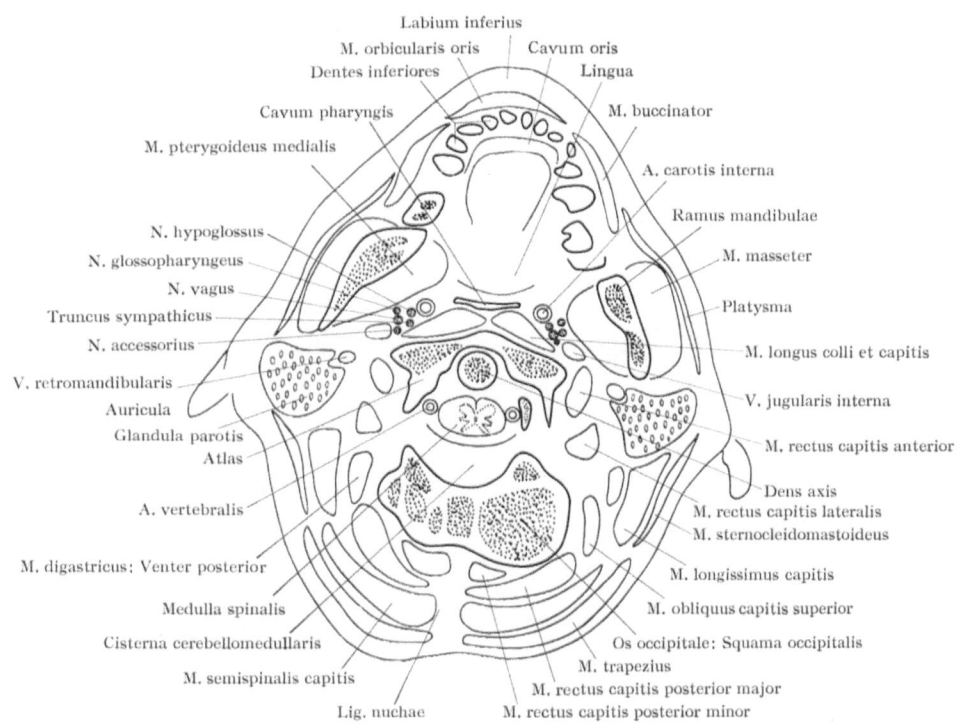

Fig. 95. Anatomical chart

Neck

Eleven axial transverse tomograms of the subject with air insufflated into the subdermal space.

Appendices:
1. Axial transverse tomograms of the parotis.
2. Axial transverse tomograms of the neck without contrast medium.

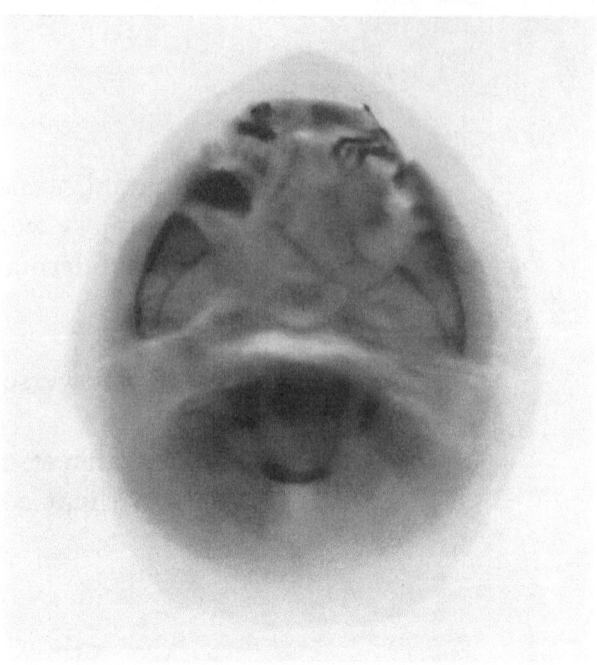

Fig. 96. Axial transverse tomogram

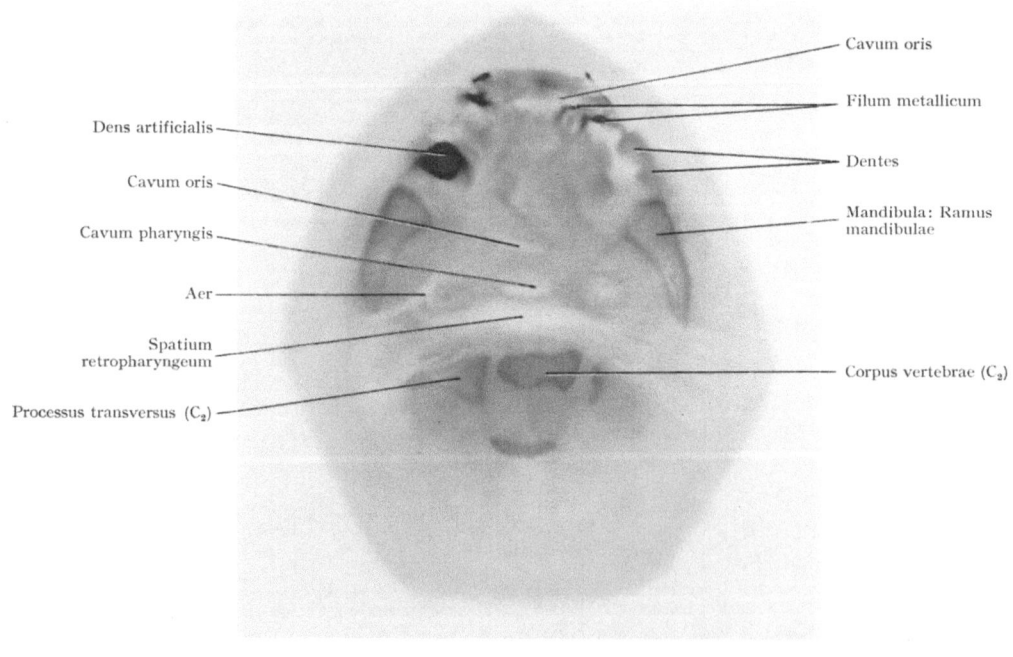

Fig. 97. Interpretation

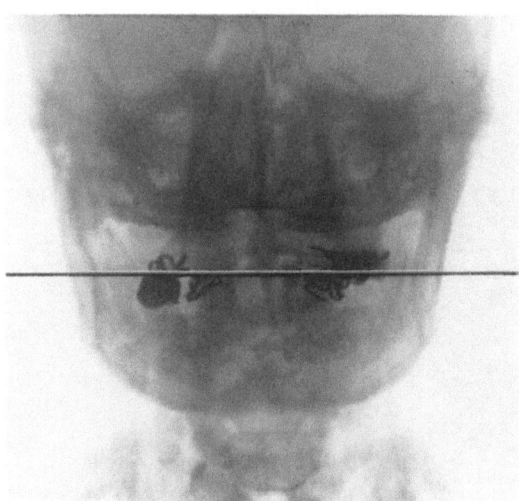

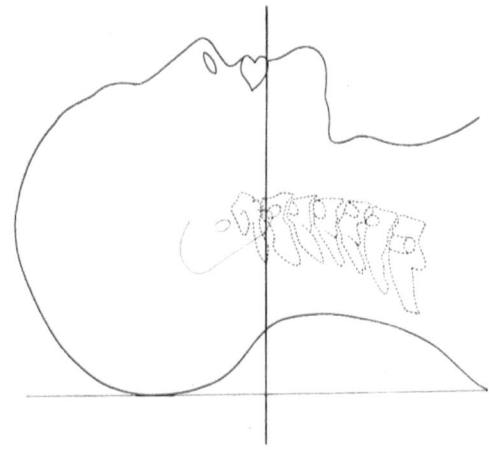

Fig. 98. Normal roentgenogram. Horizontal line showing the level tomographed

Fig. 99. Schematic drawing of the level tomographed

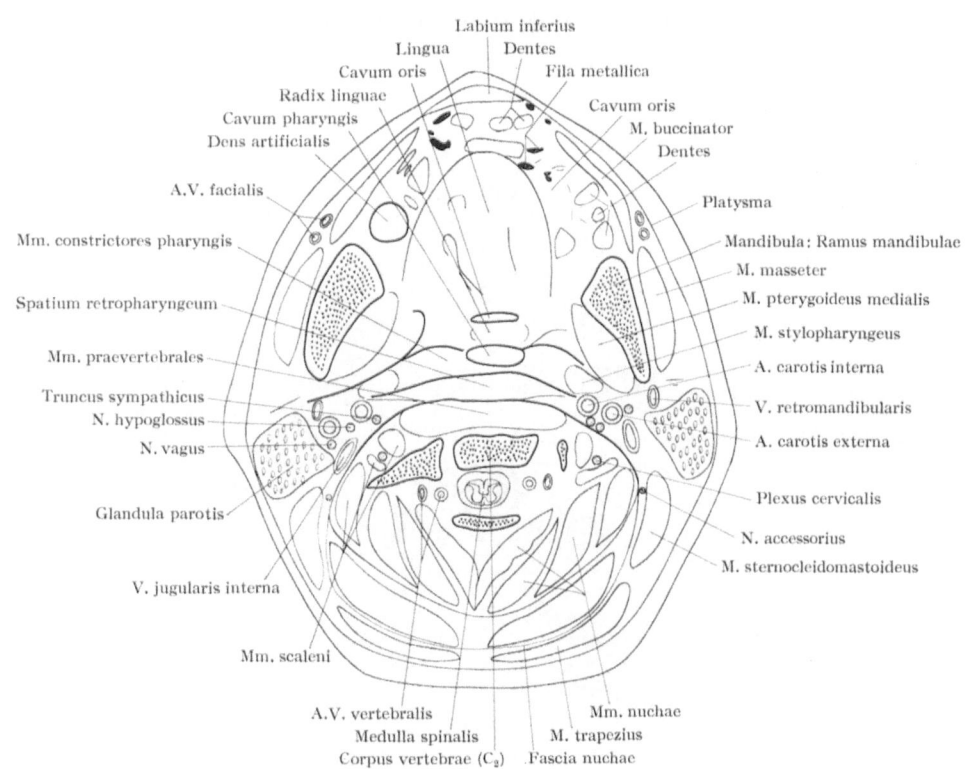

Fig. 100. Anatomical chart

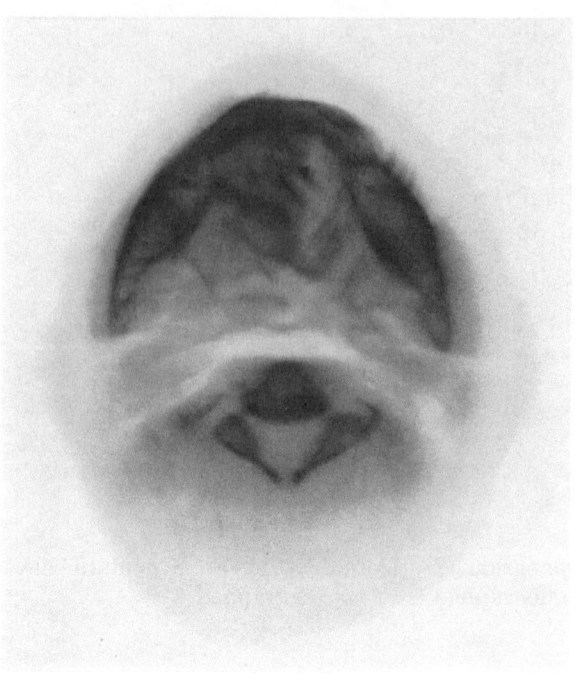

Fig. 101. Axial transverse tomogram

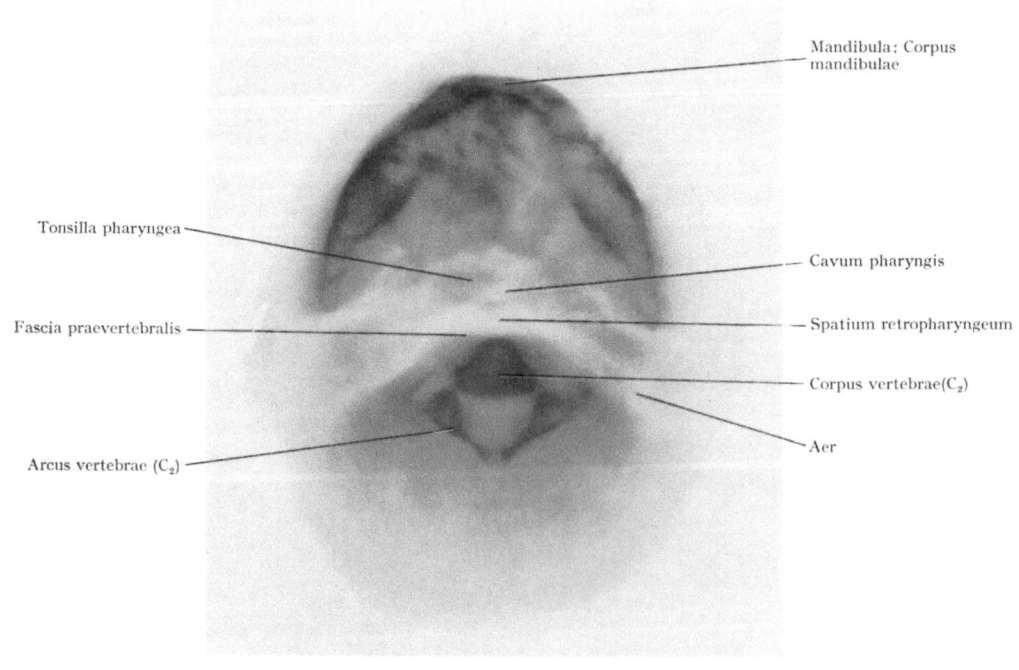

Fig. 102. Interpretation

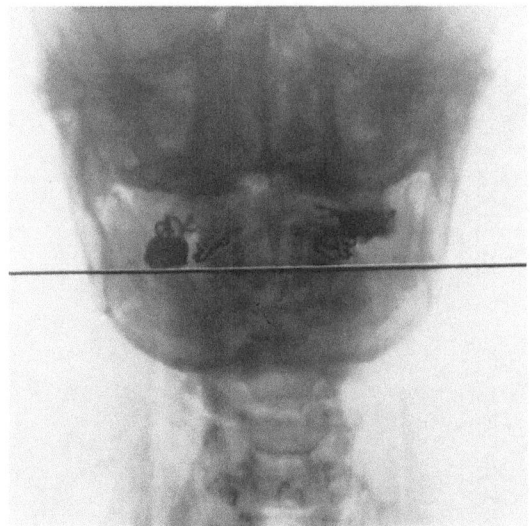

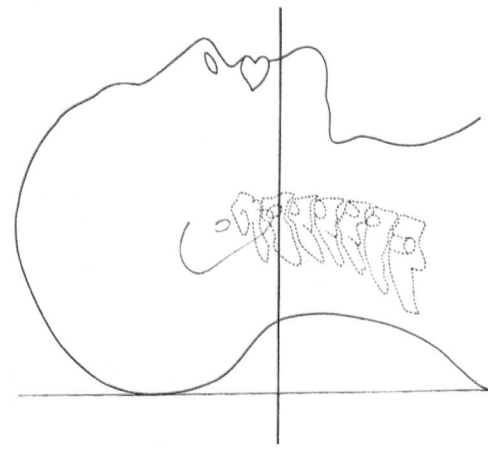

Fig. 103. Normal roentgenogram. Horizontal line showing the level tomographed

Fig. 104. Schematic drawing of the level tomographed

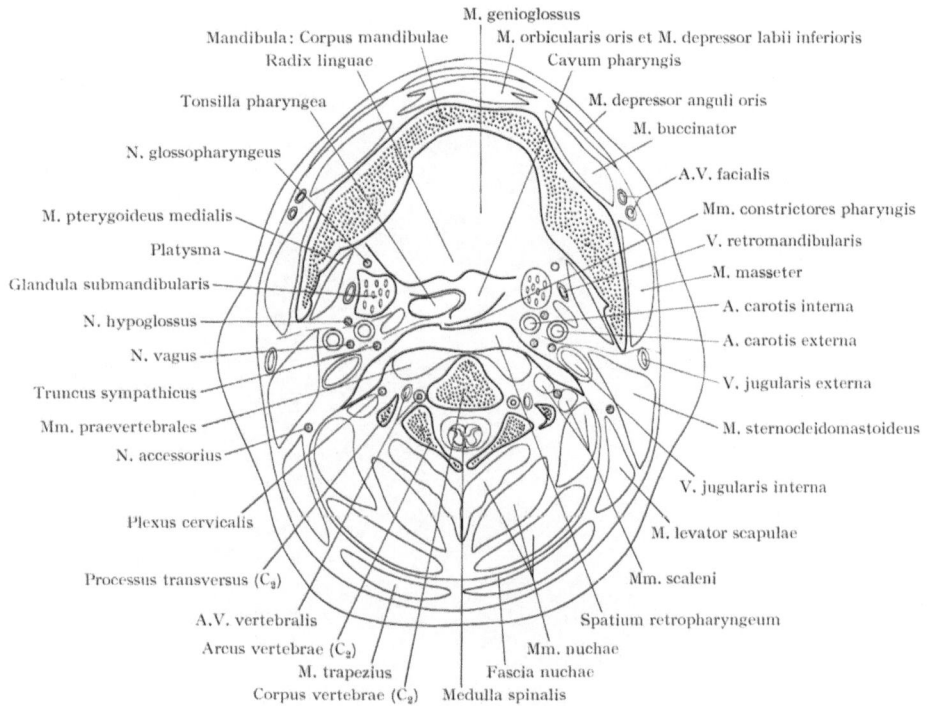

Fig. 105. Anatomical chart

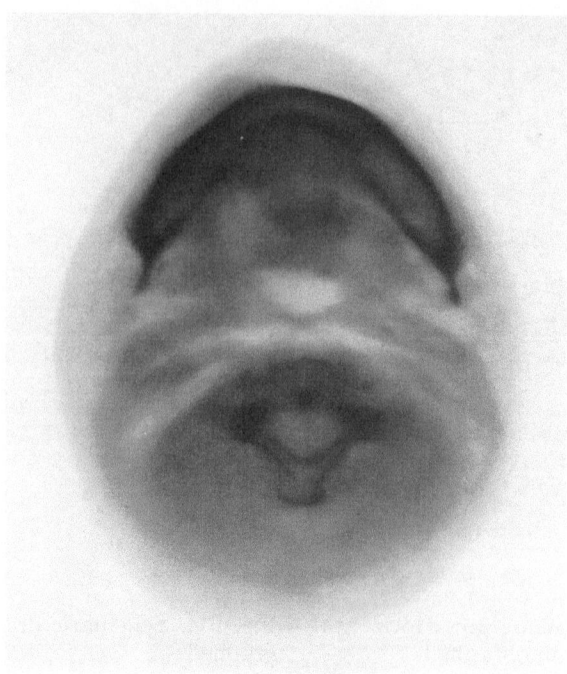

Fig. 106. Axial transverse tomogram

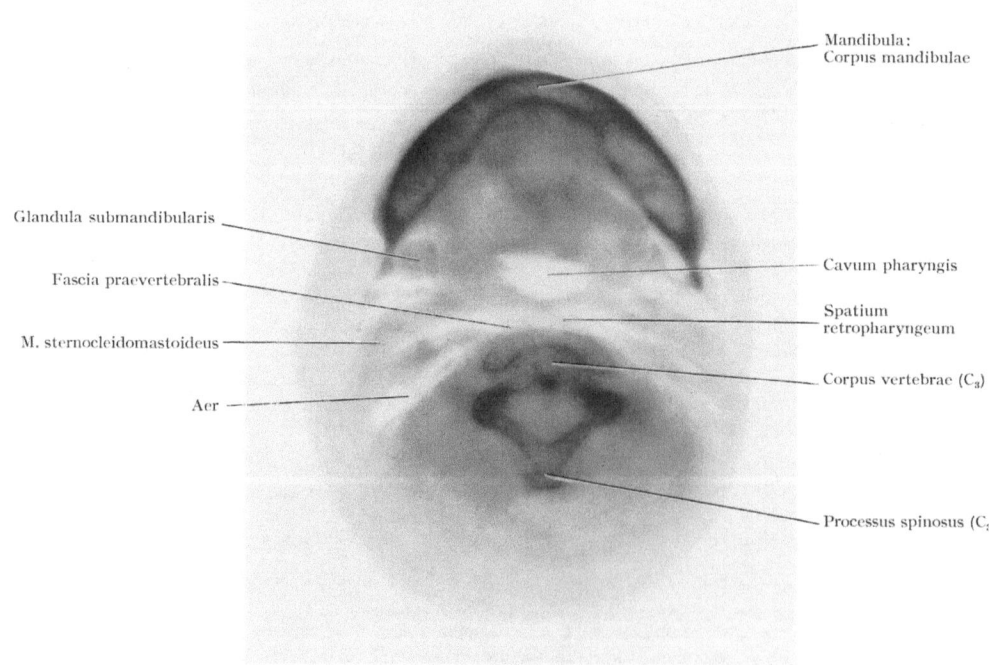

Mandibula:
Corpus mandibulae

Glandula submandibularis

Fascia praevertebralis

M. sternocleidomastoideus

Aer

Cavum pharyngis

Spatium
retropharyngeum

Corpus vertebrae (C₃)

Processus spinosus (C₃

Fig. 107. Interpretation

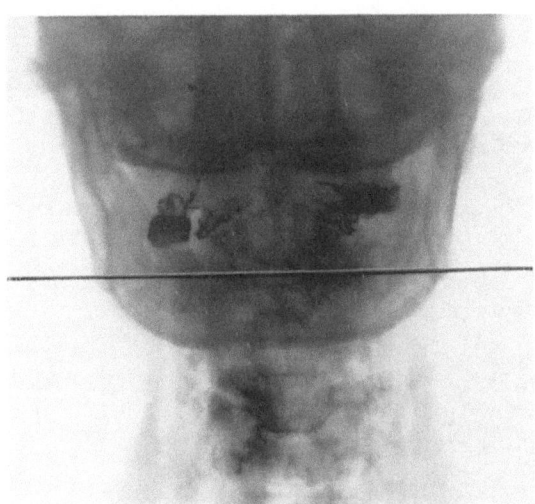
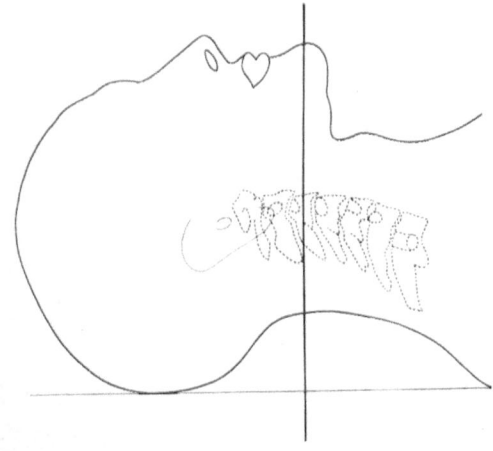

Fig. 108. Normal roentgenogram. Horizontal line showing the level tomographed

Fig. 109. Schematic drawing of the level tomographed

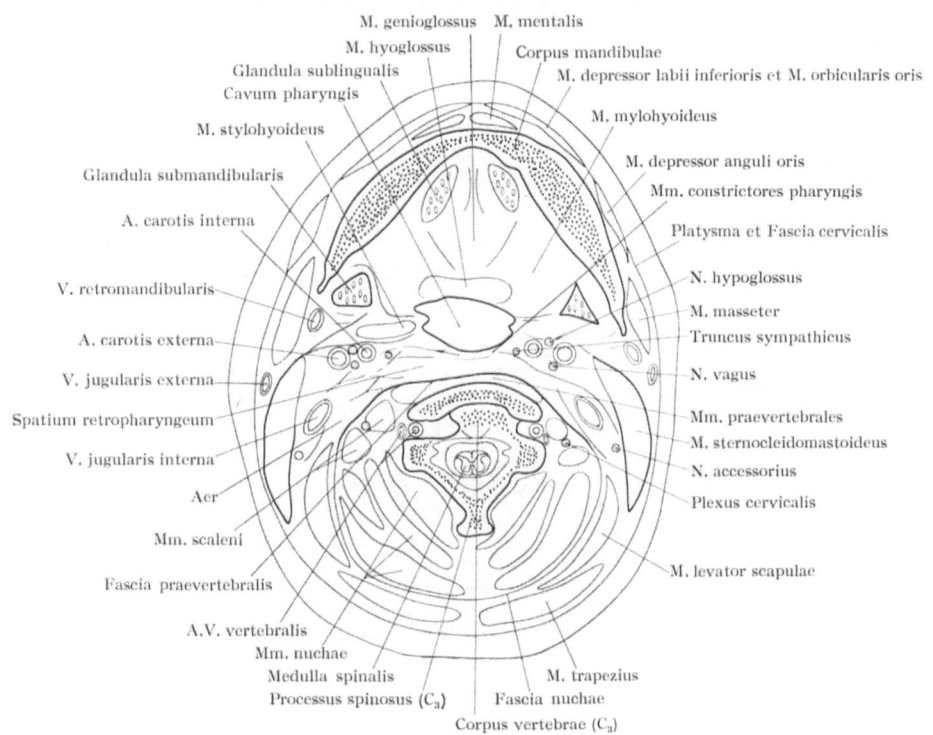

M. genioglossus M. mentalis
M. hyoglossus
Glandula sublingualis
Cavum pharyngis
M. stylohyoideus
Glandula submandibularis
A. carotis interna
V. retromandibularis
A. carotis externa
V. jugularis externa
Spatium retropharyngeum
V. jugularis interna
Aer
Mm. scaleni
Fascia praevertebralis
A.V. vertebralis
Mm. nuchae
Medulla spinalis
Processus spinosus (C₃)

Corpus mandibulae
M. depressor labii inferioris et M. orbicularis oris
M. mylohyoideus
M. depressor anguli oris
Mm. constrictores pharyngis
Platysma et Fascia cervicalis
N. hypoglossus
M. masseter
Truncus sympathicus
N. vagus
Mm. praevertebrales
M. sternocleidomastoideus
N. accessorius
Plexus cervicalis
M. levator scapulae
M. trapezius
Fascia nuchae
Corpus vertebrae (C₃)

Fig. 110. Anatomical chart

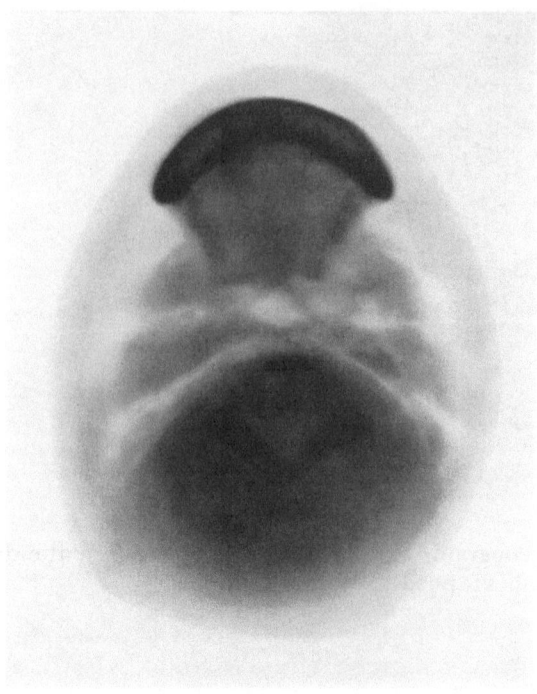

Fig. 111. Axial transverse tomogram

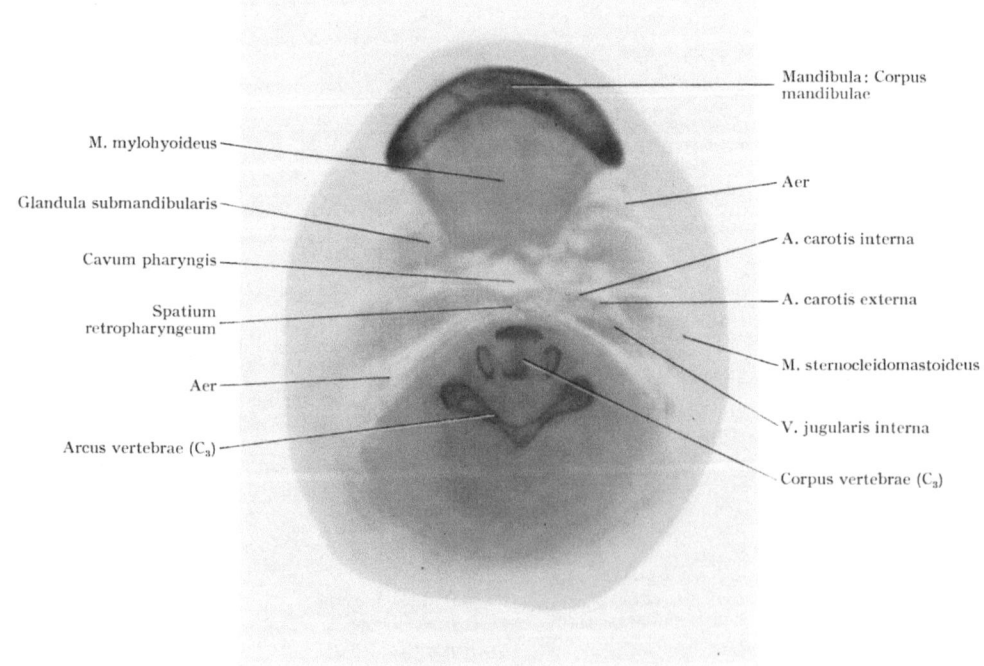

Mandibula: Corpus mandibulae

M. mylohyoideus

Glandula submandibularis

Cavum pharyngis

Spatium retropharyngeum

Aer

Arcus vertebrae (C₃)

Aer

A. carotis interna

A. carotis externa

M. sternocleidomastoideus

V. jugularis interna

Corpus vertebrae (C₃)

Fig. 112. Interpretation

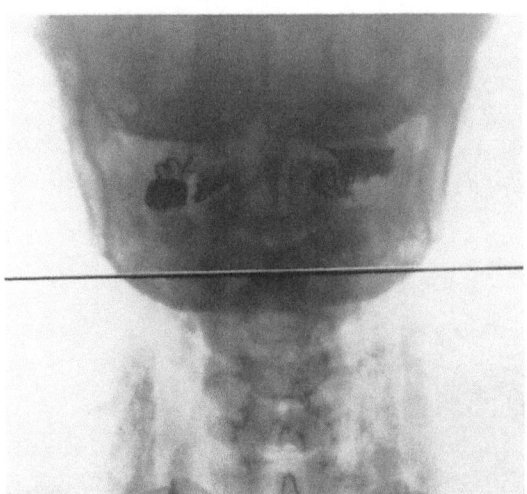

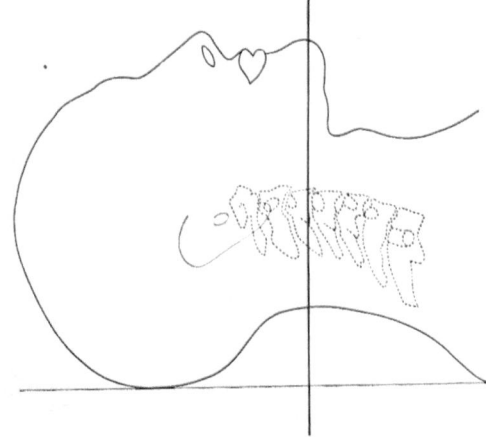

Fig. 113. Normal roentgenogram. Horizontal line showing the level tomographed

Fig. 114. Schematic drawing of the level tomographed

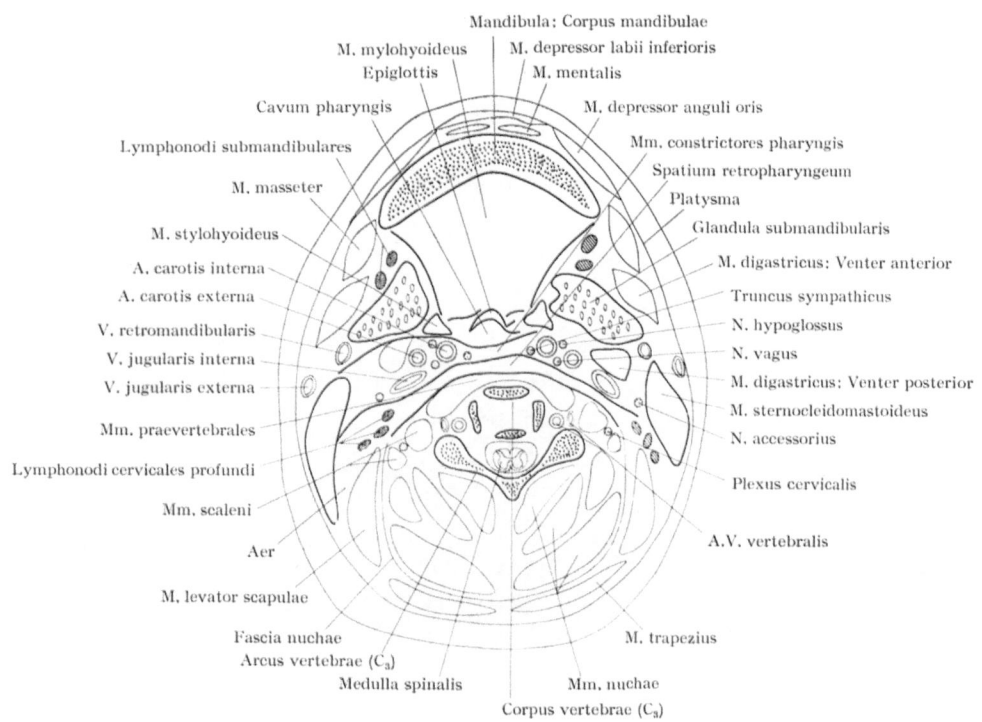

Fig. 115. Anatomical chart

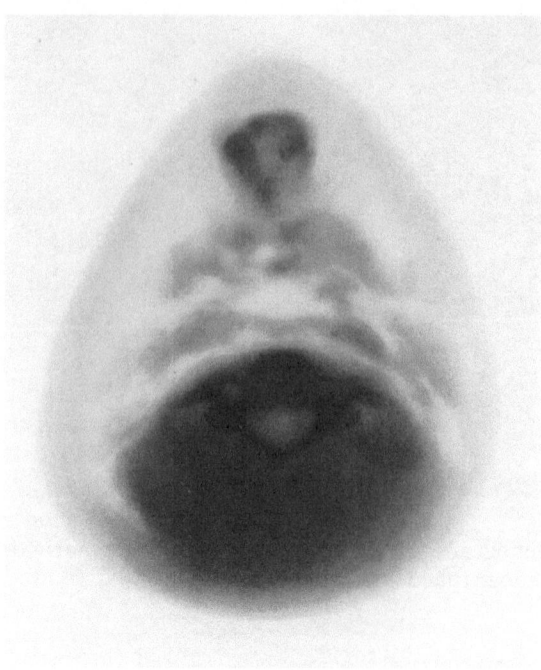

Fig. 116. Axial transverse tomogram

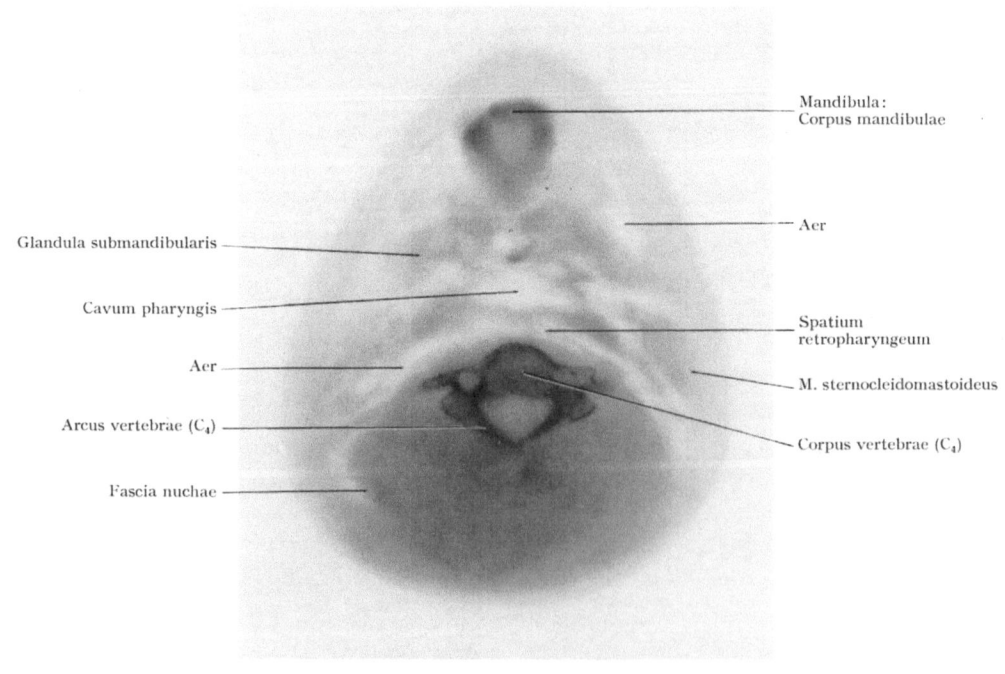

Mandibula:
Corpus mandibulae

Aer

Glandula submandibularis

Cavum pharyngis

Spatium
retropharyngeum

Aer

M. sternocleidomastoideus

Arcus vertebrae (C$_4$)

Corpus vertebrae (C$_4$)

Fascia nuchae

Fig. 117. Interpretation

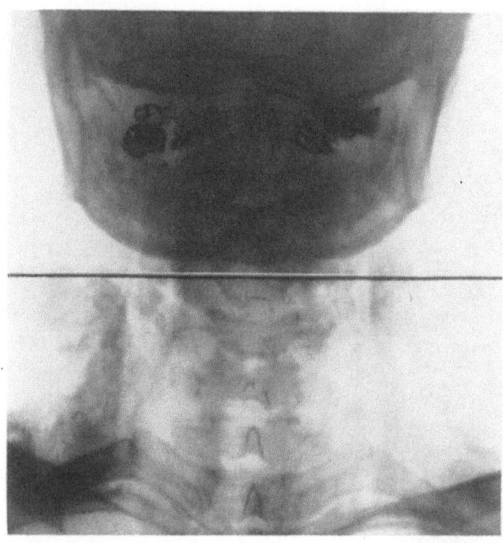

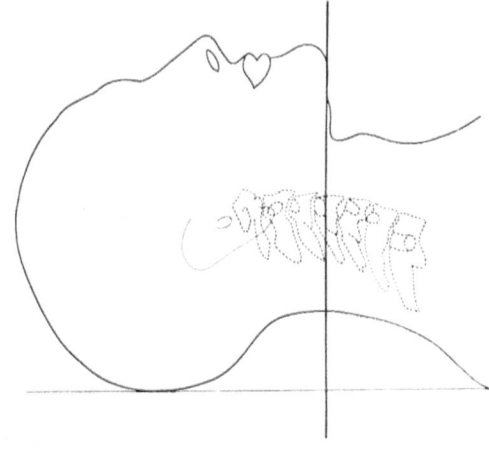

Fig. 118. Normal roentgenogram. Horizontal line showing the level tomographed

Fig. 119. Schematic drawing of the level tomographed

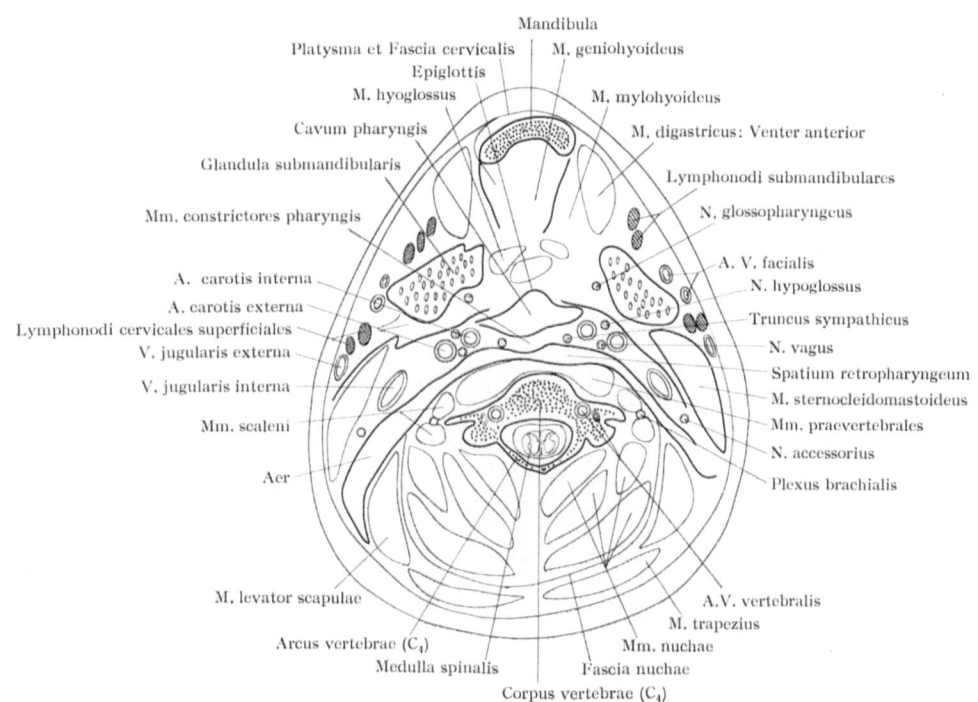

Fig. 120. Anatomical chart

63

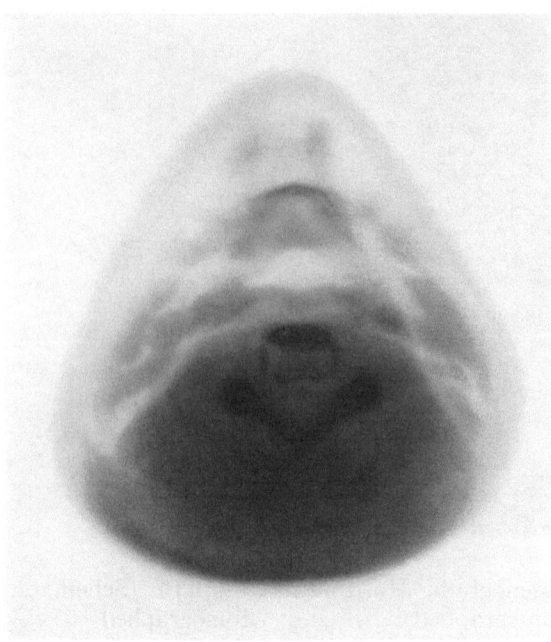

Fig. 121. Axial transverse tomogram

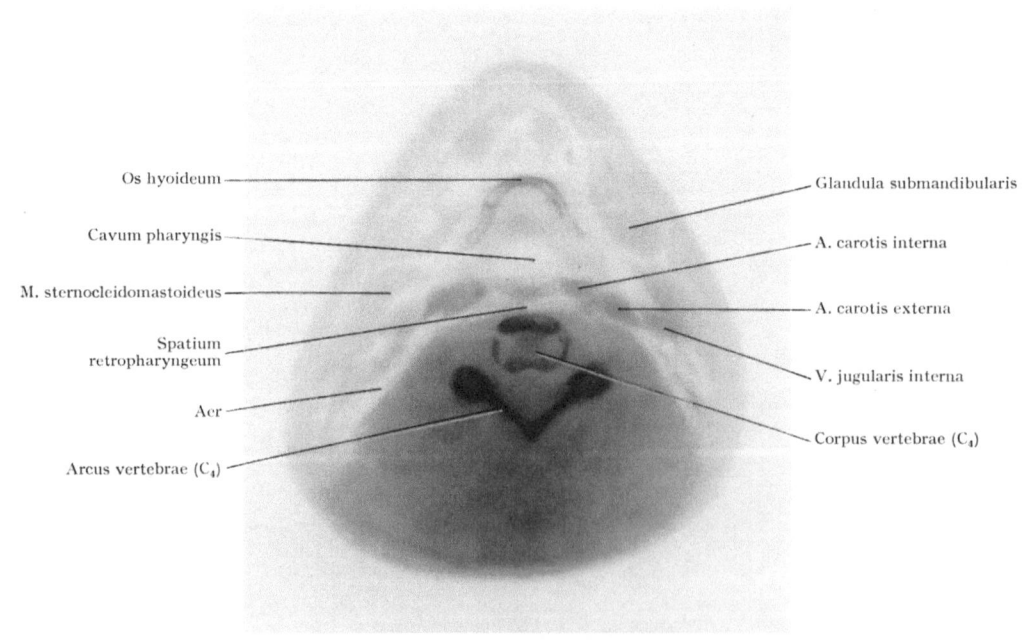

Os hyoideum — Glandula submandibularis

Cavum pharyngis — A. carotis interna

M. sternocleidomastoideus — A. carotis externa

Spatium retropharyngeum — V. jugularis interna

Aer — Corpus vertebrae (C₄)

Arcus vertebrae (C₄)

Fig. 122. Interpretation

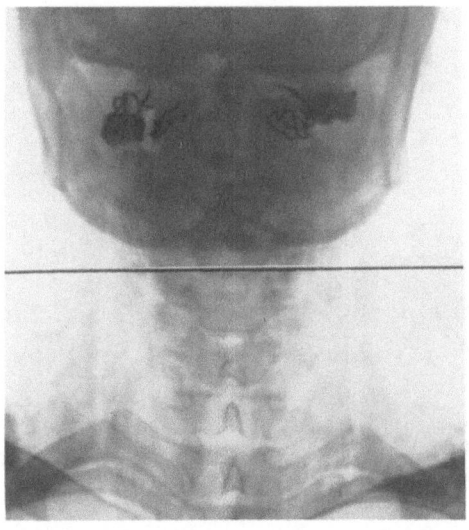

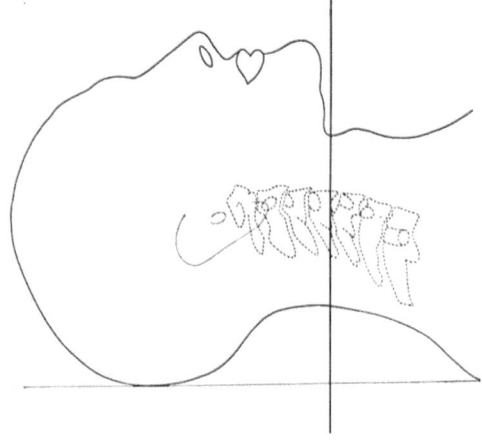

Fig. 123. Normal roentgenogram. Horizontal line showing the level tomographed

Fig. 124. Schematic drawing of the level tomographed

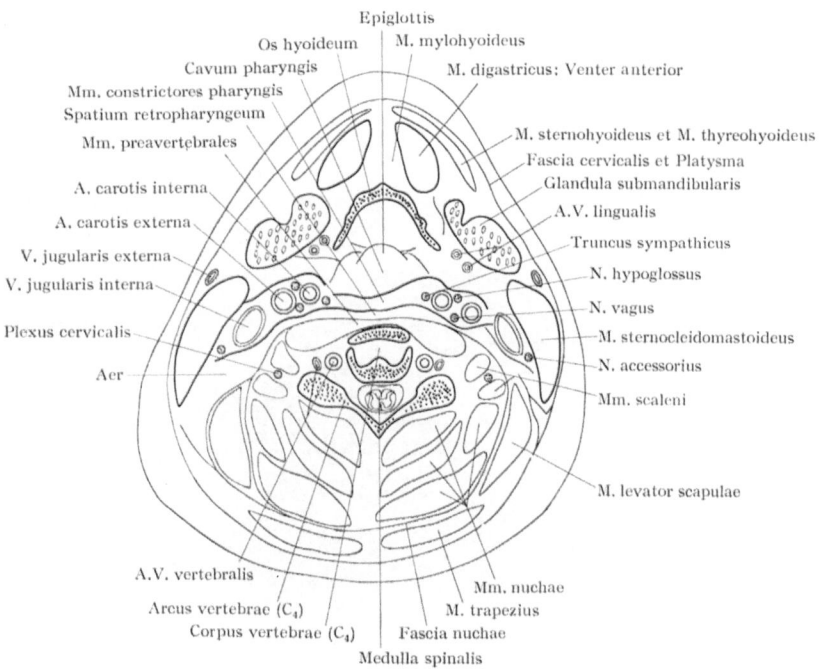

Epiglottis

Os hyoideum — M. mylohyoideus

Cavum pharyngis — M. digastricus: Venter anterior

Mm. constrictores pharyngis

Spatium retropharyngeum

Mm. preavertebrales — M. sternohyoideus et M. thyreohyoideus

Fascia cervicalis et Platysma

Glandula submandibularis

A. carotis interna — A.V. lingualis

A. carotis externa — Truncus sympathicus

V. jugularis externa — N. hypoglossus

V. jugularis interna — N. vagus

M. sternocleidomastoideus

Plexus cervicalis — N. accessorius

Mm. scaleni

Aer

M. levator scapulae

A.V. vertebralis

Arcus vertebrae (C₄) — Mm. nuchae

M. trapezius

Corpus vertebrae (C₄) — Fascia nuchae

Medulla spinalis

Fig. 125. Anatomical chart

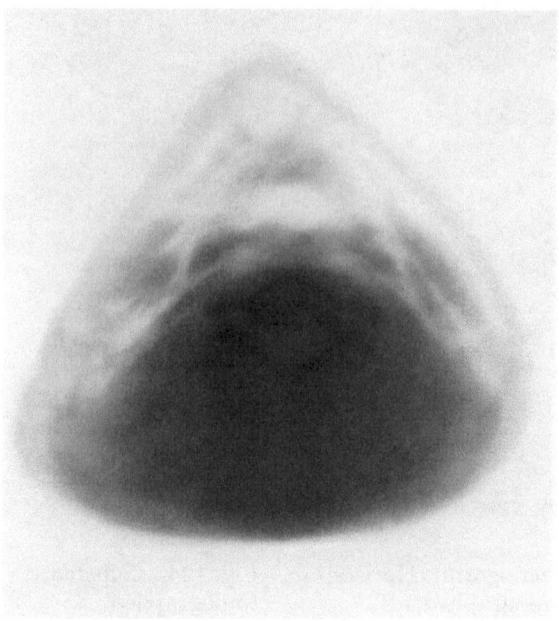

Fig. 126. Axial transverse tomogram

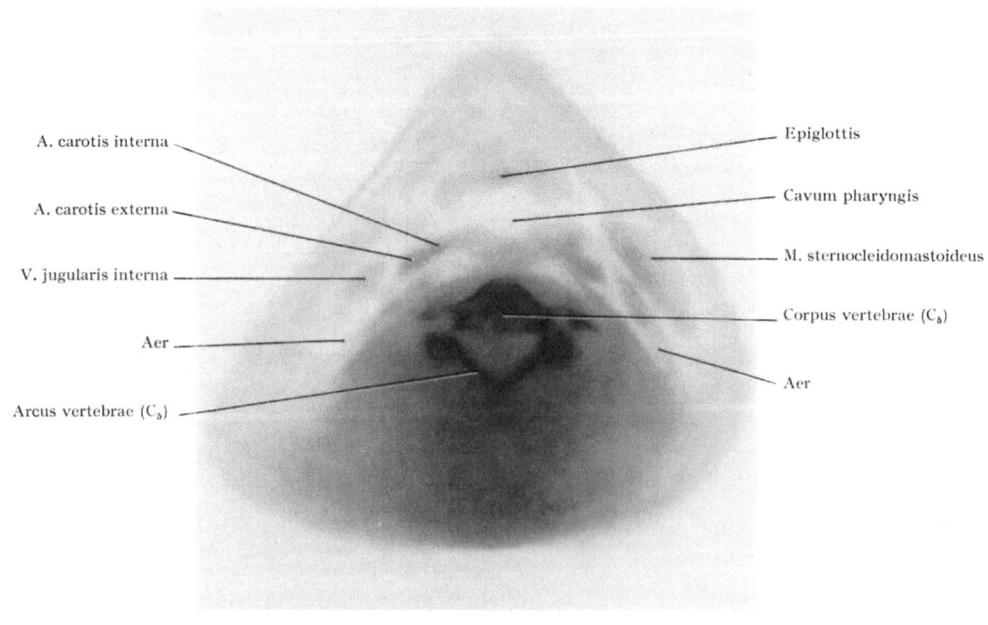

A. carotis interna

A. carotis externa

V. jugularis interna

Aer

Arcus vertebrae (C$_5$)

Epiglottis

Cavum pharyngis

M. sternocleidomastoideus

Corpus vertebrae (C$_5$)

Aer

Fig. 127. Interpretation

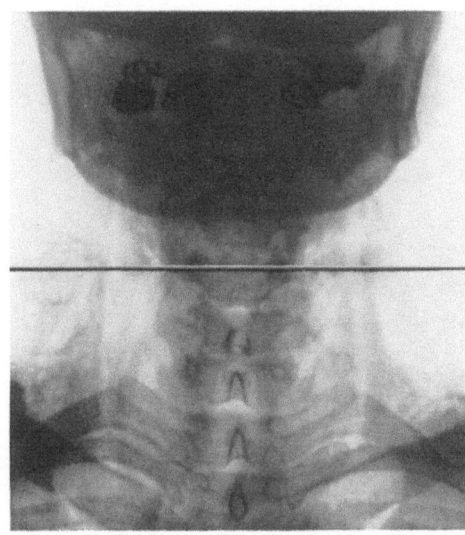

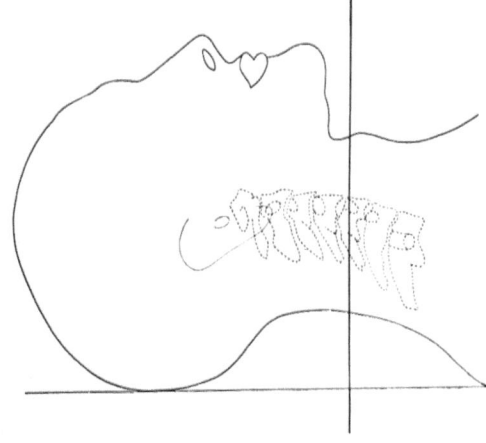

Fig. 128. Normal roentgenogram. Horizontal line showing the level tomographed

Fig. 129. Schematic drawing of the level tomographed

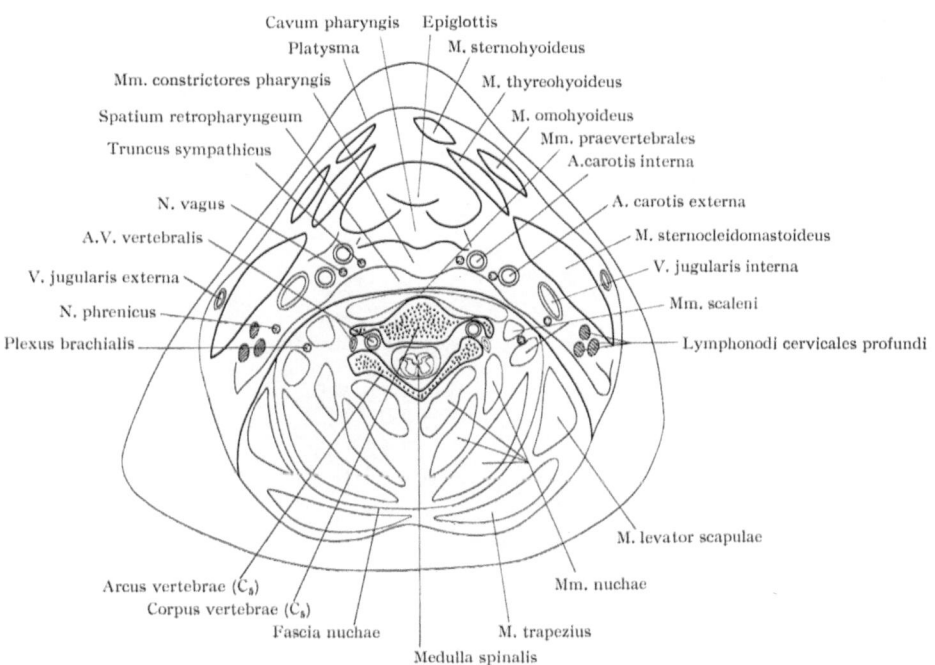

Cavum pharyngis   Epiglottis
Platysma   M. sternohyoideus
Mm. constrictores pharyngis   M. thyreohyoideus
Spatium retropharyngeum   M. omohyoideus
Truncus sympathicus   Mm. praevertebrales
    A. carotis interna
N. vagus   A. carotis externa
A.V. vertebralis   M. sternocleidomastoideus
V. jugularis externa   V. jugularis interna
N. phrenicus   Mm. scaleni
Plexus brachialis   Lymphonodi cervicales profundi
    M. levator scapulae
Arcus vertebrae (C₅)   Mm. nuchae
Corpus vertebrae (C₅)
Fascia nuchae   M. trapezius
Medulla spinalis

Fig. 130. Anatomical chart

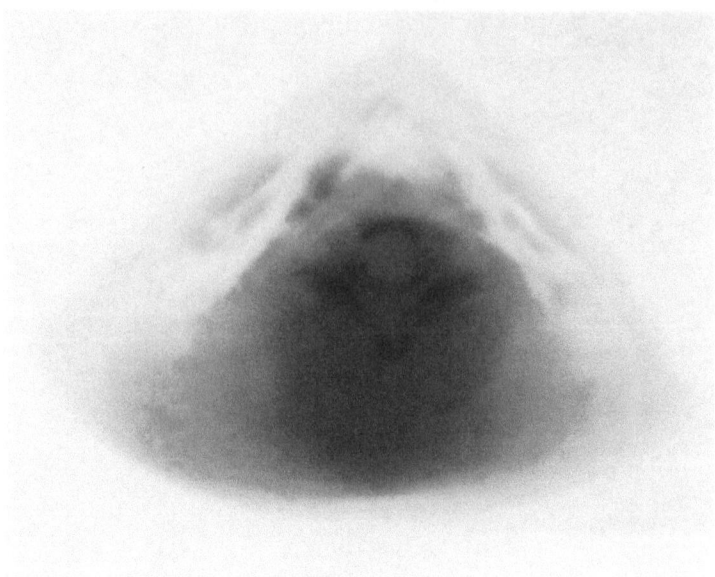

Fig. 131. Axial transverse tomogram

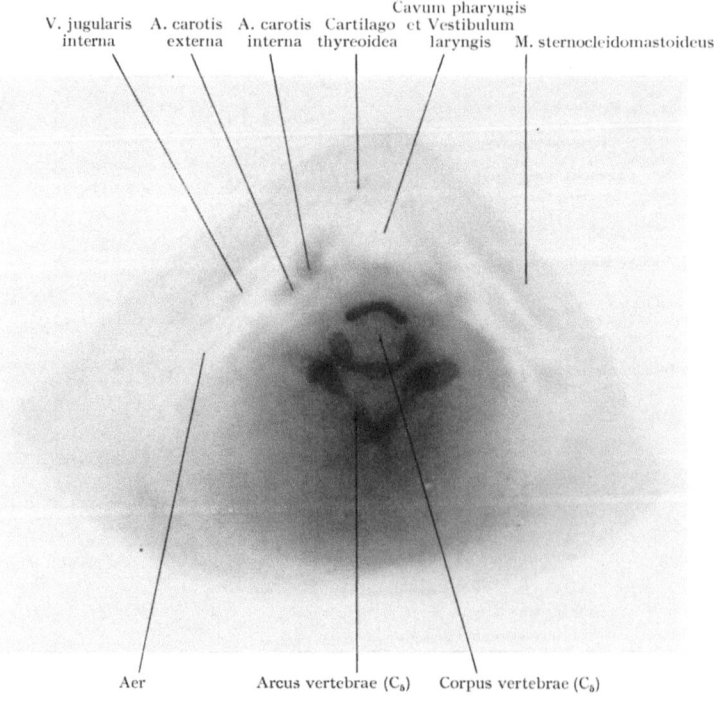

Fig. 132. Interpretation

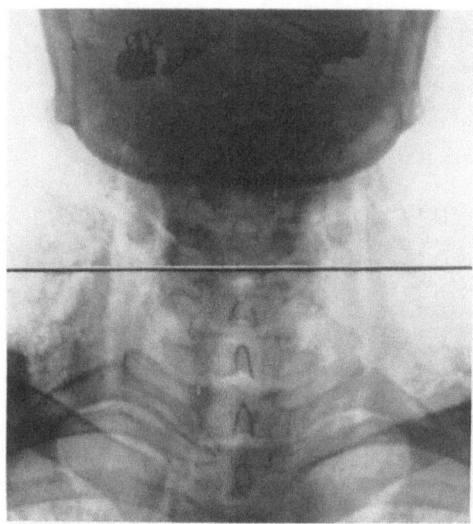
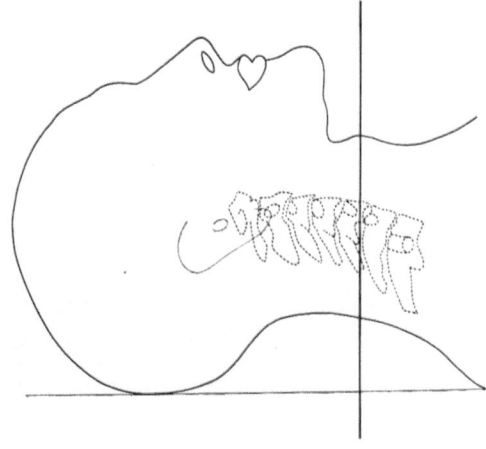

Fig. 133. Normal roentgenogram. Horizontal line showing the level tomographed

Fig. 134. Schematic drawing of the level tomographed

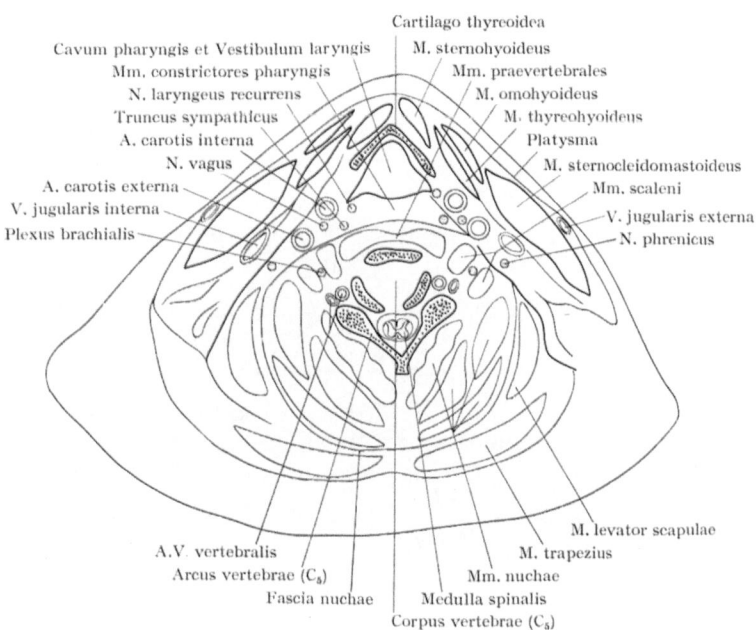

Fig. 135. Anatomical chart

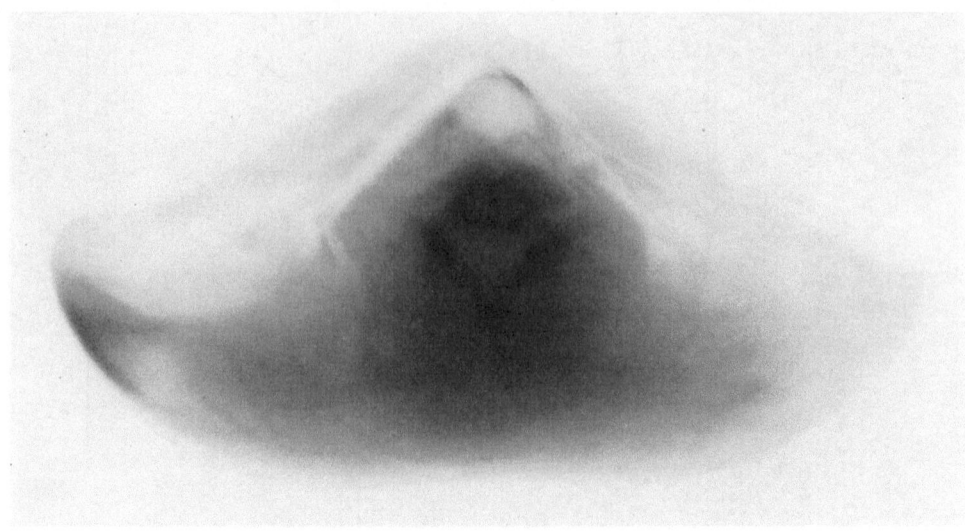

Fig. 136. Axial transverse tomogram

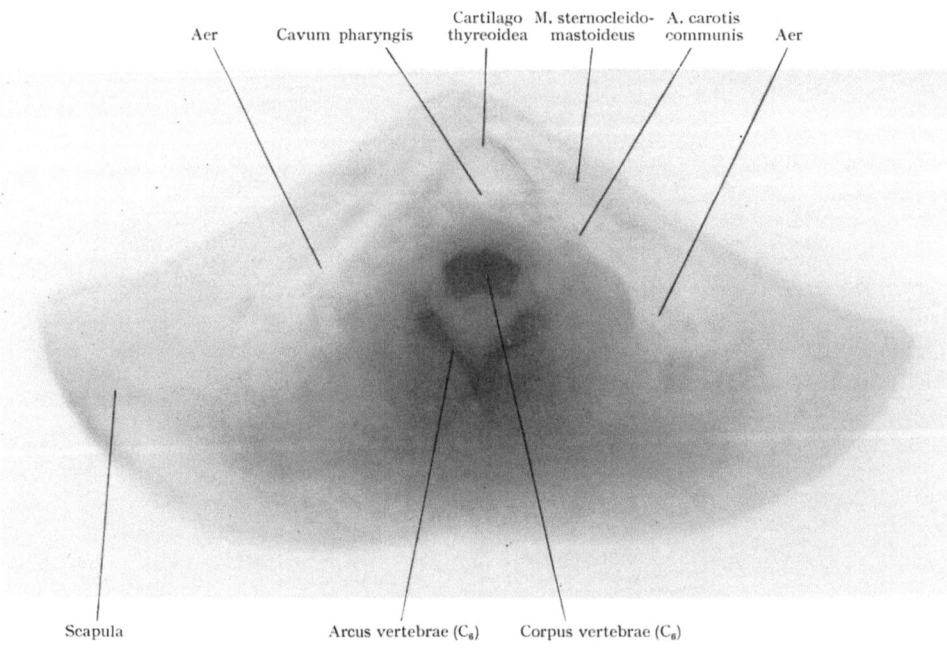

Aer Cavum pharyngis Cartilago thyreoidea M. sternocleido-mastoideus A. carotis communis Aer

Scapula Arcus vertebrae (C$_6$) Corpus vertebrae (C$_6$)

Fig. 137. Interpretation

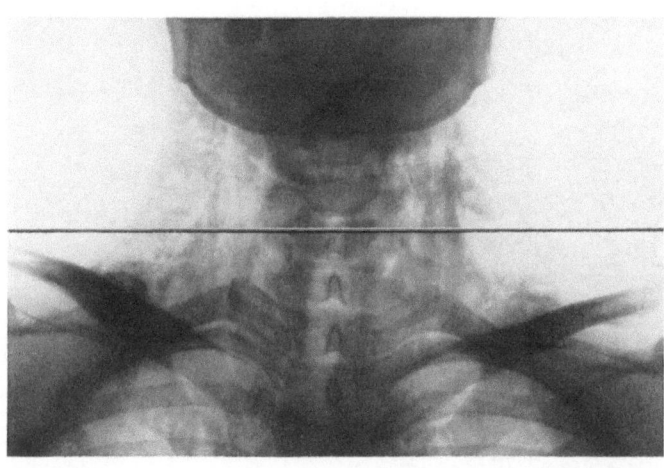

Fig. 138. Normal roentgenogram. Horizontal line showing the level tomographed

Fig. 139. Schematic drawing of the level tomographed

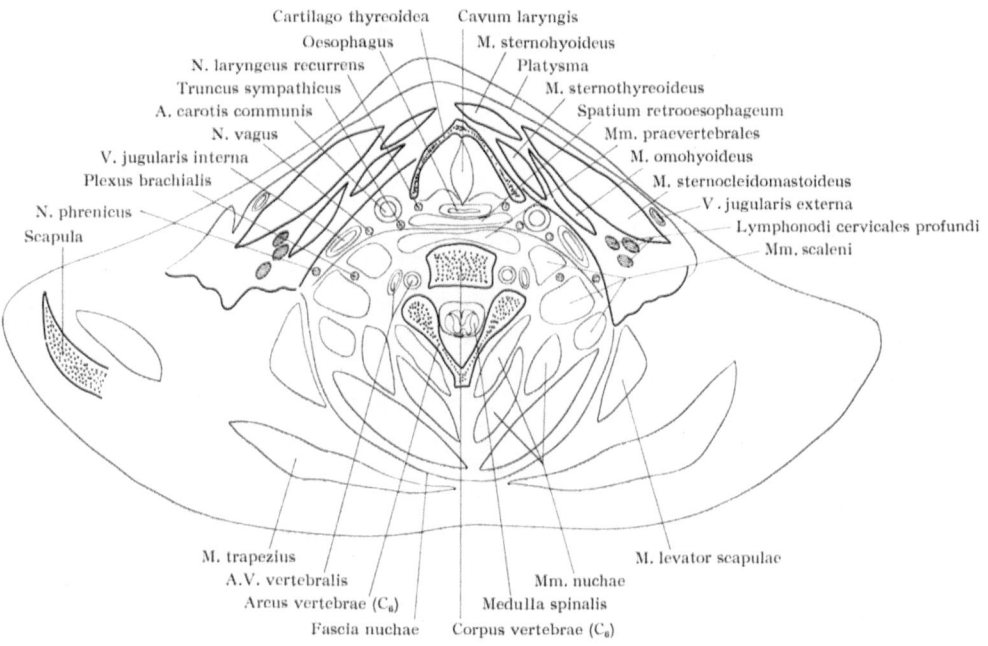

Cartilago thyreoidea
Oesophagus
N. laryngeus recurrens
Truncus sympathicus
A. carotis communis
N. vagus
V. jugularis interna
Plexus brachialis
N. phrenicus
Scapula

Cavum laryngis
M. sternohyoideus
Platysma
M. sternothyreoideus
Spatium retrooesophageum
Mm. praevertebrales
M. omohyoideus
M. sternocleidomastoideus
V. jugularis externa
Lymphonodi cervicales profundi
Mm. scaleni

M. trapezius
A.V. vertebralis
Arcus vertebrae (C$_6$)
Fascia nuchae

Mm. nuchae
Medulla spinalis
Corpus vertebrae (C$_6$)

M. levator scapulae

Fig. 140. Anatomical chart

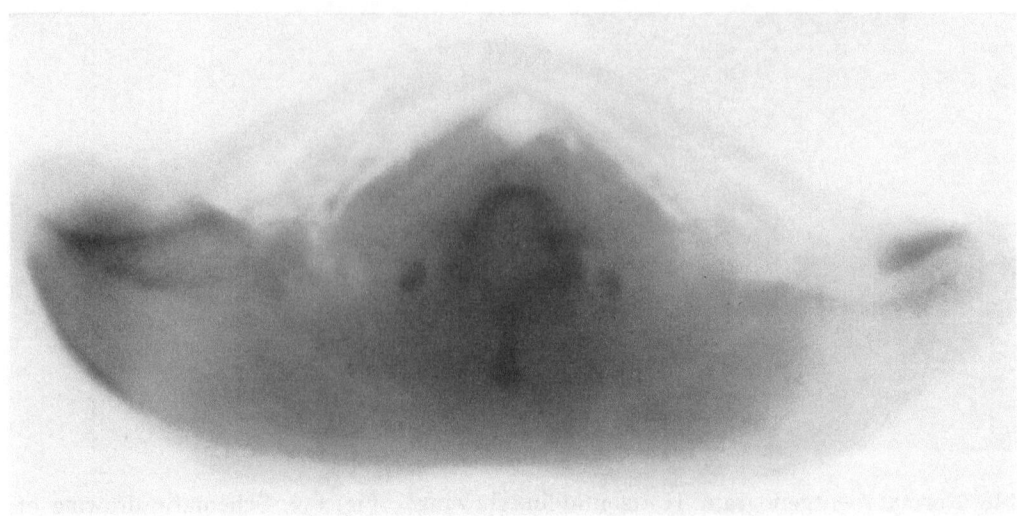

Fig. 141. Axial transverse tomogram

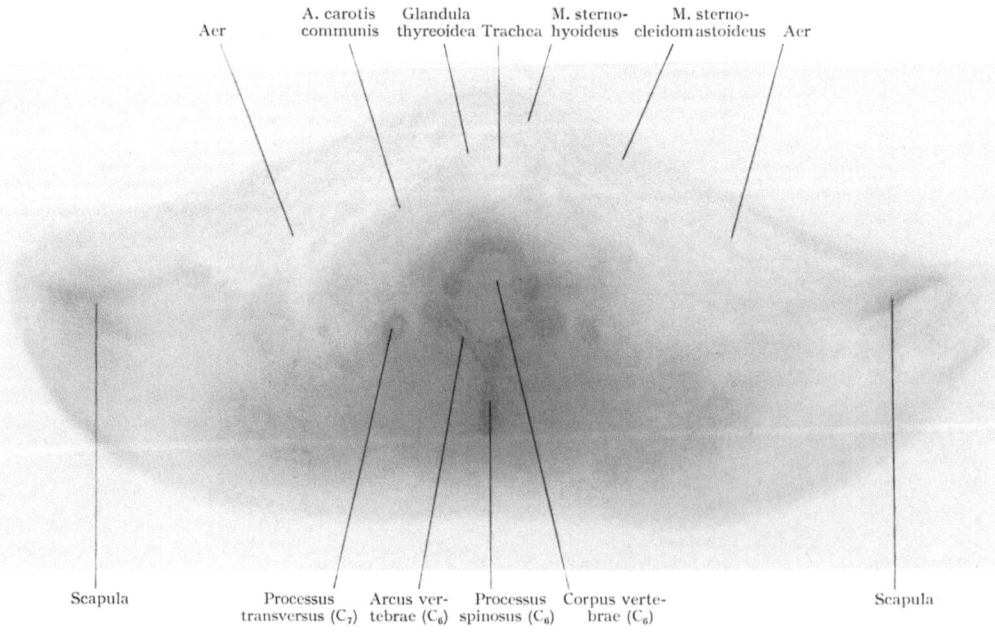

Fig. 142. Interpretation

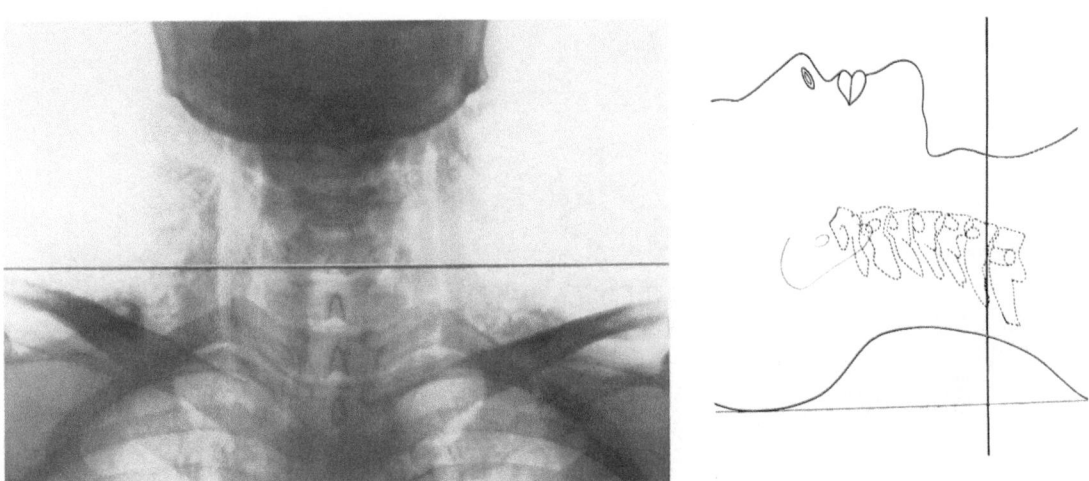

Fig. 143. Normal roentgenogram. Horizontal line showing the level tomographed

Fig. 144. Schematic drawing of the level tomographed

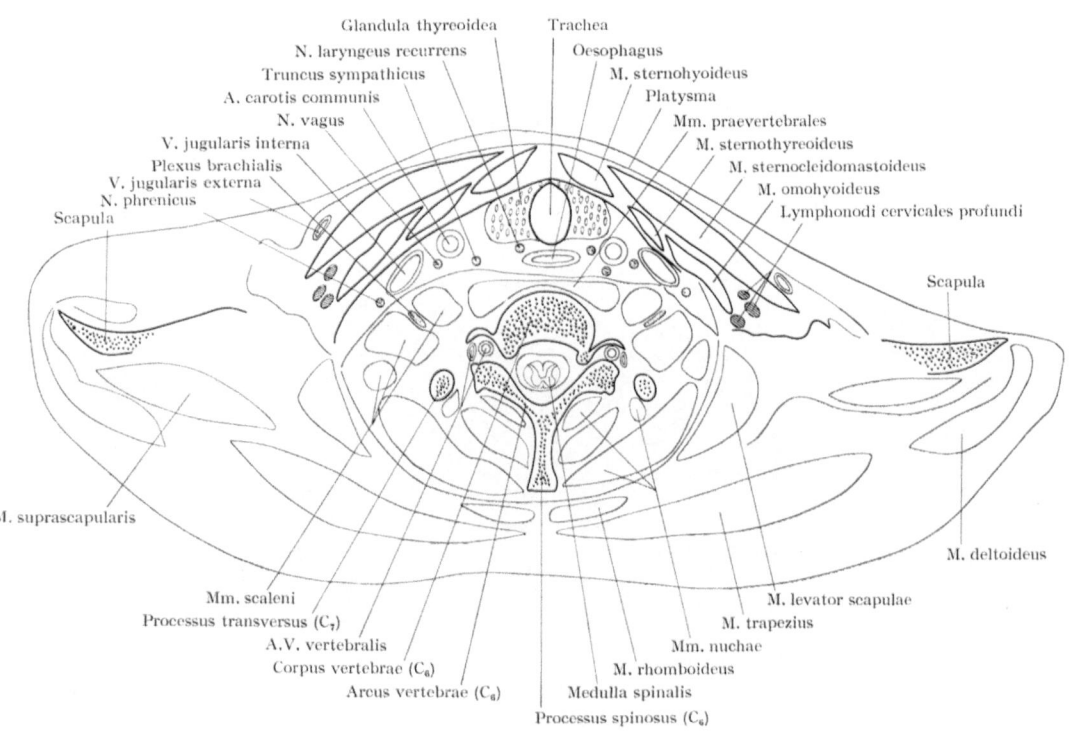

Glandula thyreoidea
N. laryngeus recurrens
Truncus sympathicus
A. carotis communis
N. vagus
V. jugularis interna
Plexus brachialis
V. jugularis externa
N. phrenicus
Scapula

Trachea
Oesophagus
M. sternohyoideus
Platysma
Mm. praevertebrales
M. sternothyreoideus
M. sternocleidomastoideus
M. omohyoideus
Lymphonodi cervicales profundi

Scapula

M. suprascapularis

M. deltoideus

Mm. scaleni
Processus transversus (C₇)
A.V. vertebralis
Corpus vertebrae (C₆)
Arcus vertebrae (C₆)

M. levator scapulae
M. trapezius
Mm. nuchae
M. rhomboideus
Medulla spinalis
Processus spinosus (C₆)

Fig. 145. Anatomical chart

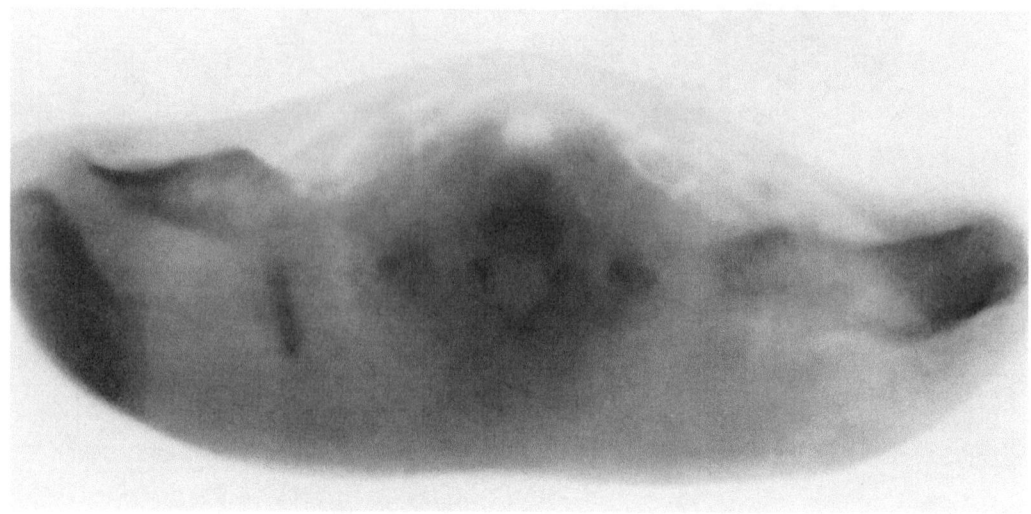

Fig. 146. Axial transverse tomogram

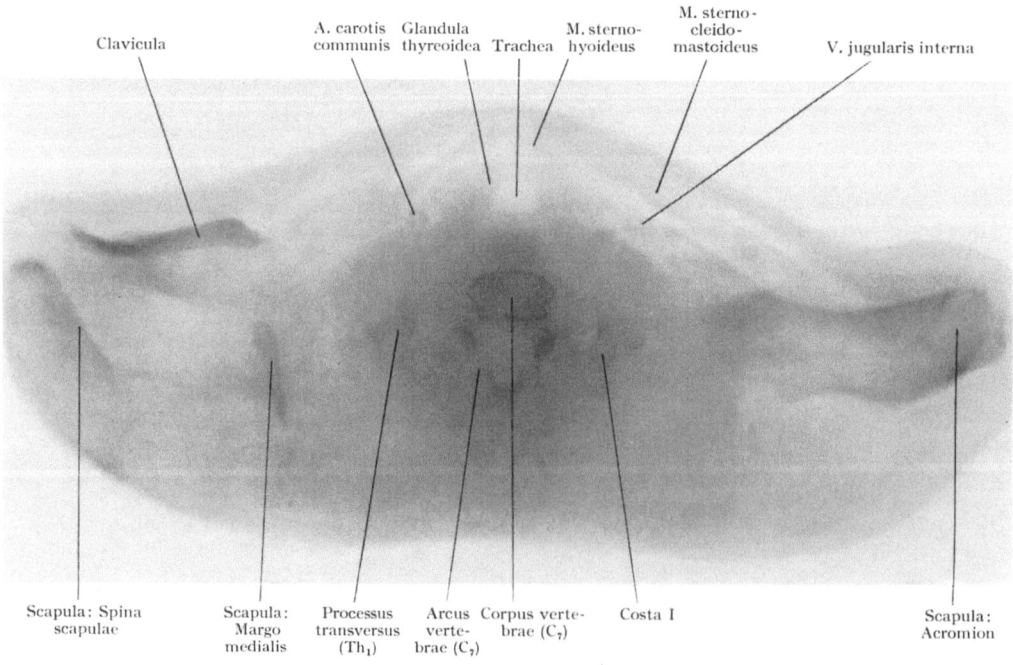

Clavicula   A. carotis Glandula Trachea M. sterno- M. sterno- V. jugularis interna
             communis   thyreoidea   hyoideus   cleido-
                                                       mastoideus

Scapula: Spina   Scapula: Processus   Arcus   Corpus verte-   Costa I   Scapula:
scapulae   Margo   transversus verte-   brae (C₇)   Acromion
                  medialis   (Th₁)   brae (C₇)

Fig. 147. Interpretation

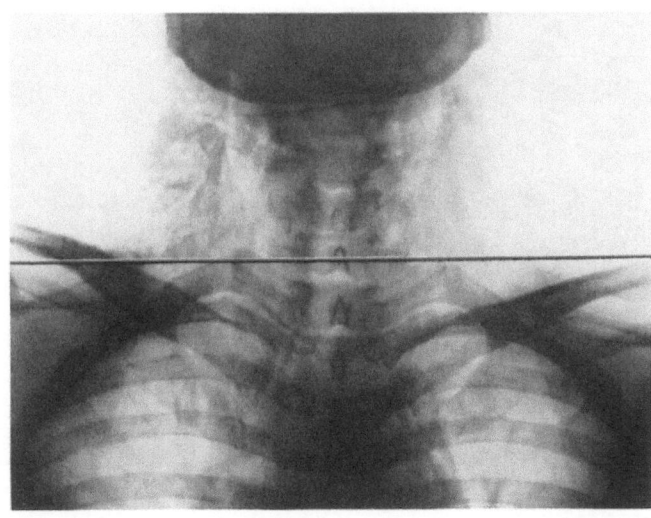

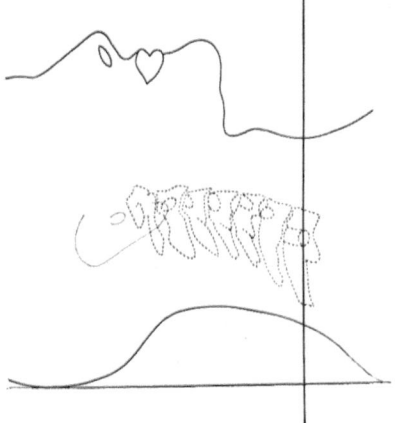

Fig. 148. Normal roentgenogram. Horizontal line show-ing the level tomographed

Fig. 149. Schematic drawing of the level tomographed

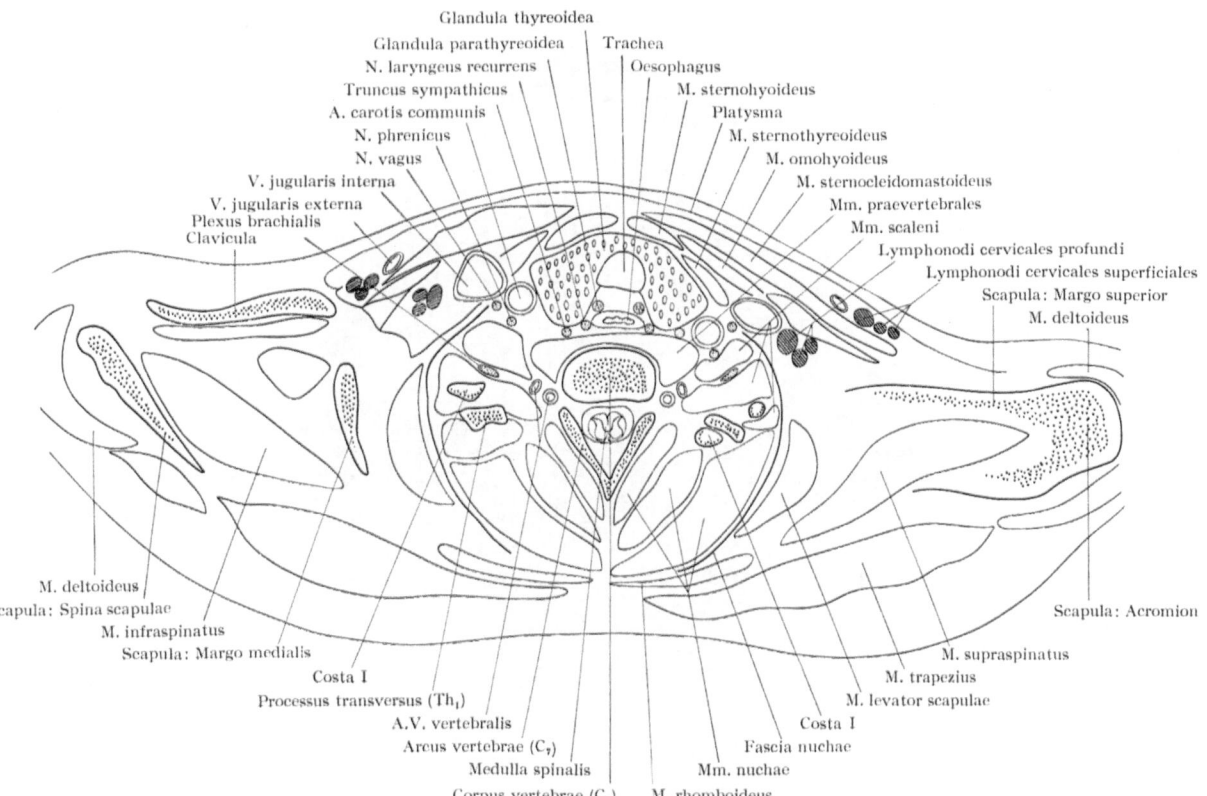

Fig. 150. Anatomical chart

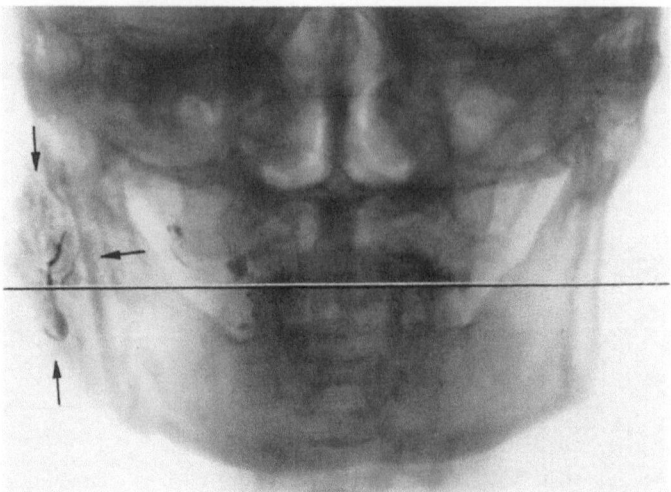

Fig. 151. Normal roentgenogram of the parotis (↗). Horizontal line showing the level tomographed

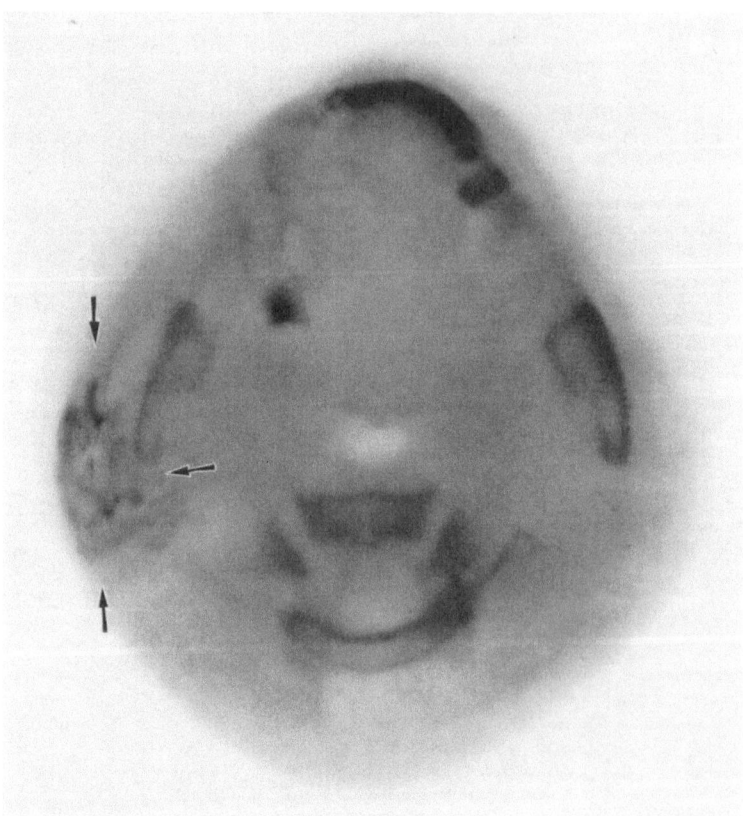

Fig. 152. Axial transverse tomogram of the parotis (↗) (see Figs. 96 and 97)

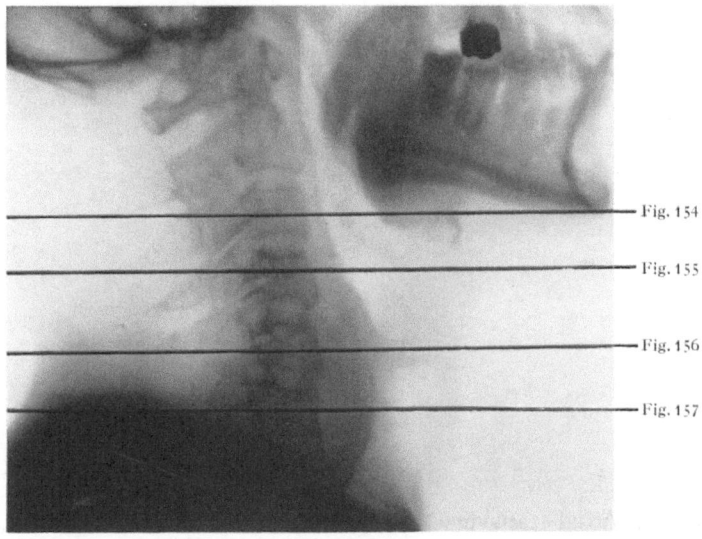

Fig. 153. Normal roentgenogram of the neck without contrast medium. Horizontal lines showing the level tomographed

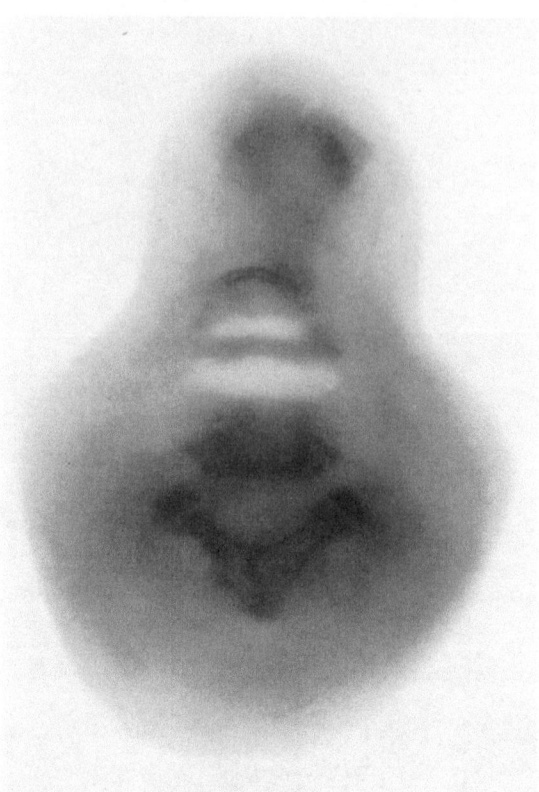

Fig. 154. Axial transverse tomogram of the neck (see Figs. 121 and 122)

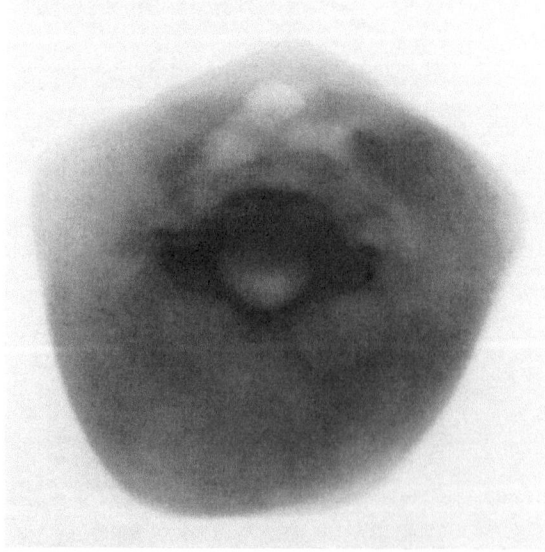

Fig. 155. Axial transverse tomogram of the neck (see Figs. 126 and 127)

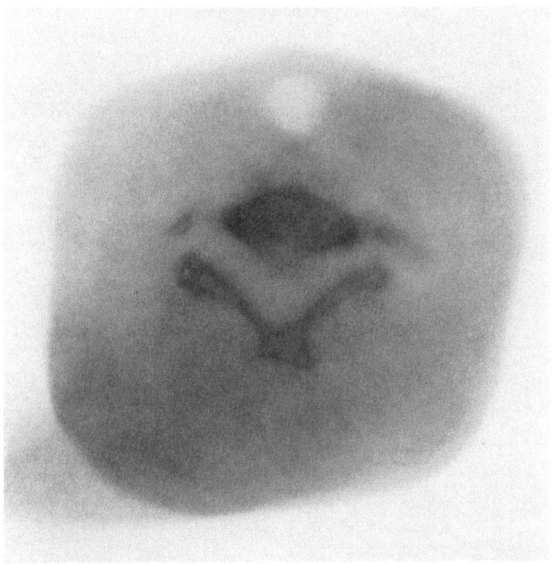

Fig. 156. Axial transverse tomogram of the neck (see Figs. 141 and 142)

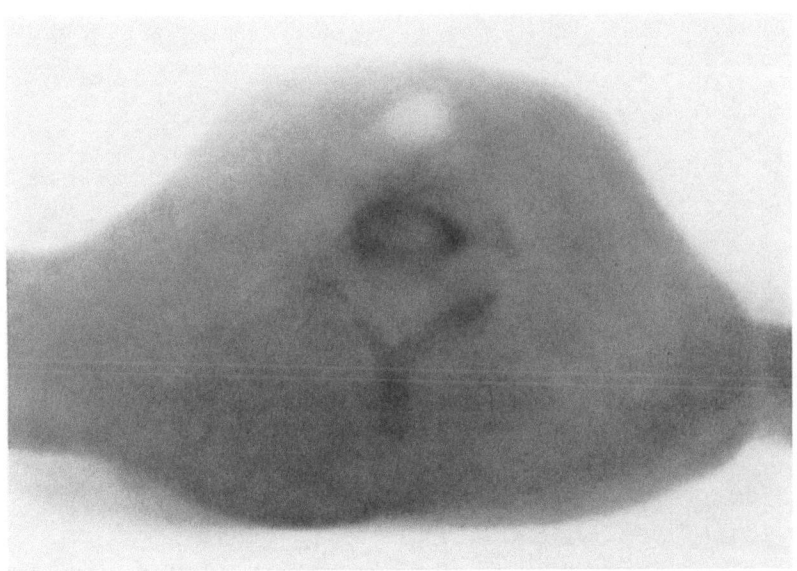

Fig. 157. Axial transverse tomogram of the neck (see Figs. 142 and 147)

Chest

Twenty three axial transverse tomograms.

Appendices:
1. Axial transverse tomograms of the esophagus.
2. Axial transverse tomograms of the thoracic duct and lymph nodes.

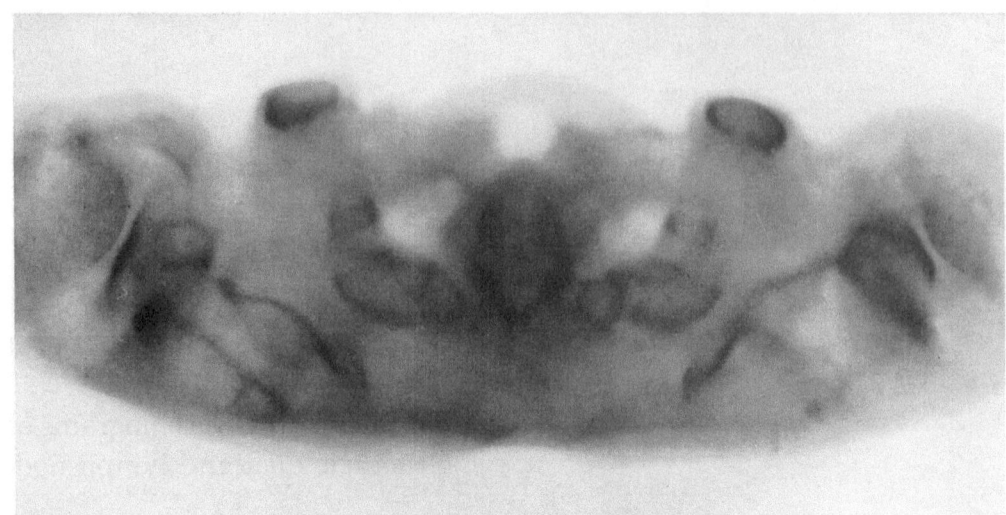

Fig. 158. Axial transverse tomogram

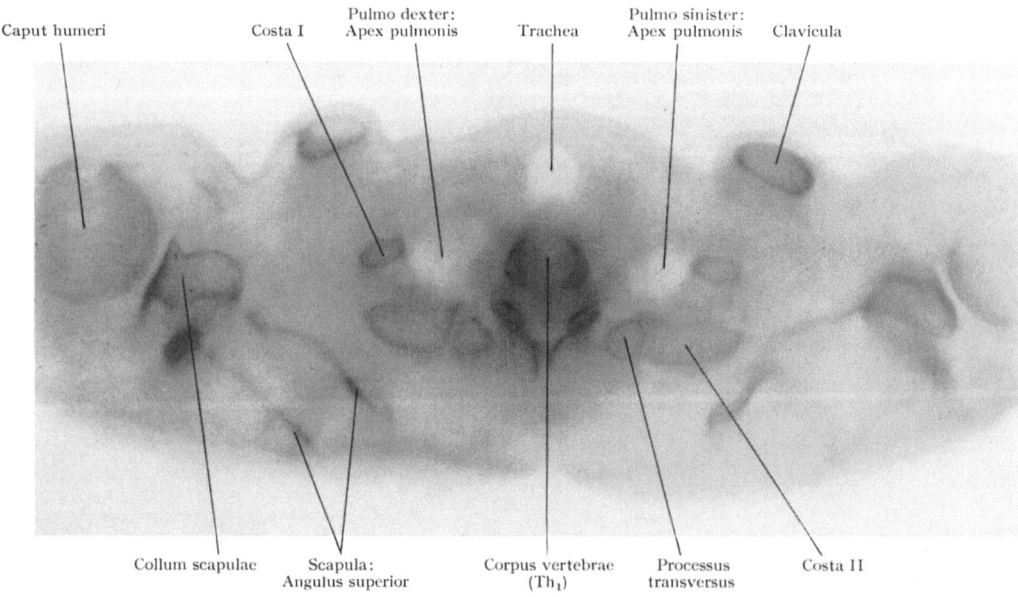

Fig. 159. Interpretation

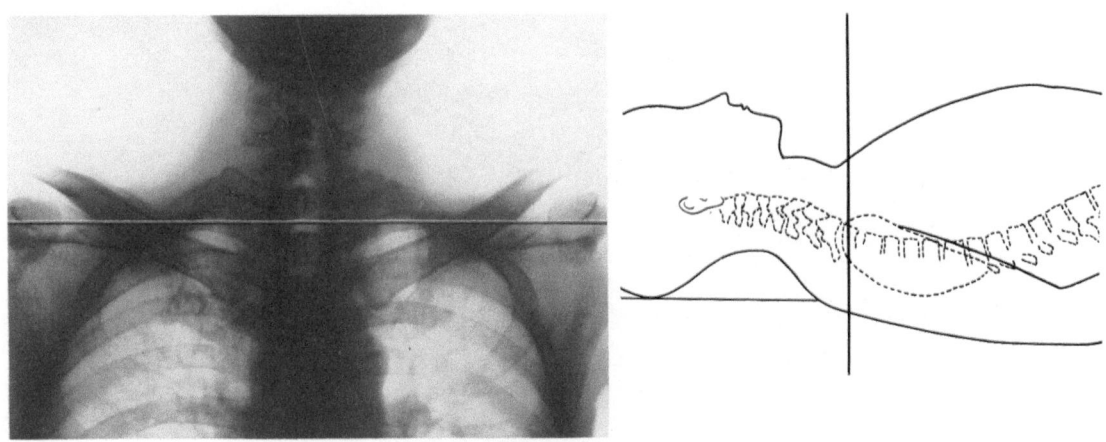

Fig. 160. Normal roentgenogram. Horizontal line showing the level tomographed

Fig. 161. Schematic drawing of the level tomographed. Subject supine with arms parallel to body axis

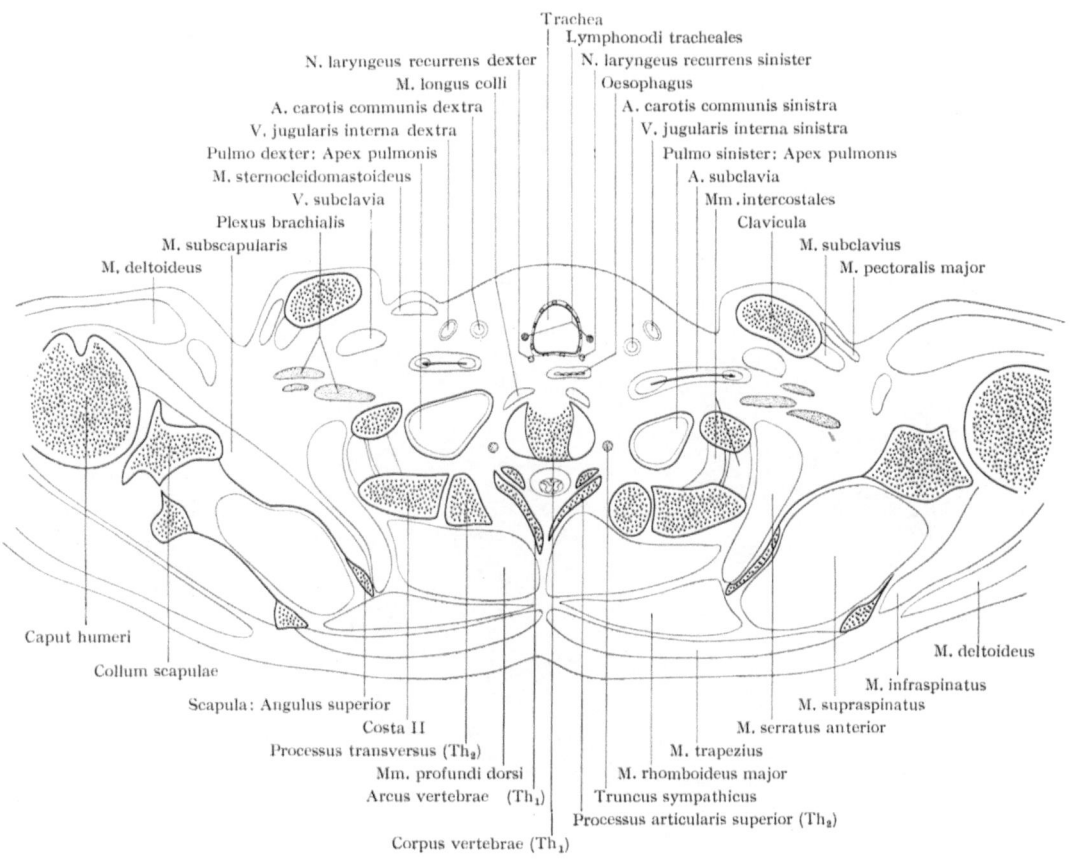

Trachea
Lymphonodi tracheales
N. laryngeus recurrens dexter
N. laryngeus recurrens sinister
M. longus colli
Oesophagus
A. carotis communis dextra
A. carotis communis sinistra
V. jugularis interna dextra
V. jugularis interna sinistra
Pulmo dexter: Apex pulmonis
Pulmo sinister: Apex pulmonis
M. sternocleidomastoideus
A. subclavia
V. subclavia
Mm. intercostales
Plexus brachialis
Clavicula
M. subscapularis
M. subclavius
M. deltoideus
M. pectoralis major

Caput humeri
M. deltoideus
Collum scapulae
M. infraspinatus
Scapula: Angulus superior
M. supraspinatus
Costa II
M. serratus anterior
Processus transversus (Th₂)
M. trapezius
Mm. profundi dorsi
M. rhomboideus major
Arcus vertebrae (Th₁)
Truncus sympathicus
Processus articularis superior (Th₂)
Corpus vertebrae (Th₁)

Fig. 162. Anatomical chart

83

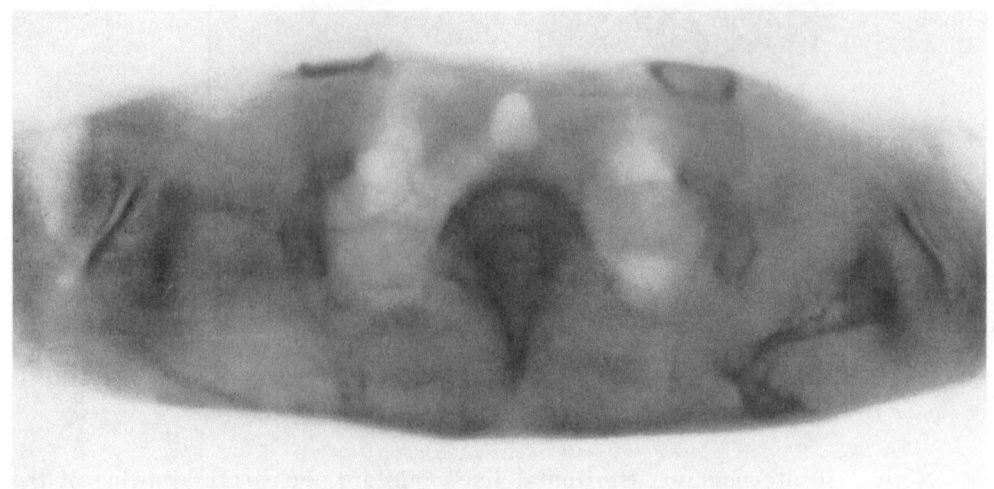

Fig. 163. Axial transverse tomogram

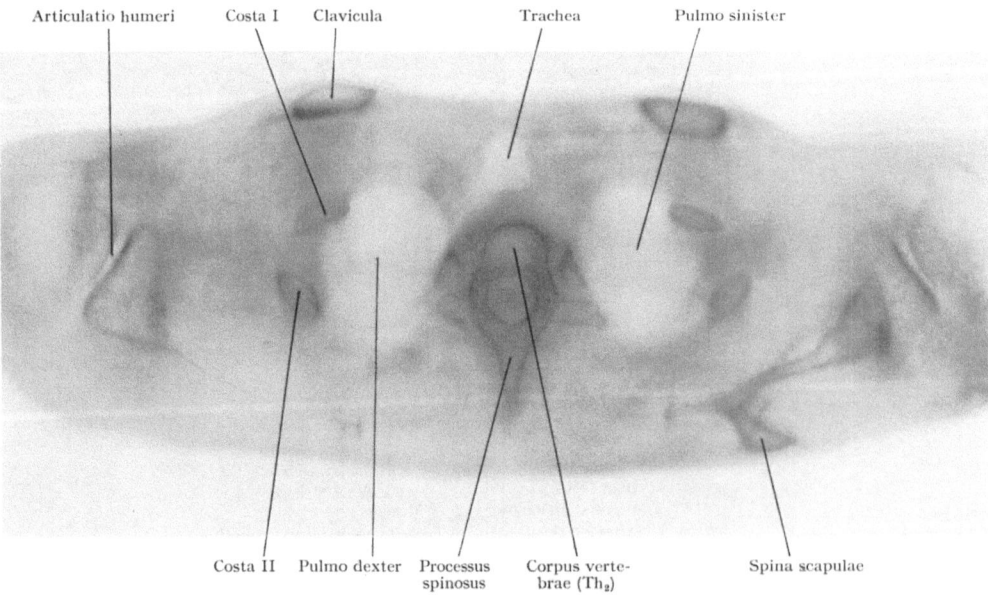

Fig. 164. Interpretation

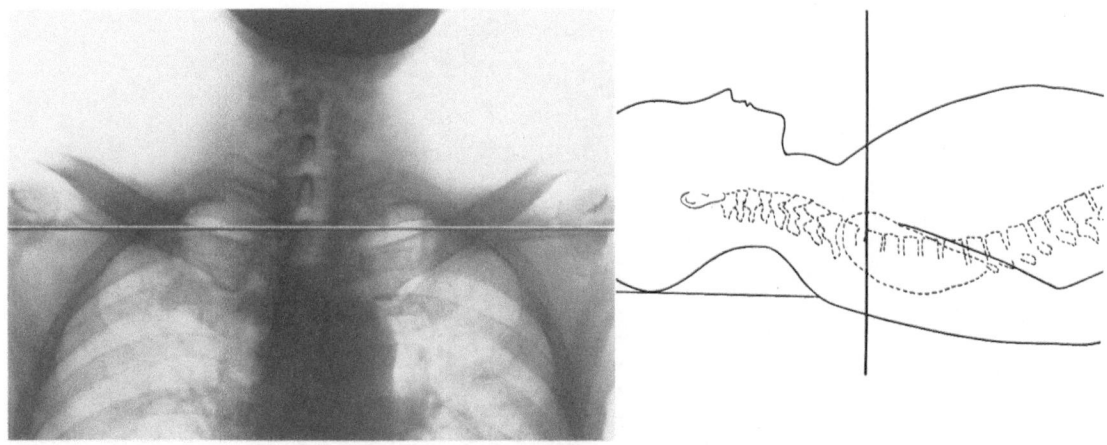

Fig. 165. Normal roentgenogram. Horizontal line showing the level tomographed

Fig. 166. Schematic drawing of the level tomographed. Subject supine with arms parallel to body axis

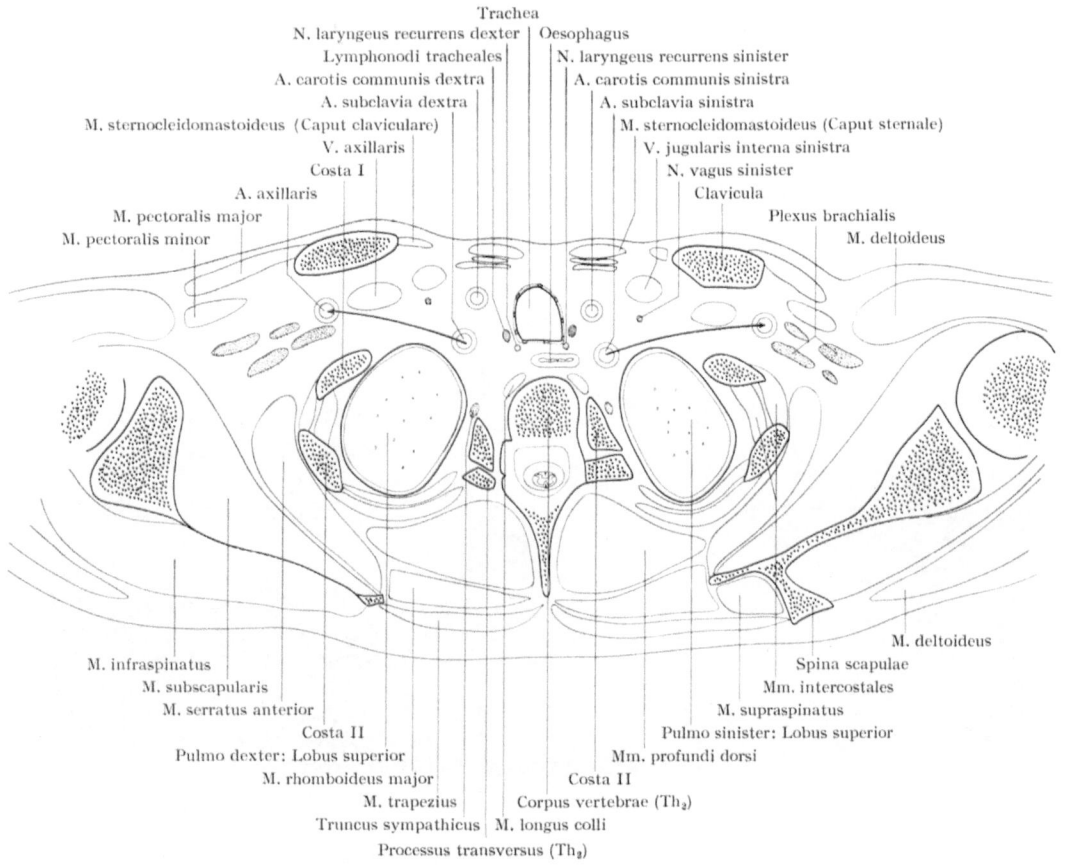

Fig. 167. Anatomical chart

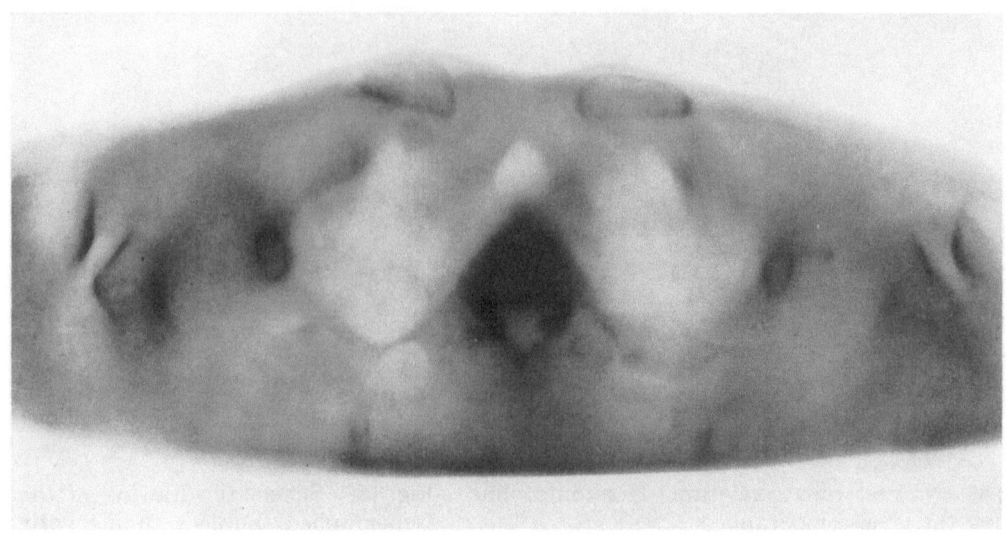

Fig. 168. Axial transverse tomogram

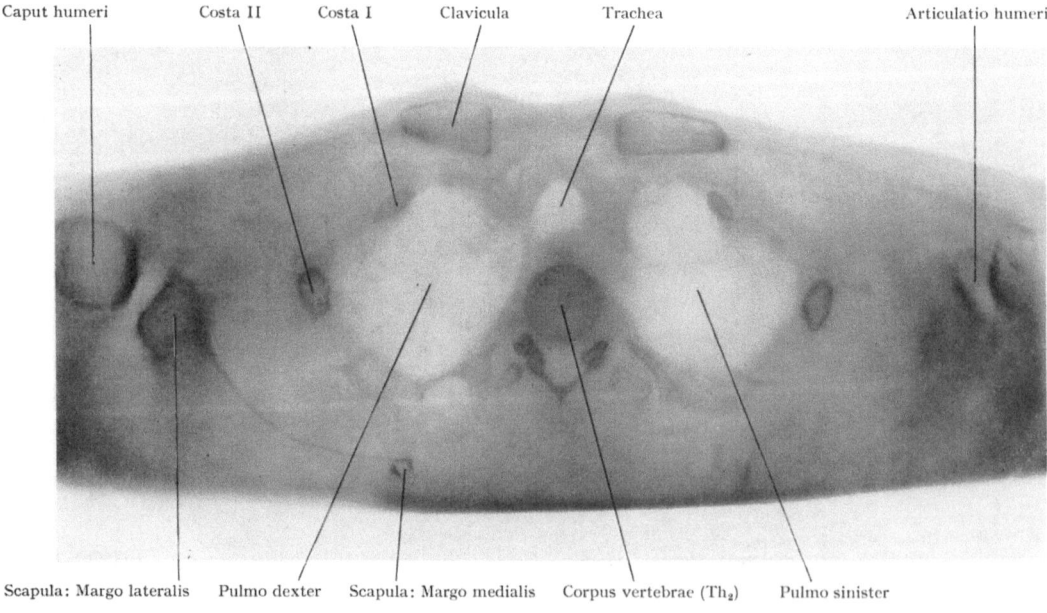

Fig. 169. Interpretation

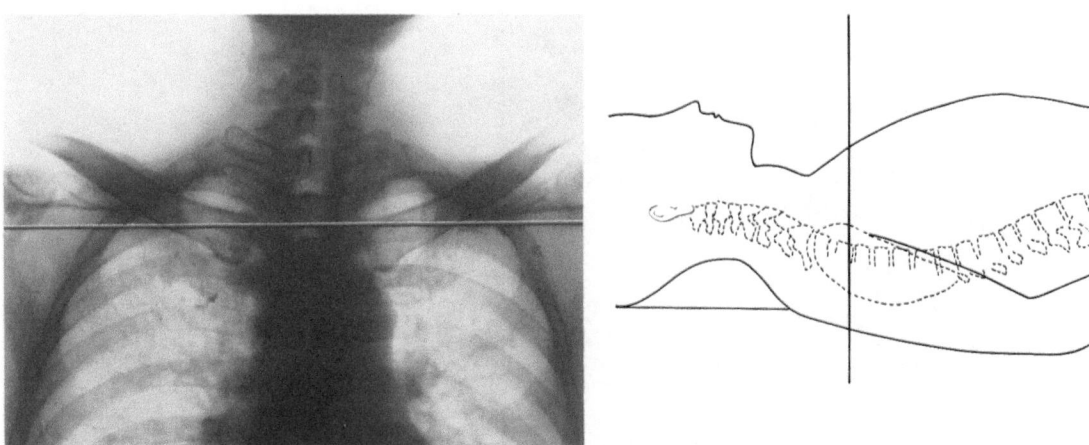

Fig. 170. Normal roentgenogram. Horizontal line showing the level tomographed

Fig. 171. Schematic drawing of the level tomographed. Subject supine with arms parallel to body axis

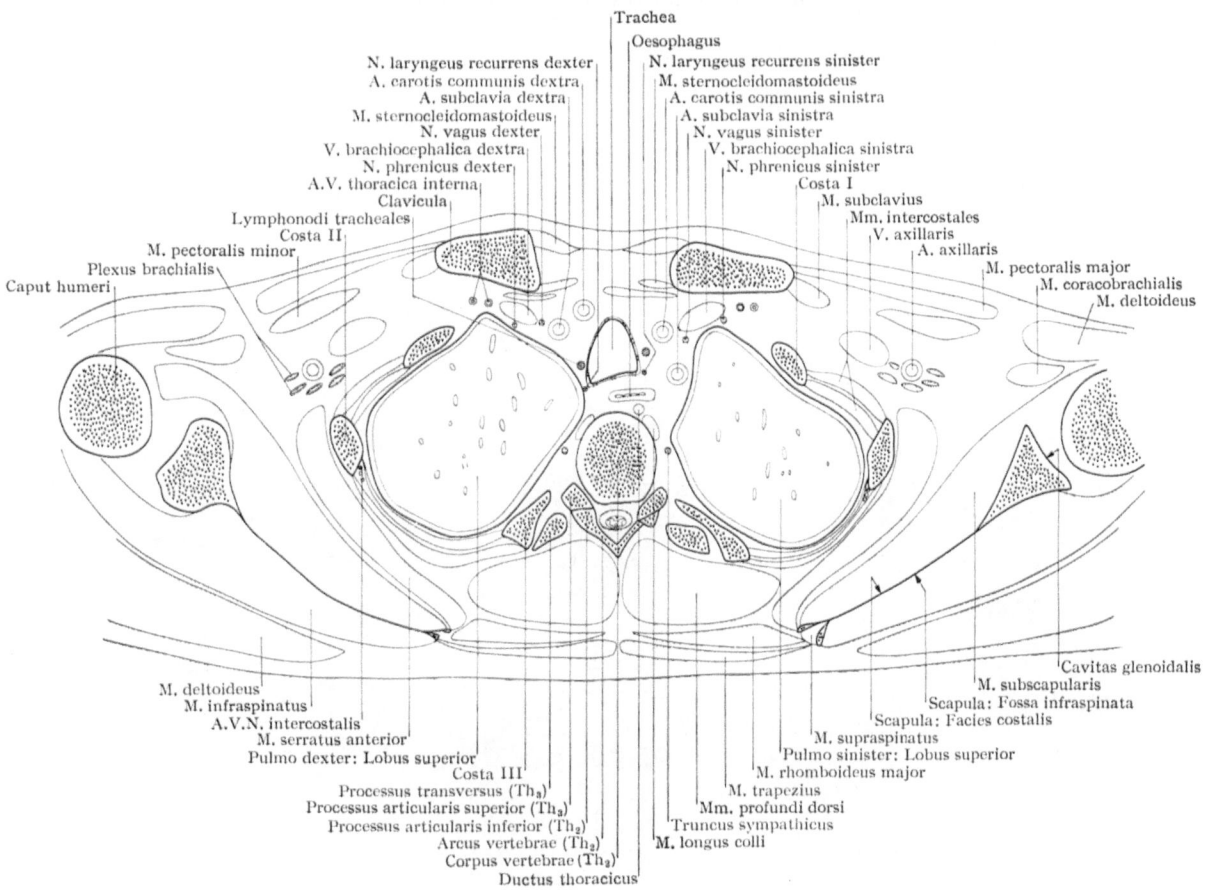

Trachea
Oesophagus
N. laryngeus recurrens dexter
A. carotis communis dextra
A. subclavia dextra
M. sternocleidomastoideus
N. vagus dexter
V. brachiocephalica dextra
N. phrenicus dexter
A.V. thoracica interna
Clavicula
Lymphonodi tracheales
Costa II
M. pectoralis minor
Plexus brachialis
Caput humeri

N. laryngeus recurrens sinister
M. sternocleidomastoideus
A. carotis communis sinistra
A. subclavia sinistra
N. vagus sinister
V. brachiocephalica sinistra
N. phrenicus sinister
Costa I
M. subclavius
Mm. intercostales
V. axillaris
A. axillaris
M. pectoralis major
M. coracobrachialis
M. deltoideus

Cavitas glenoidalis
M. subscapularis
Scapula: Fossa infraspinata
Scapula: Facies costalis
M. supraspinatus
Pulmo sinister: Lobus superior
M. rhomboideus major
M. trapezius
Mm. profundi dorsi
Truncus sympathicus
M. longus colli

M. deltoideus
M. infraspinatus
A.V.N. intercostalis
M. serratus anterior
Pulmo dexter: Lobus superior
Costa III
Processus transversus (Th₃)
Processus articularis superior (Th₃)
Processus articularis inferior (Th₂)
Arcus vertebrae (Th₃)
Corpus vertebrae (Th₄)
Ductus thoracicus

Fig. 172. Anatomical chart

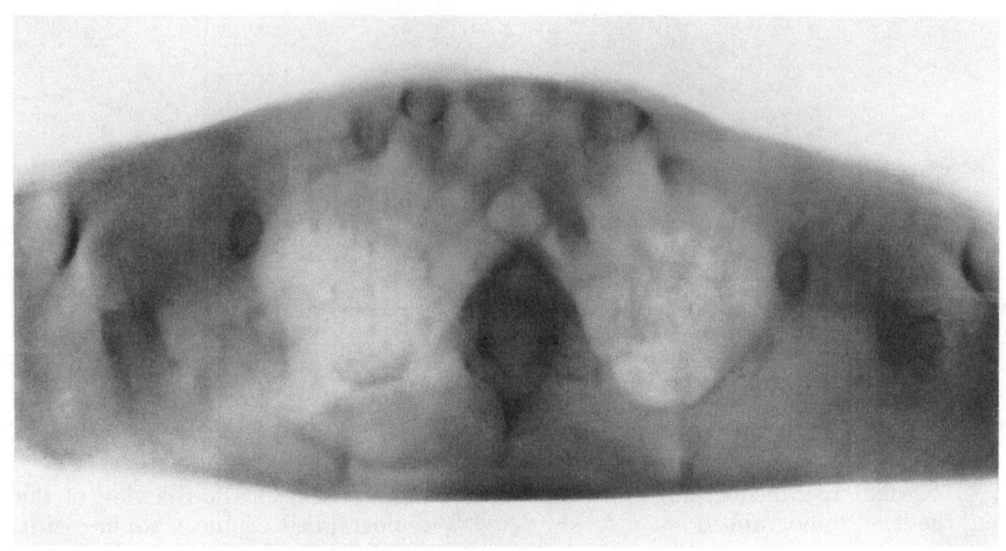

Fig. 173. Axial transverse tomogram

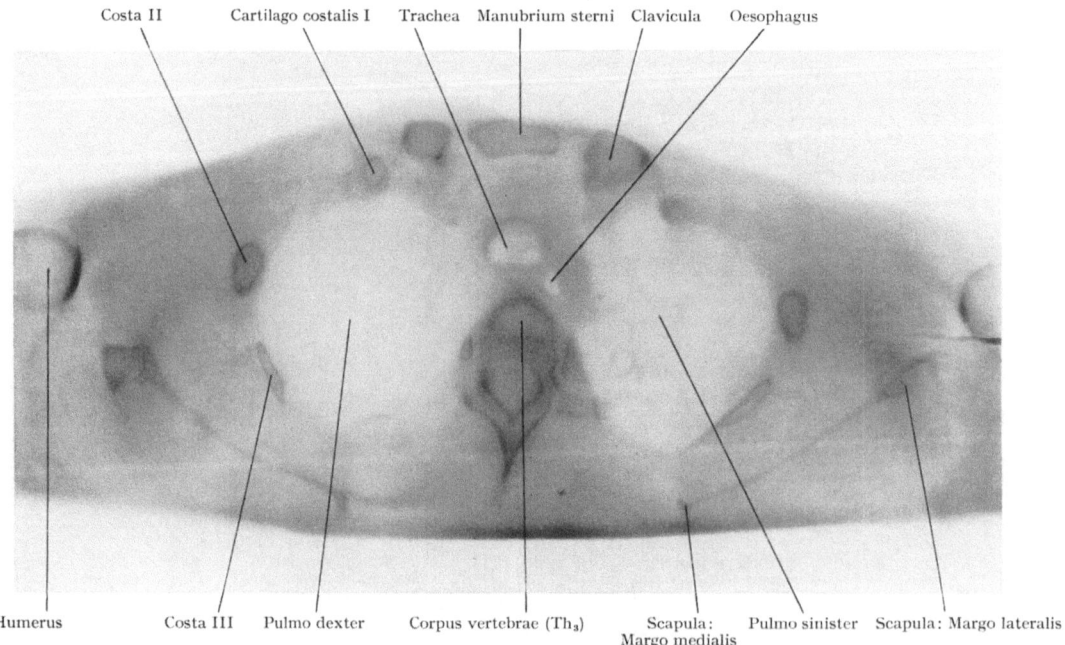

Fig. 174. Interpretation

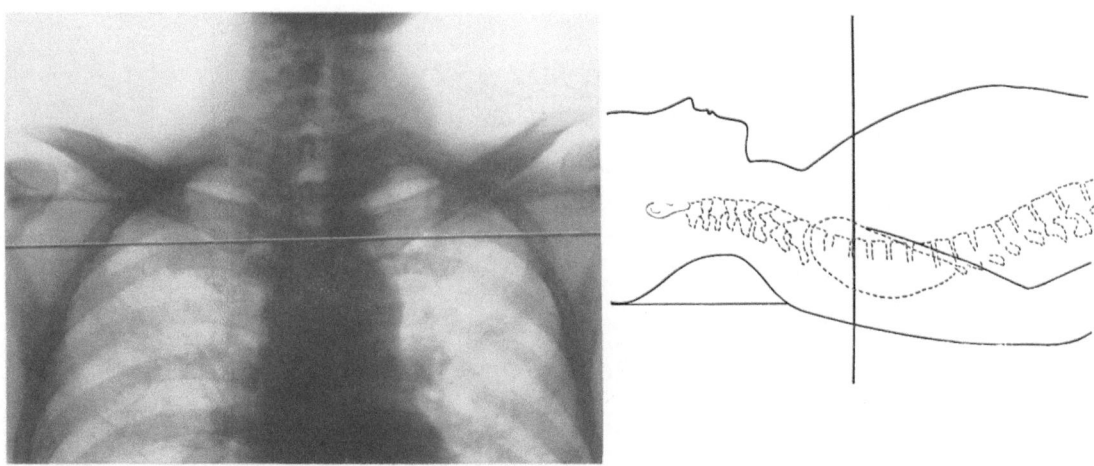

Fig. 175. Normal roentgenogram. Horizontal line showing the level tomographed

Fig. 176. Schematic drawing of the level tomographed. Subject supine with arms parallel to body axis

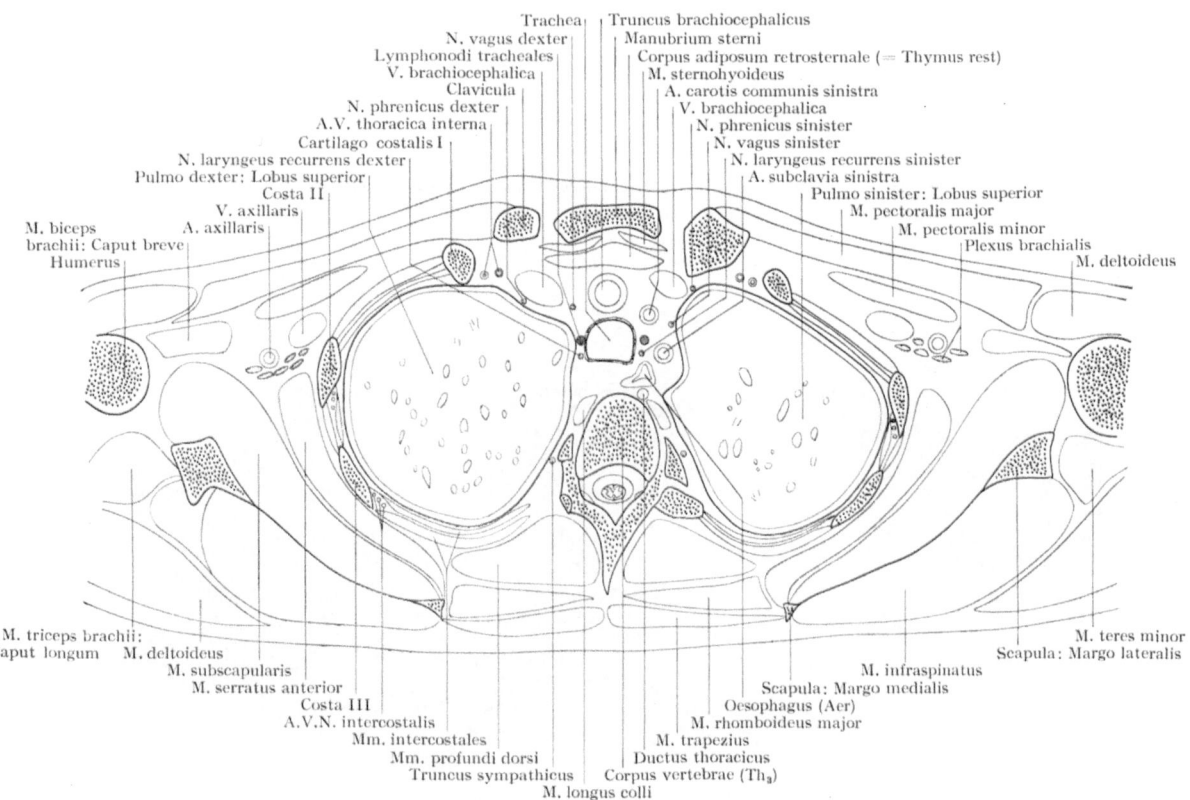

Fig. 177. Anatomical chart

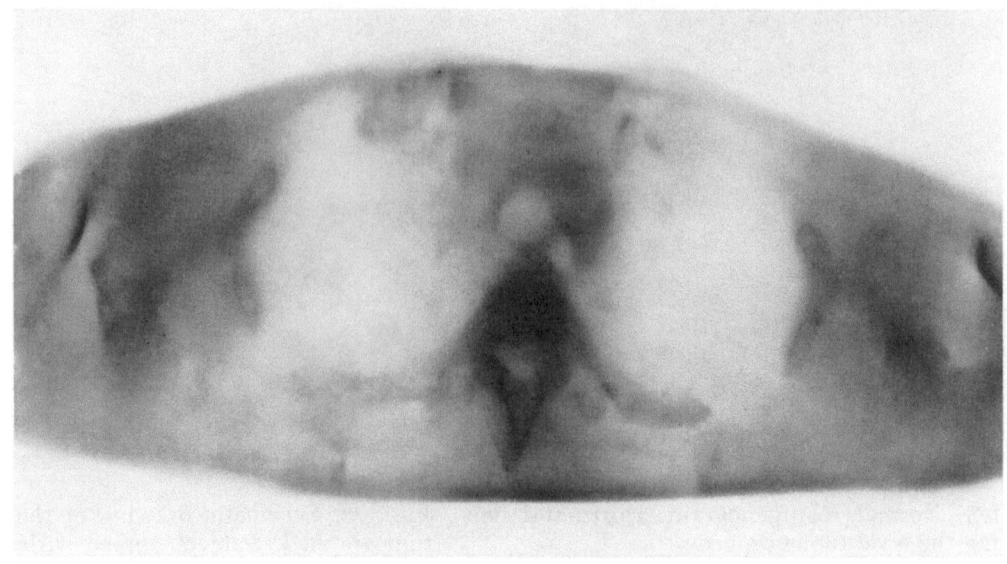

Fig. 178. Axial transverse tomogram

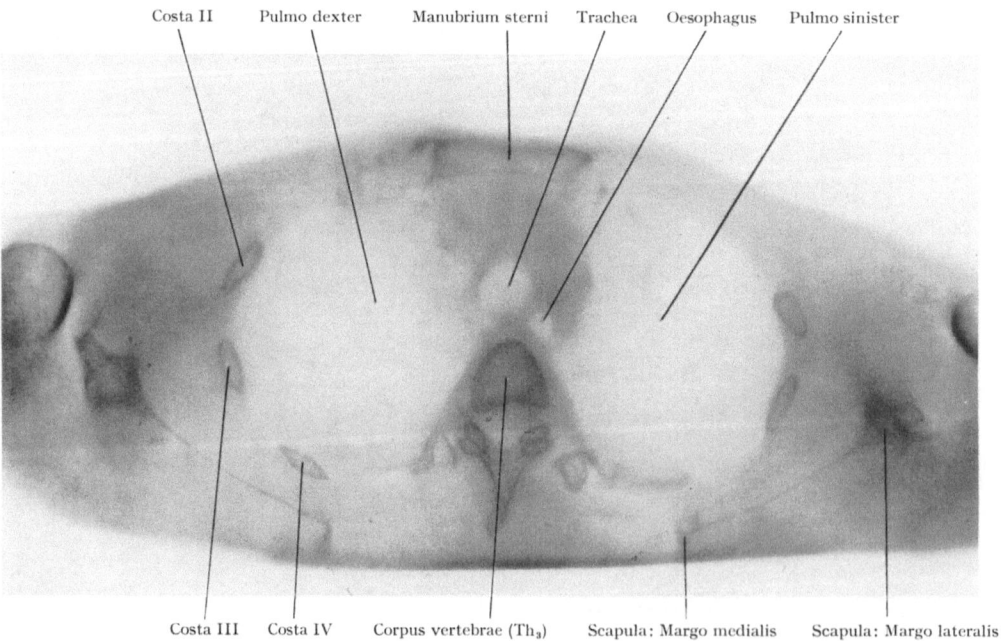

Costa II   Pulmo dexter   Manubrium sterni   Trachea   Oesophagus   Pulmo sinister

Costa III   Costa IV   Corpus vertebrae (Th$_3$)   Scapula: Margo medialis   Scapula: Margo lateralis

Fig. 179. Interpretation

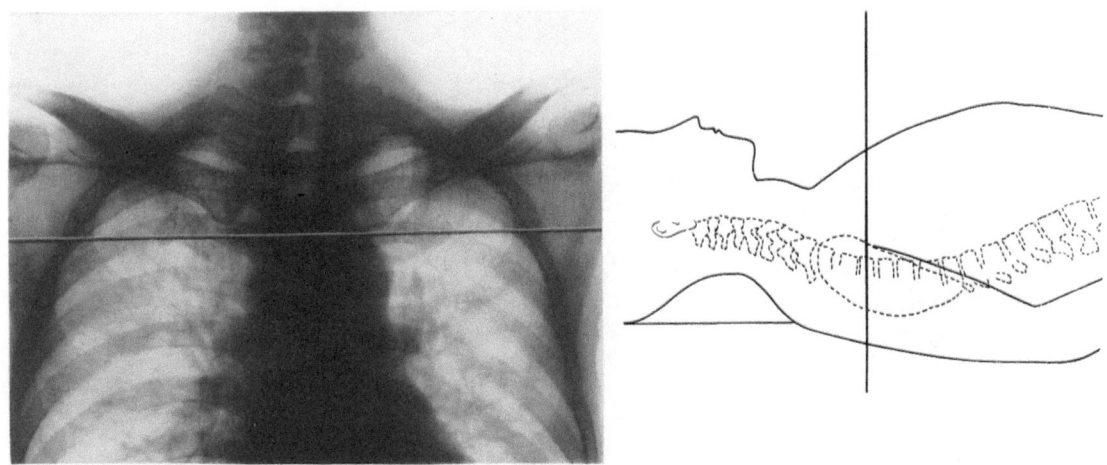

Fig. 180. Normal roentgenogram. Horizontal line showing the level tomographed

Fig. 181. Schematic drawing of the level tomographed. Subject supine with arms parallel to body axis

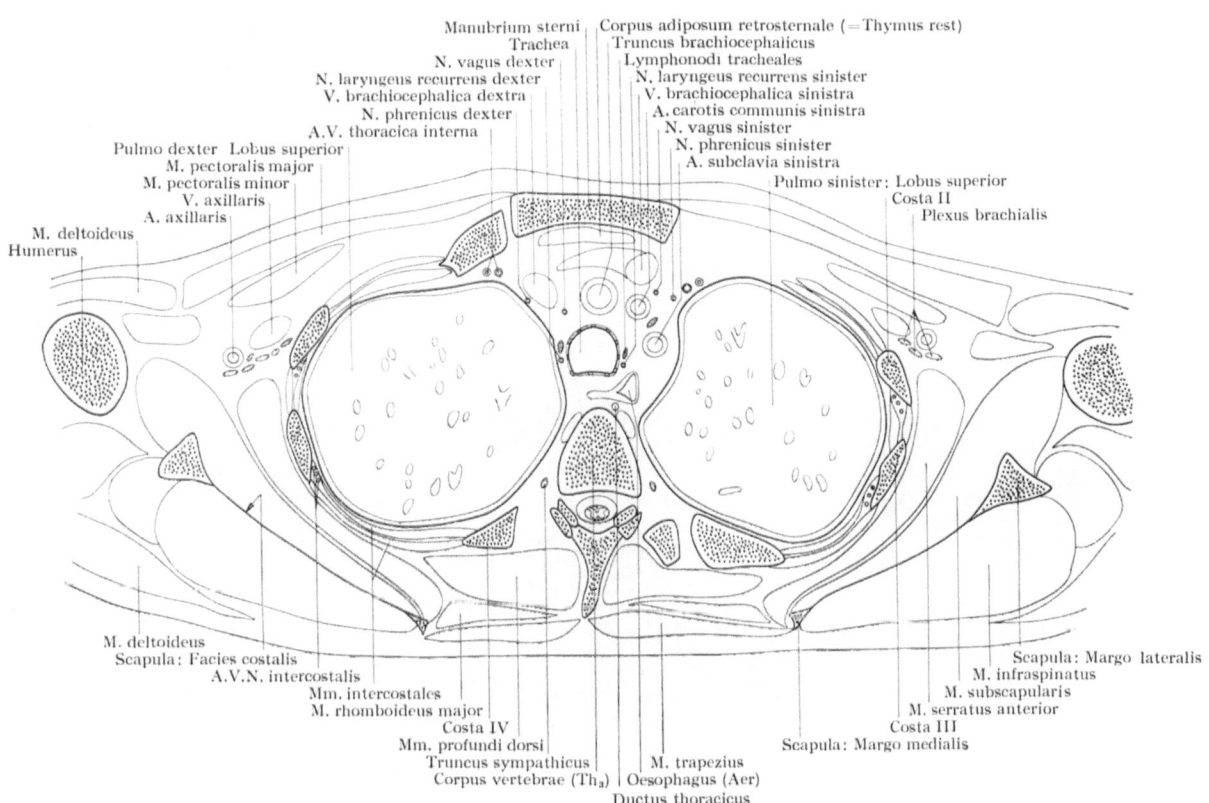

Manubrium sterni | Corpus adiposum retrosternale (=Thymus rest)
Trachea | Truncus brachiocephalicus
N. vagus dexter | Lymphonodi tracheales
N. laryngeus recurrens dexter | N. laryngeus recurrens sinister
V. brachiocephalica dextra | V. brachiocephalica sinistra
N. phrenicus dexter | A. carotis communis sinistra
A.V. thoracica interna | N. vagus sinister
| N. phrenicus sinister
Pulmo dexter Lobus superior | A. subclavia sinistra
M. pectoralis major | Pulmo sinister: Lobus superior
M. pectoralis minor | Costa II
V. axillaris | Plexus brachialis
A. axillaris

M. deltoideus
Humerus

M. deltoideus
Scapula: Facies costalis | Scapula: Margo lateralis
A.V.N. intercostalis | M. infraspinatus
Mm. intercostales | M. subscapularis
M. rhomboideus major | M. serratus anterior
Costa IV | Costa III
Mm. profundi dorsi | Scapula: Margo medialis
Truncus sympathicus | M. trapezius
Corpus vertebrae (Th₃) | Oesophagus (Aer)
Ductus thoracicus

Fig. 182. Anatomical chart

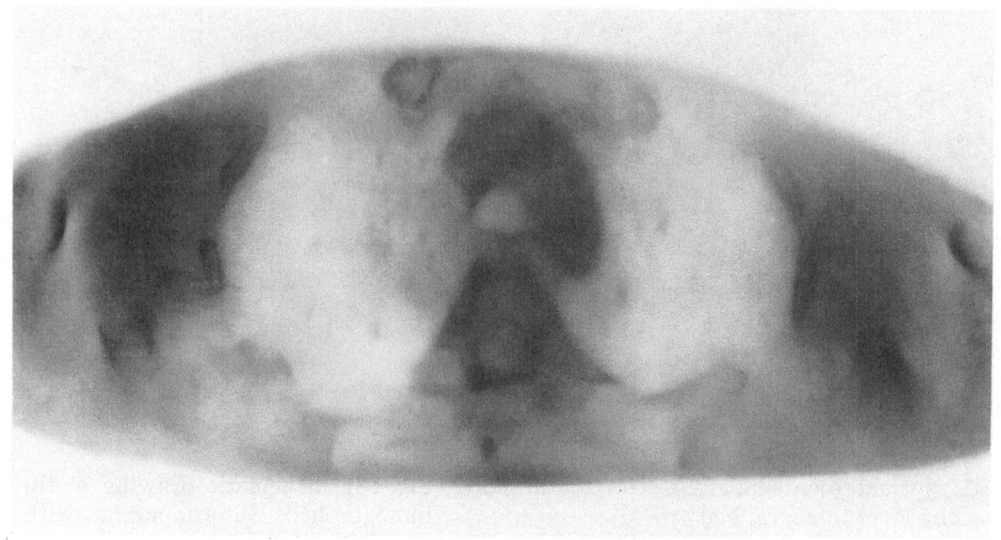

Fig. 183. Axial transverse tomogram

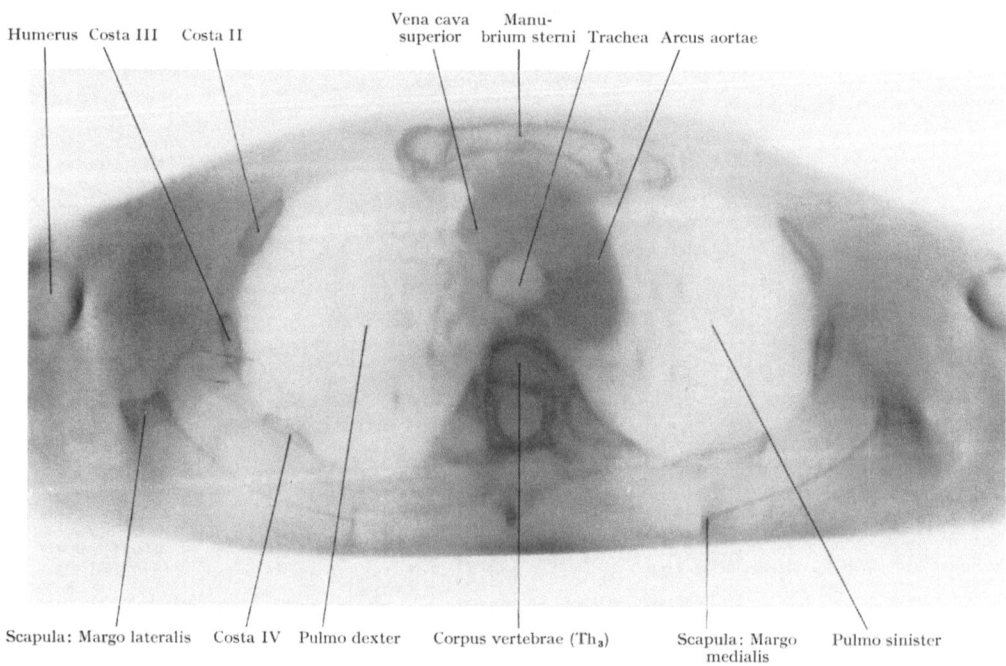

Fig. 184. Interpretation

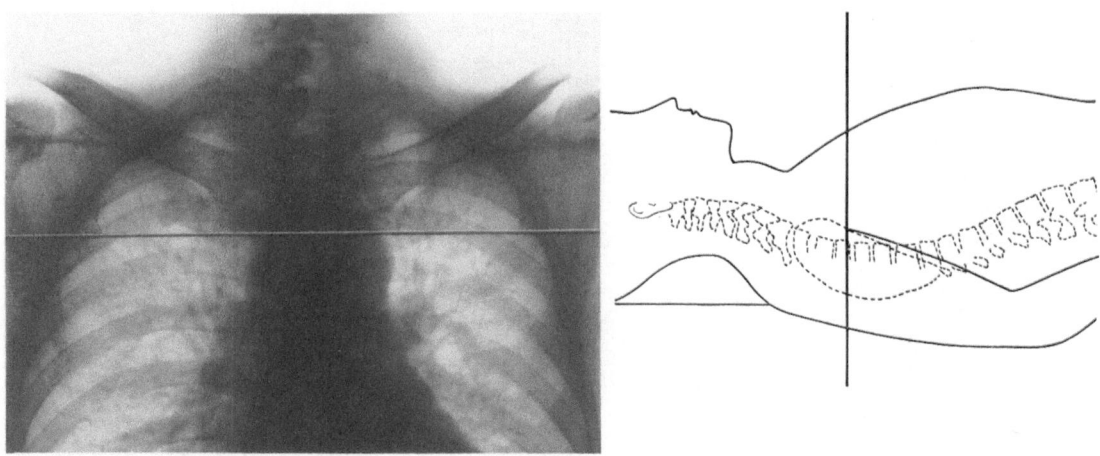

Fig. 185. Normal roentgenogram. Horizontal line showing the level tomographed

Fig. 186. Schematic drawing of the level tomographed. Subject supine with arms parallel to body axis

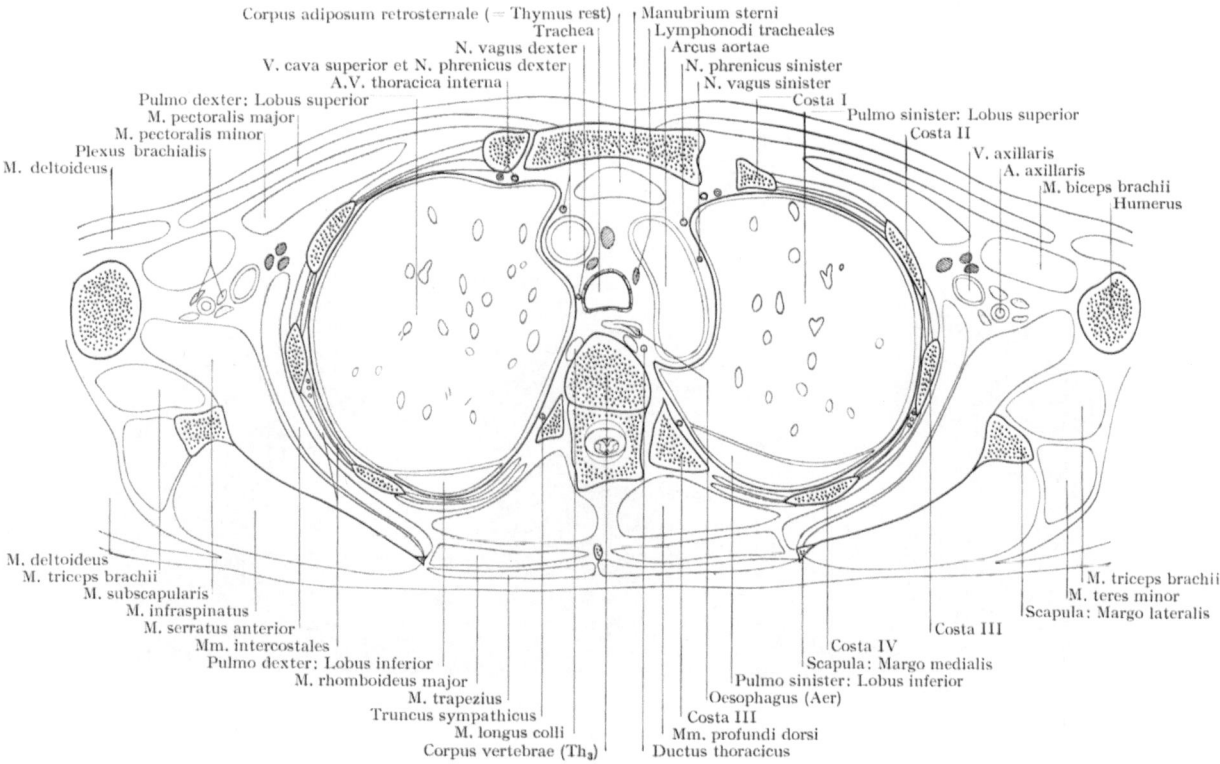

Fig. 187. Anatomical chart

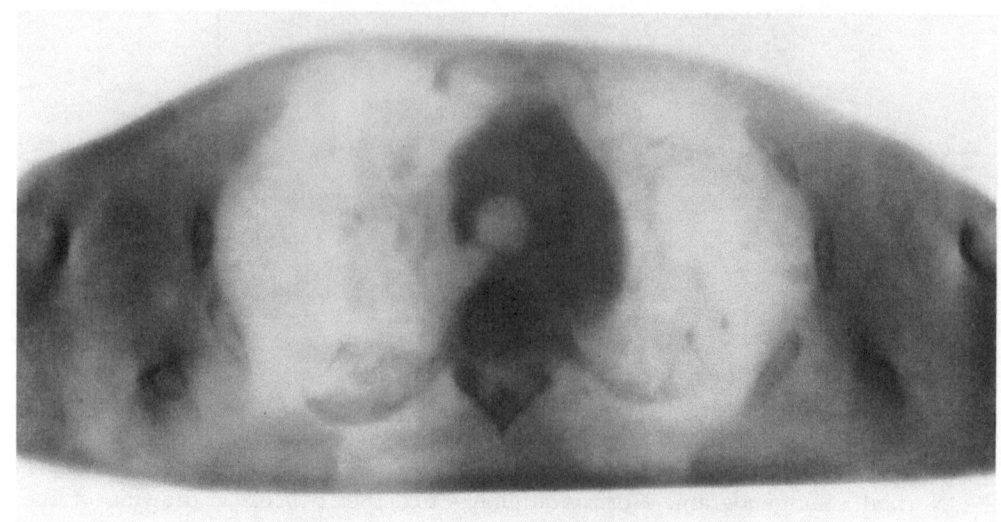

Fig. 188. Axial transverse tomogram

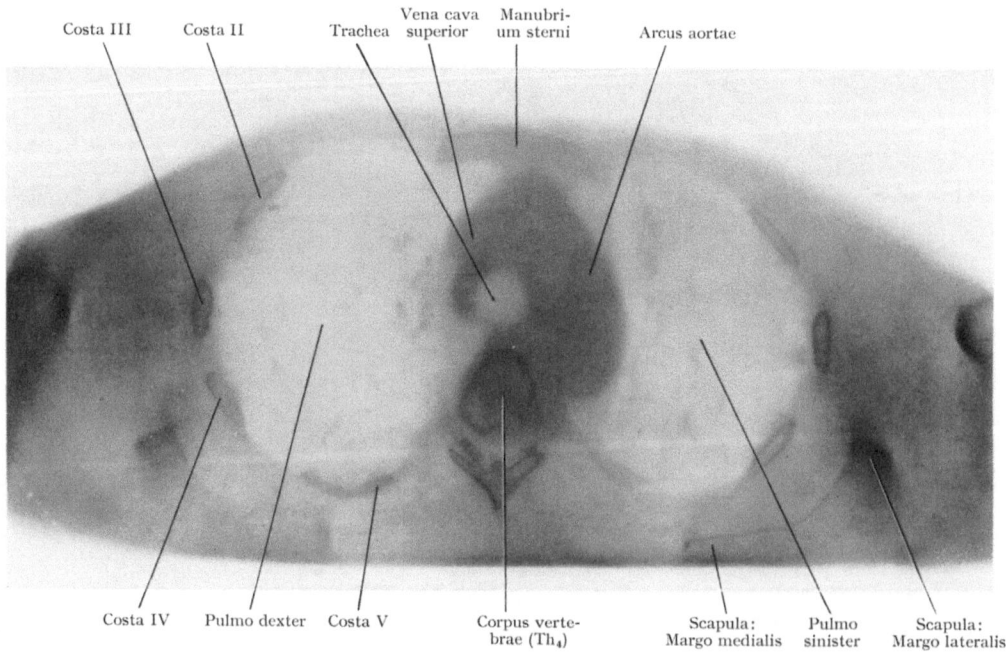

Fig. 189. Interpretation

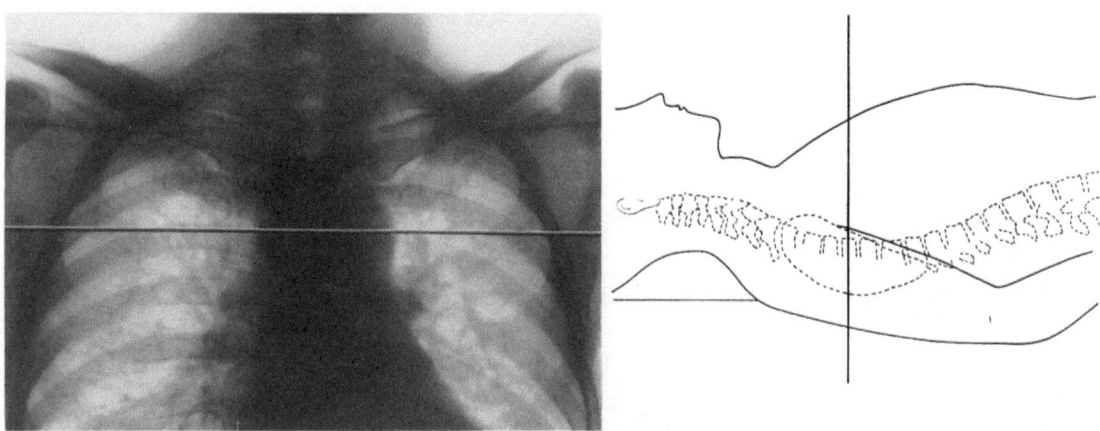

Fig. 190. Normal roentgenogram. Horizontal line showing the level tomographed

Fig. 191. Schematic drawing of the level tomographed. Subject supine with arms parallel to body axis

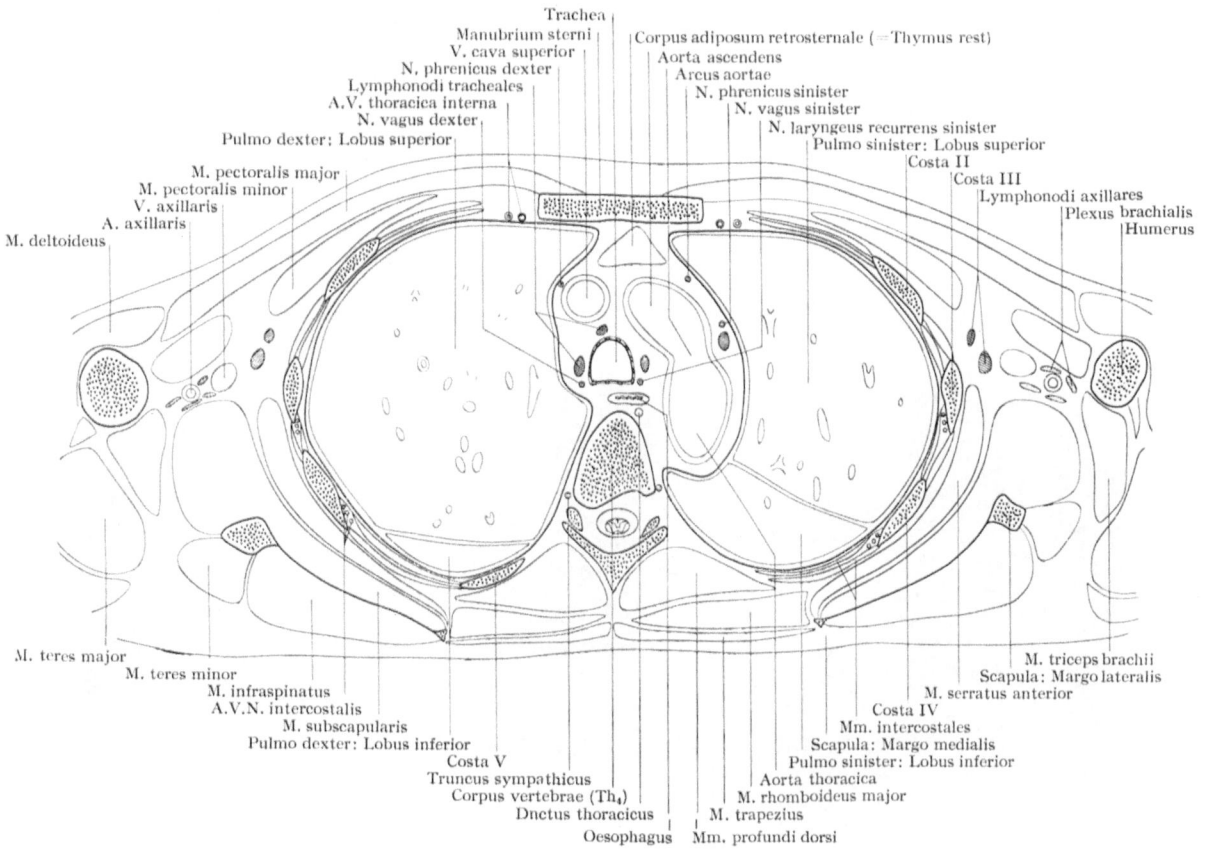

Trachea
Manubrium sterni
V. cava superior
N. phrenicus dexter
Lymphonodi tracheales
A.V. thoracica interna
N. vagus dexter
Pulmo dexter: Lobus superior
M. pectoralis major
M. pectoralis minor
V. axillaris
A. axillaris
M. deltoideus

Corpus adiposum retrosternale (= Thymus rest)
Aorta ascendens
Arcus aortae
N. phrenicus sinister
N. vagus sinister
N. laryngeus recurrens sinister
Pulmo sinister: Lobus superior
Costa II
Costa III
Lymphonodi axillares
Plexus brachialis
Humerus

M. teres major
M. teres minor
M. infraspinatus
A.V.N. intercostalis
M. subscapularis
Pulmo dexter: Lobus inferior
Costa V
Truncus sympathicus
Corpus vertebrae (Th₄)
Dnctus thoracicus
Oesophagus

M. triceps brachii
Scapula: Margo lateralis
M. serratus anterior
Costa IV
Mm. intercostales
Scapula: Margo medialis
Pulmo sinister: Lobus inferior
Aorta thoracica
M. rhomboideus major
M. trapezius
Mm. profundi dorsi

Fig. 192. Anatomical chart

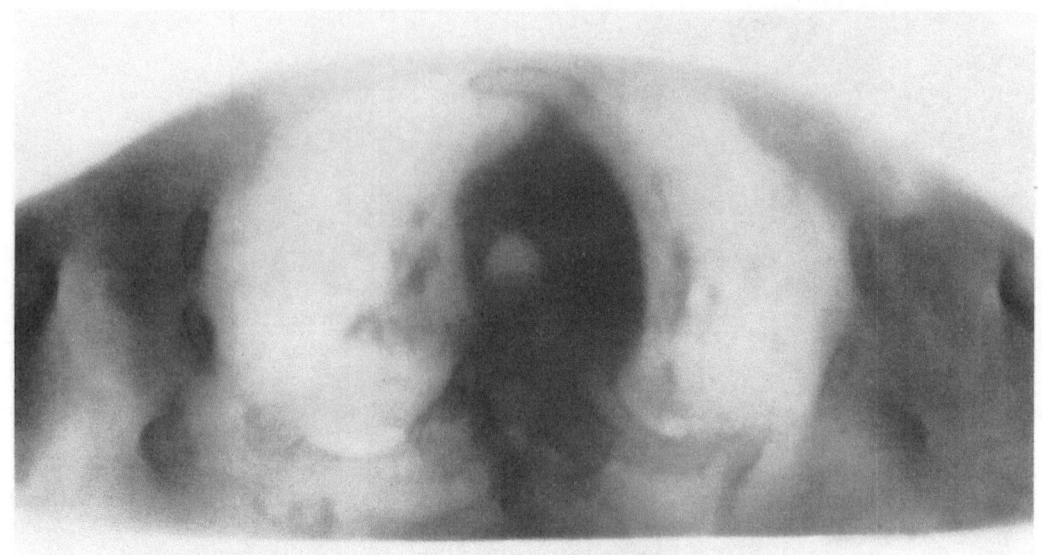

Fig. 193. Axial transverse tomogram

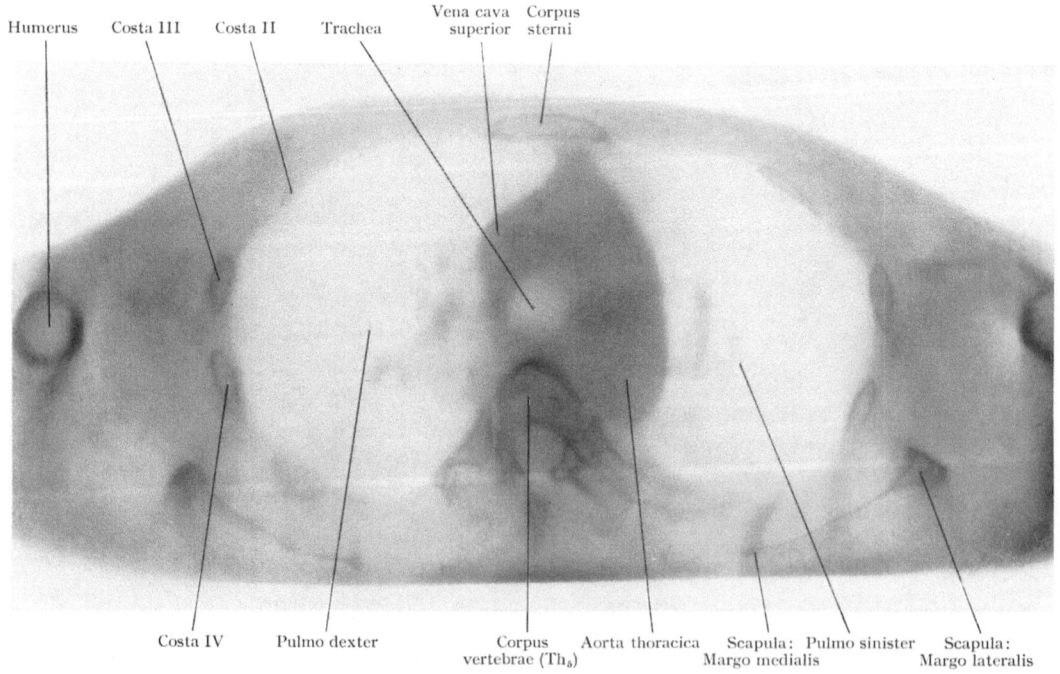

Fig. 194. Interpretation

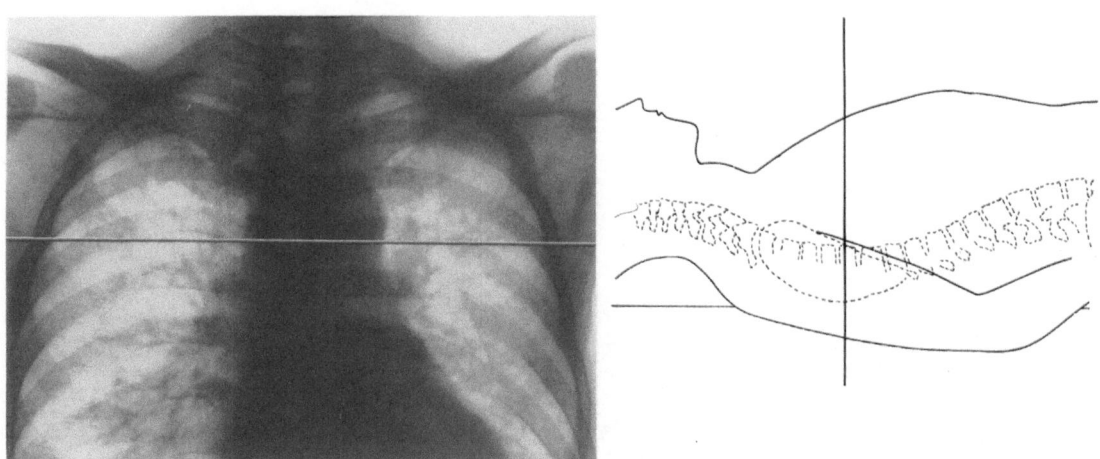

Fig. 195. Normal roentgenogram. Horizontal line showing the level tomographed

Fig. 196. Schematic drawing of the level tomographed. Subject supine with arms parallel to body axis

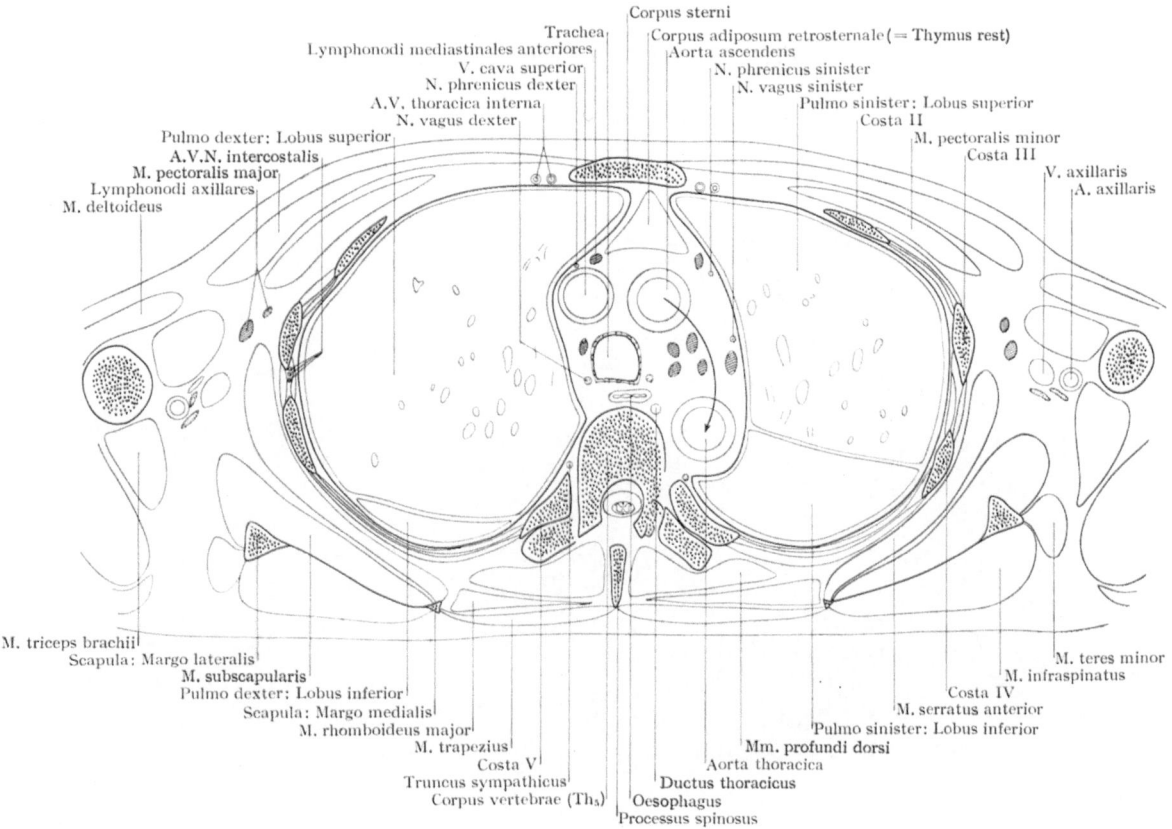

Corpus sterni
Corpus adiposum retrosternale (= Thymus rest)
Trachea
Lymphonodi mediastinales anteriores
V. cava superior
N. phrenicus dexter
A.V. thoracica interna
N. vagus dexter
Pulmo dexter: Lobus superior
A.V.N. intercostalis
M. pectoralis major
Lymphonodi axillares
M. deltoideus
Aorta ascendens
N. phrenicus sinister
N. vagus sinister
Pulmo sinister: Lobus superior
Costa II
M. pectoralis minor
Costa III
V. axillaris
A. axillaris

M. triceps brachii
Scapula: Margo lateralis
M. subscapularis
Pulmo dexter: Lobus inferior
Scapula: Margo medialis
M. rhomboideus major
M. trapezius
Costa V
Truncus sympathicus
Corpus vertebrae (Th₅)
M. teres minor
M. infraspinatus
Costa IV
M. serratus anterior
Pulmo sinister: Lobus inferior
Mm. profundi dorsi
Aorta thoracica
Ductus thoracicus
Oesophagus
Processus spinosus

Fig. 197. Anatomical chart

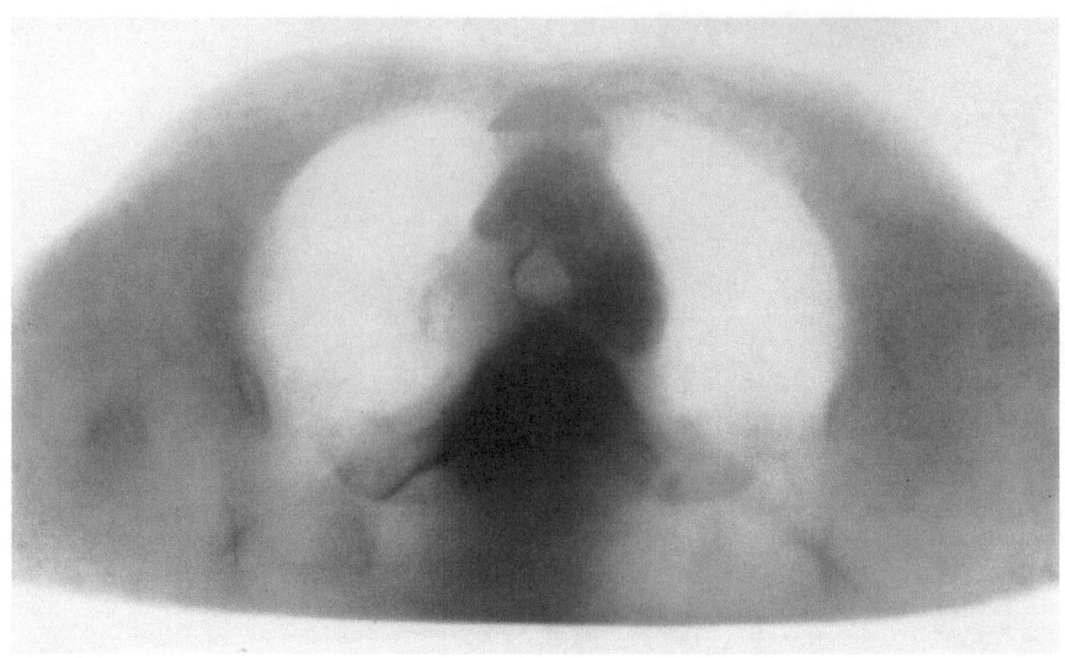

Fig. 198. Axial transverse tomogram

Scapula:
Margo lateralis   Pulmo dexter   Costa II   Vena cava superior   Corpus sterni   Trachea   Arcus aortae

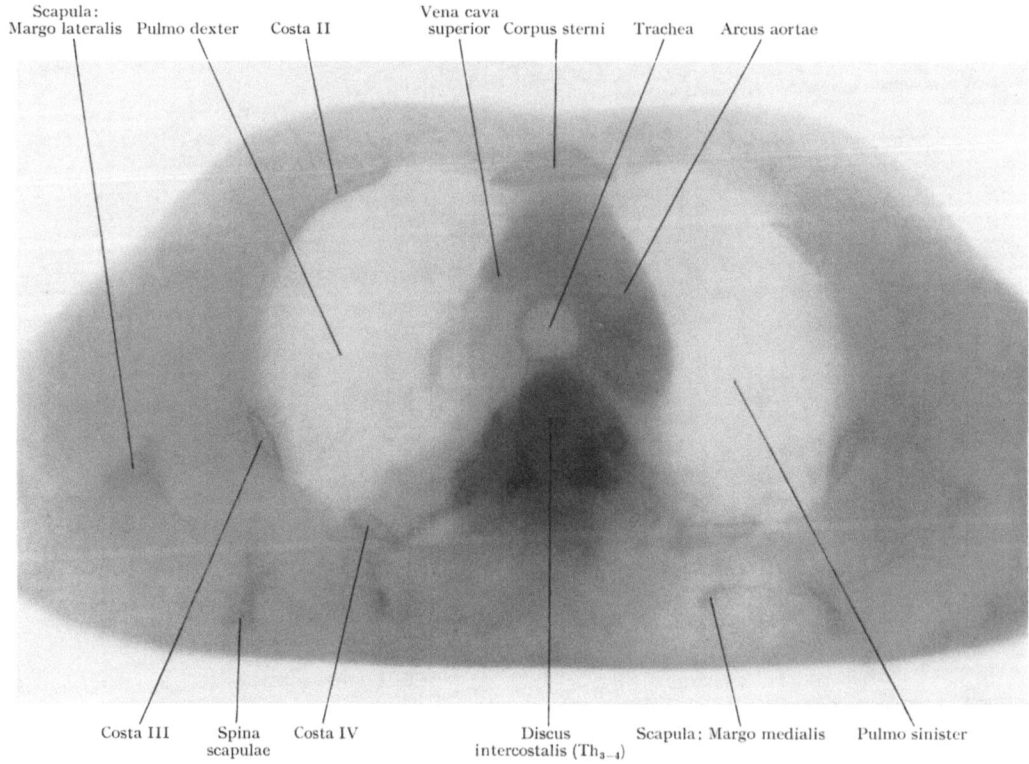

Costa III   Spina scapulae   Costa IV   Discus intercostalis (Th$_{3-4}$)   Scapula: Margo medialis   Pulmo sinister

Fig. 199. Interpretation

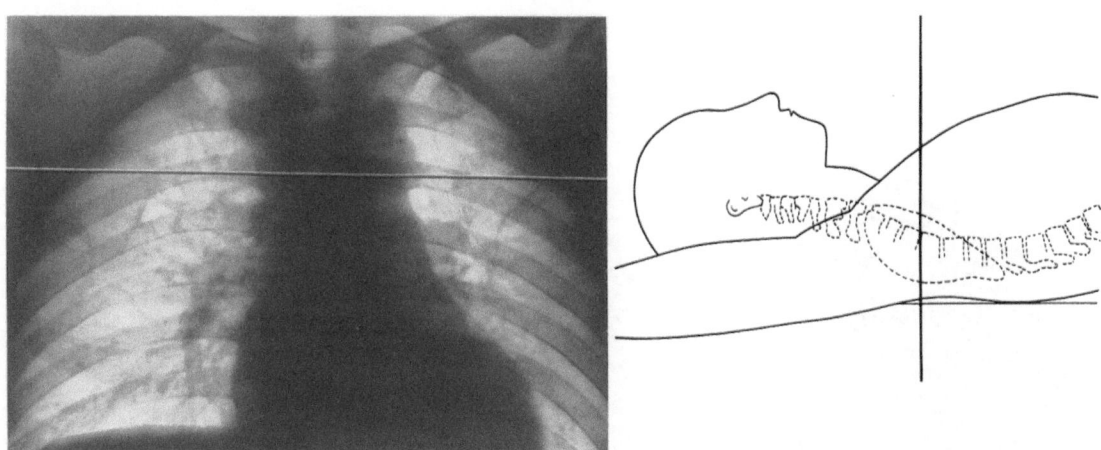

Fig. 200. Normal roentgenogram. Horizontal line showing the level tomographed

Fig. 201. Schematic drawing of the level tomographed. Subject supine with hands folded behind the head

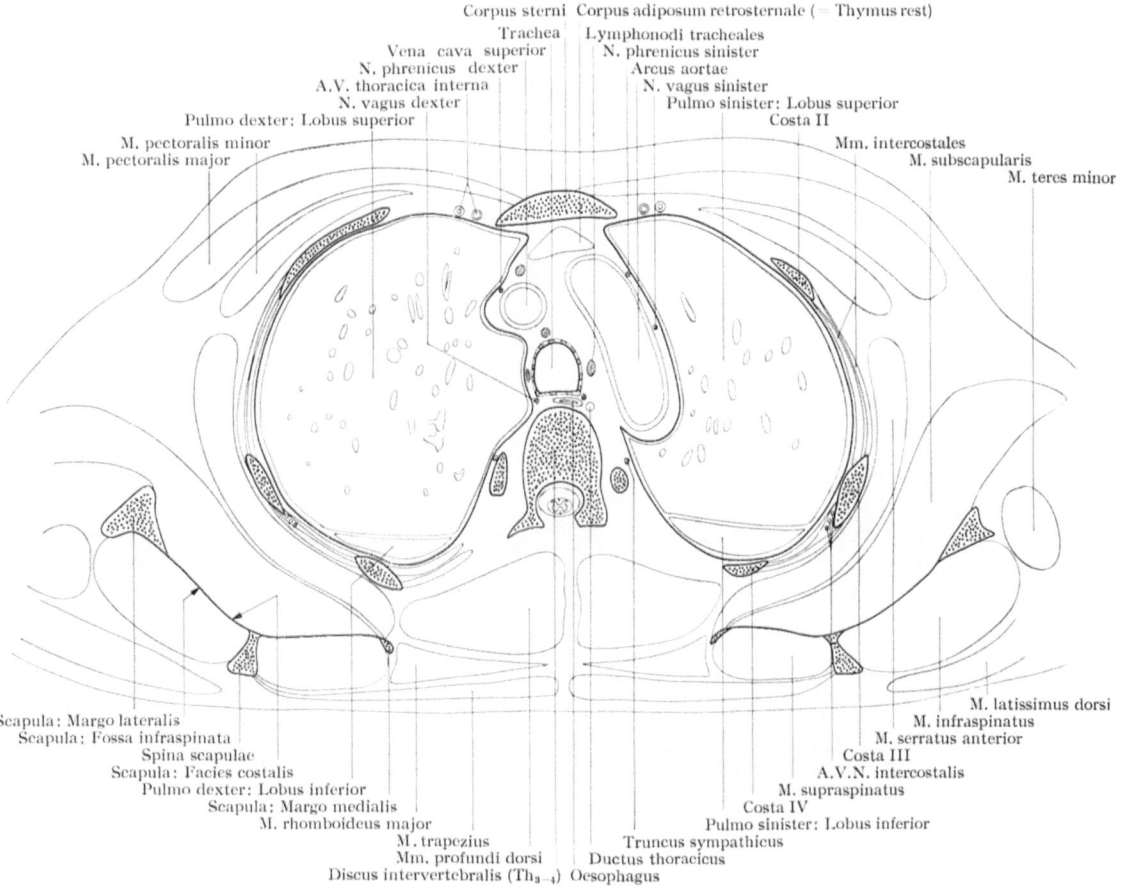

Fig. 202. Anatomical chart

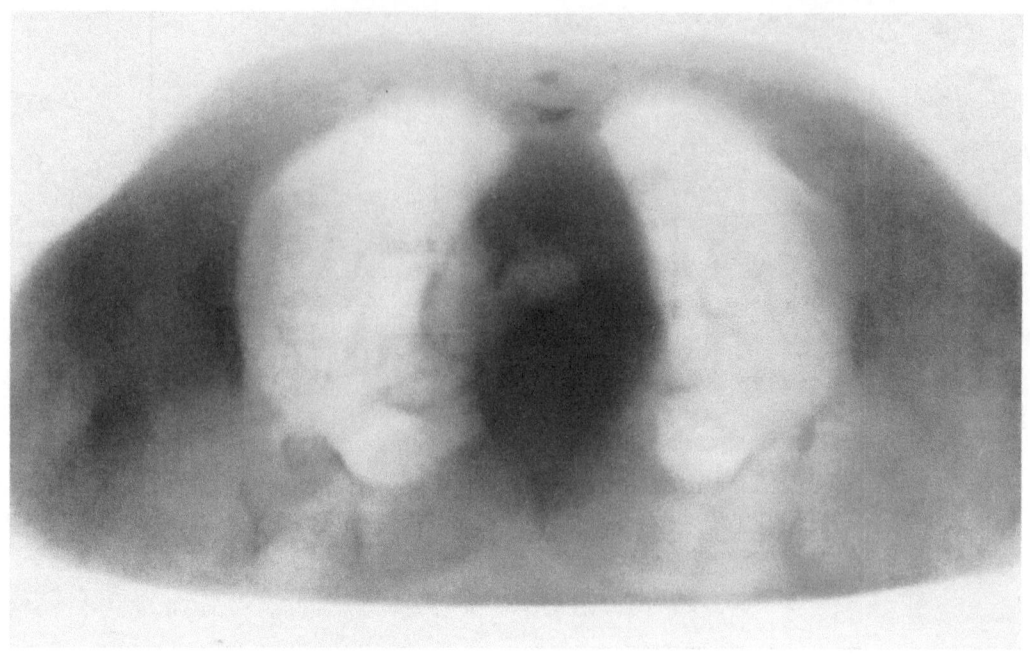

Fig. 203. Axial transverse tomogram

Pulmo dexter   Costa II   Vena cava superior   Corpus sterni   Bifurcatio tracheae   Pulmo sinister

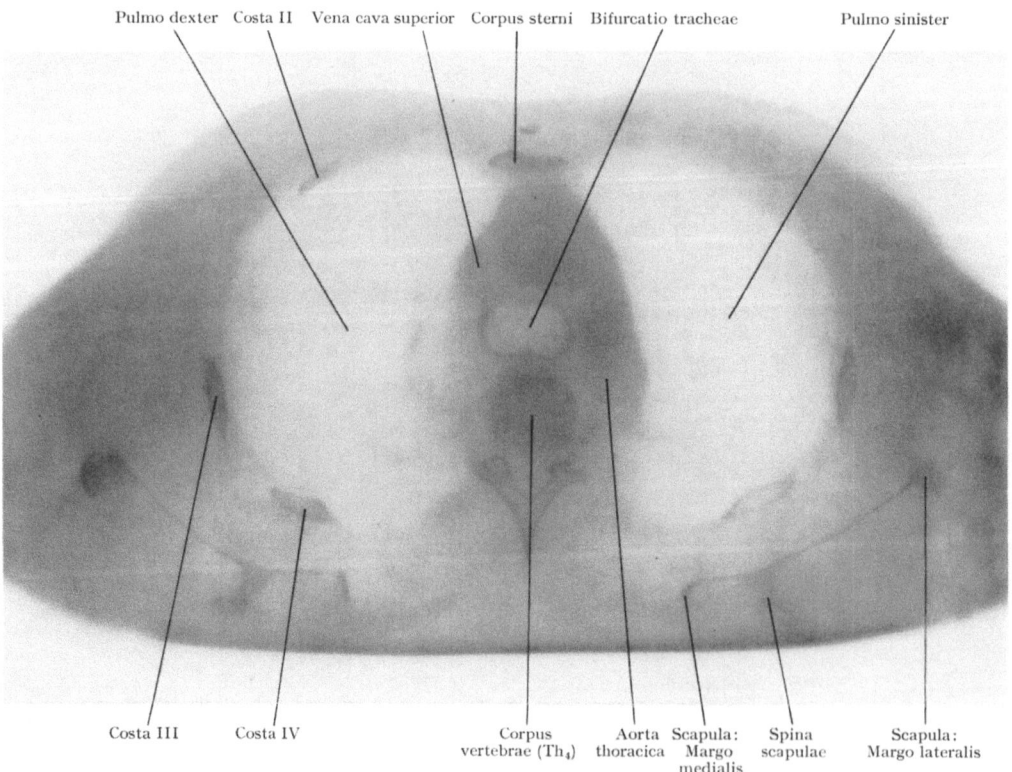

Costa III   Costa IV   Corpus vertebrae (Th$_4$)   Aorta thoracica   Scapula: Margo medialis   Spina scapulae   Scapula: Margo lateralis

Fig. 204. Interpretation

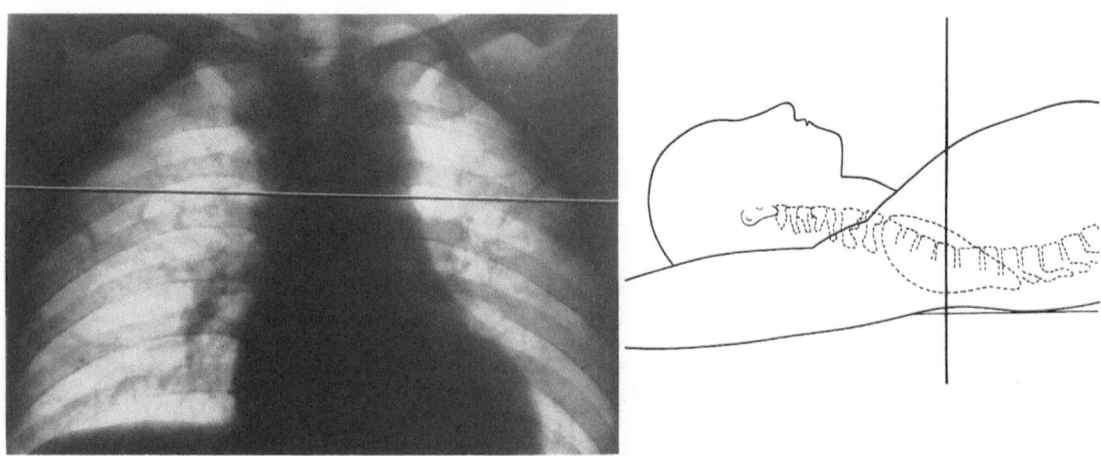

Fig. 205. Normal roentgenogram. Horizontal line showing the level tomographed

Fig. 206. Schematic drawing of the level tomographed. Subject supine with hands folded behind the head

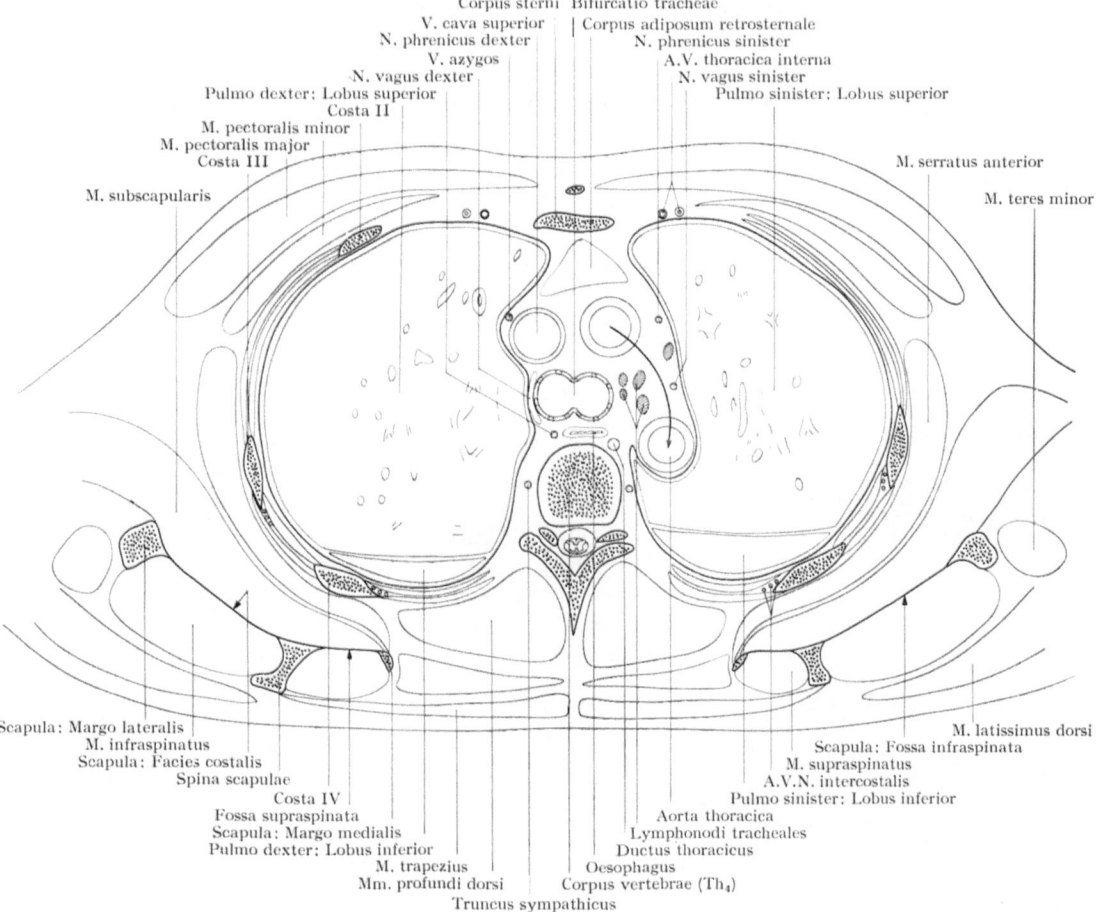

Corpus sterni Bifurcatio tracheae
V. cava superior | Corpus adiposum retrosternale
N. phrenicus dexter | N. phrenicus sinister
V. azygos A.V. thoracica interna
N. vagus dexter N. vagus sinister
Pulmo dexter: Lobus superior Pulmo sinister: Lobus superior
Costa II
M. pectoralis minor
M. pectoralis major
Costa III

M. serratus anterior

M. subscapularis M. teres minor

Scapula: Margo lateralis M. latissimus dorsi
M. infraspinatus Scapula: Fossa infraspinata
Scapula: Facies costalis M. supraspinatus
Spina scapulae A.V.N. intercostalis
Costa IV Pulmo sinister: Lobus inferior
Fossa supraspinata Aorta thoracica
Scapula: Margo medialis Lymphonodi tracheales
Pulmo dexter: Lobus inferior Ductus thoracicus
M. trapezius Oesophagus
Mm. profundi dorsi Corpus vertebrae (Th$_4$)
Truncus sympathicus

Fig. 207. Anatomical chart

101

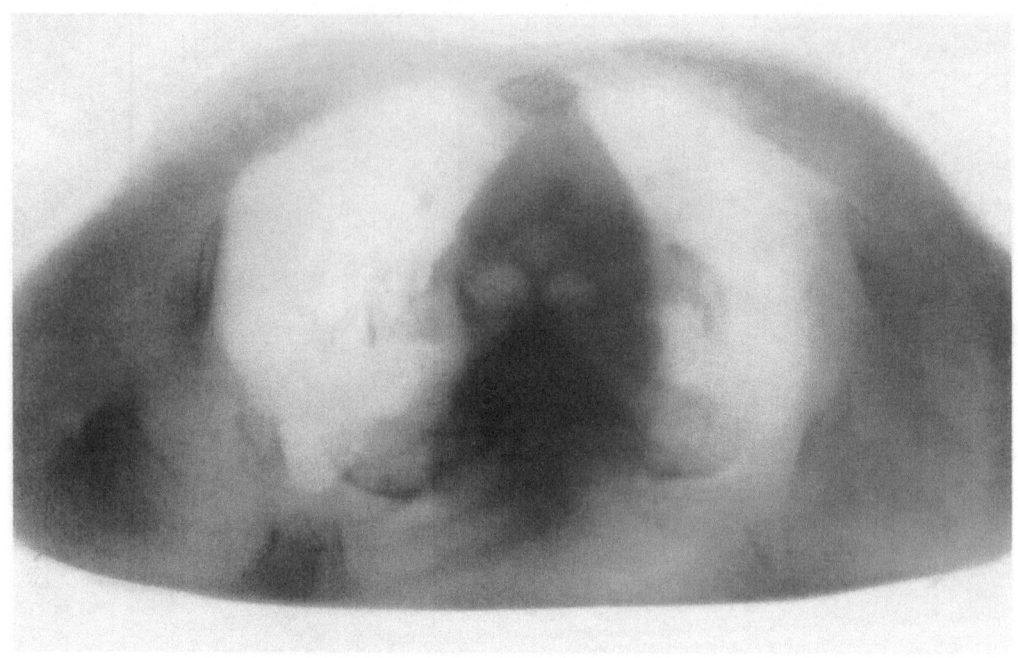

Fig. 208. Axial transverse tomogram

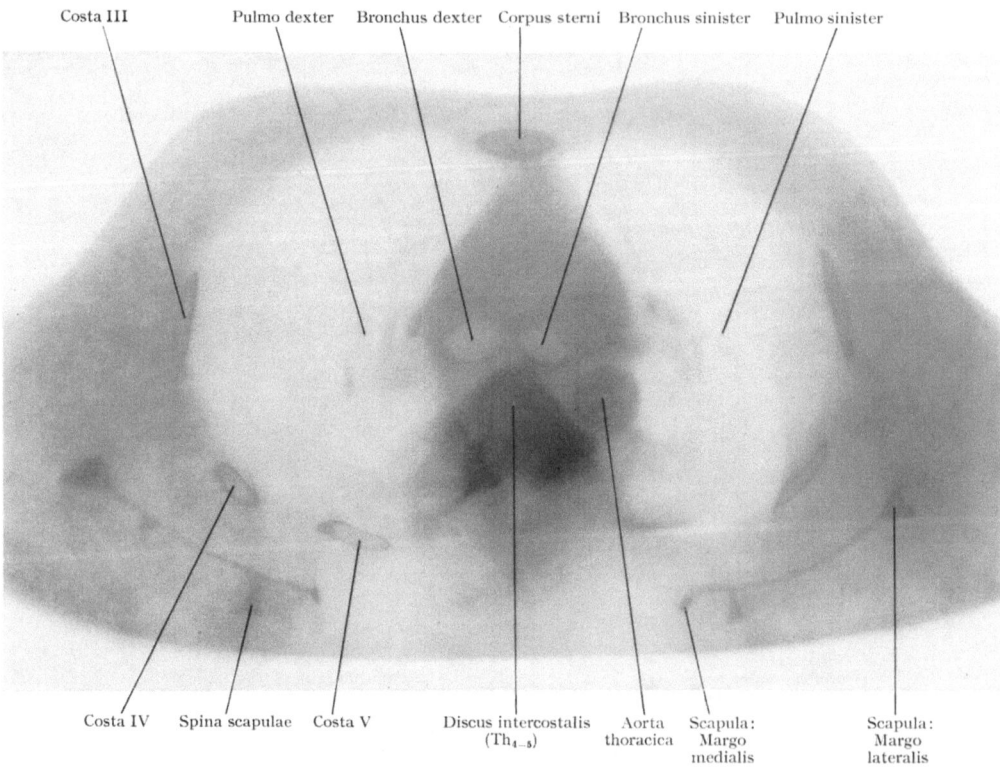

Fig. 209. Interpretation

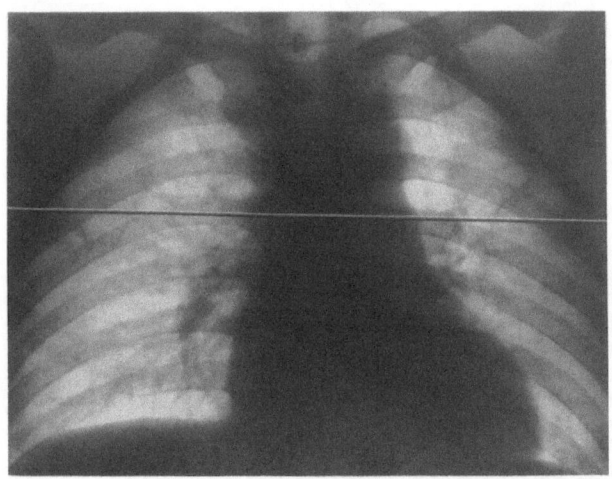

Fig. 210. Normal roentgenogram. Horizontal line showing the level tomographed

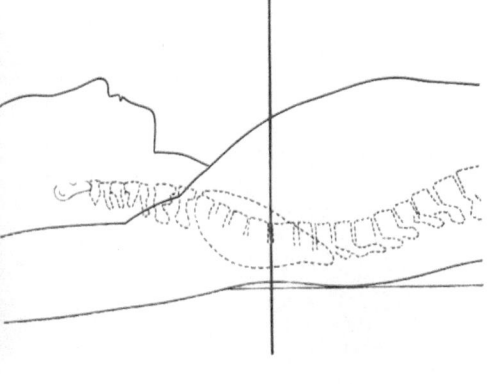

Fig. 211. Schematic drawing of the level tomographed. Subject supine with hands folded behind the head

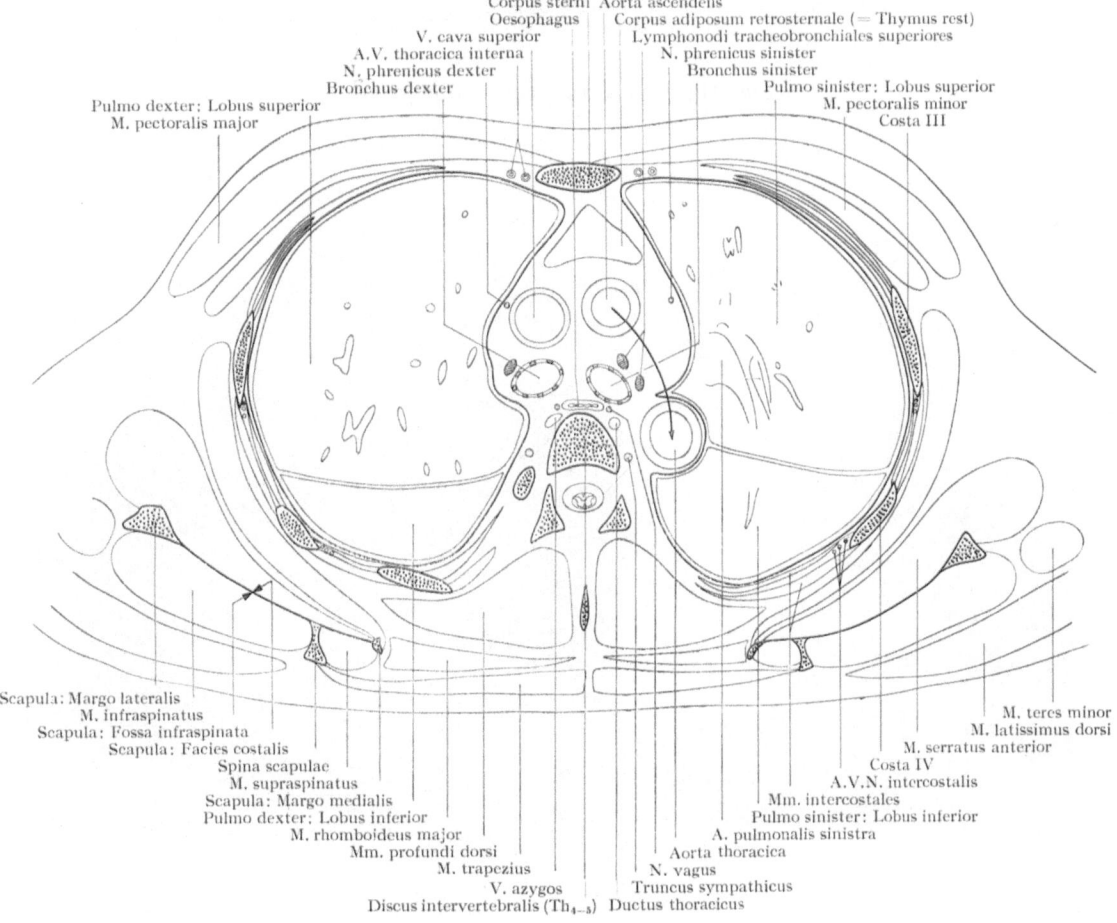

Corpus sterni Aorta ascendens
Oesophagus Corpus adiposum retrosternale (= Thymus rest)
V. cava superior Lymphonodi tracheobronchiales superiores
A.V. thoracica interna N. phrenicus sinister
N. phrenicus dexter Bronchus sinister
Bronchus dexter Pulmo sinister; Lobus superior
Pulmo dexter; Lobus superior M. pectoralis minor
M. pectoralis major Costa III

Scapula; Margo lateralis M. teres minor
M. infraspinatus M. latissimus dorsi
Scapula; Fossa infraspinata M. serratus anterior
Scapula; Facies costalis Costa IV
Spina scapulae A.V.N. intercostalis
M. supraspinatus Mm. intercostales
Scapula; Margo medialis Pulmo sinister; Lobus inferior
Pulmo dexter; Lobus inferior A. pulmonalis sinistra
M. rhomboideus major Aorta thoracica
Mm. profundi dorsi N. vagus
M. trapezius Truncus sympathicus
V. azygos Ductus thoracicus
Discus intervertebralis (Th$_{4-5}$)

Fig. 212. Anatomical chart

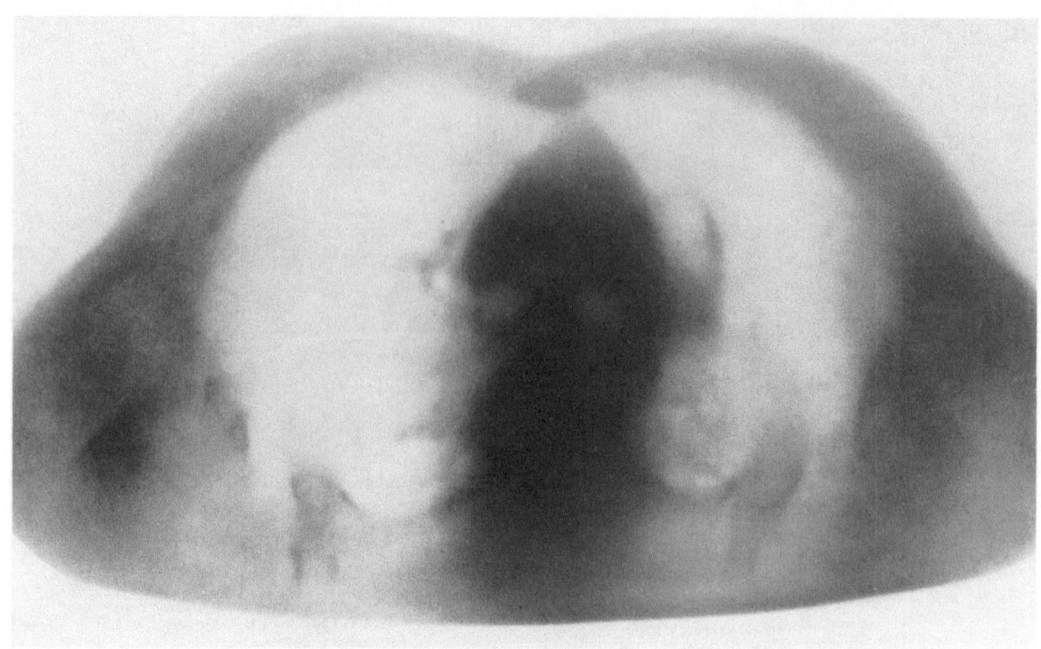

Fig. 213. Axial transverse tomogram

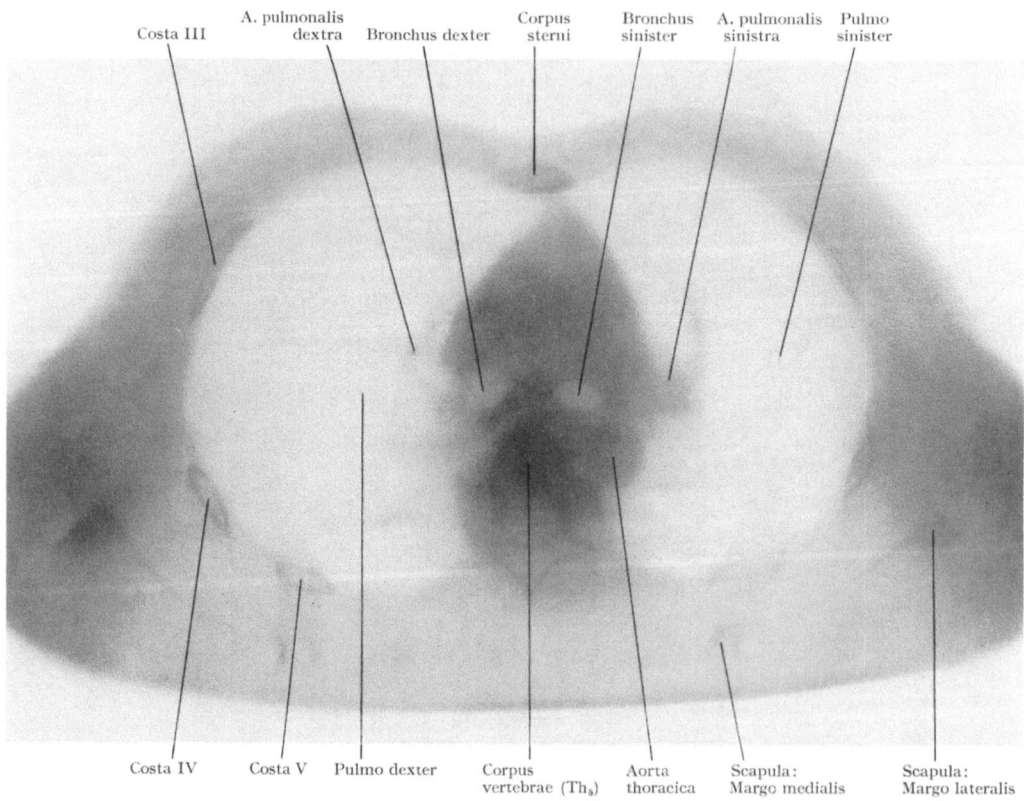

Fig. 214. Interpretation

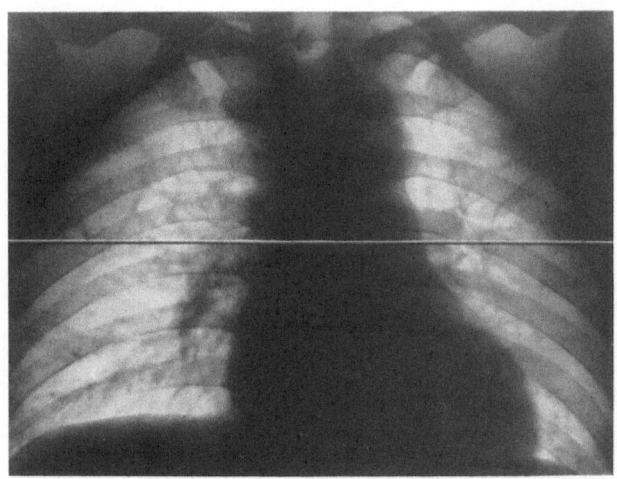

Fig. 215. Normal roentgenogram. Horizontal line showing the level tomographed

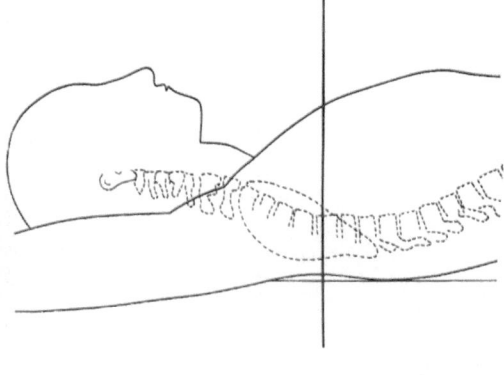

Fig. 216. Schematic drawing of the level tomographed. Subject supine with hands folded behind the head

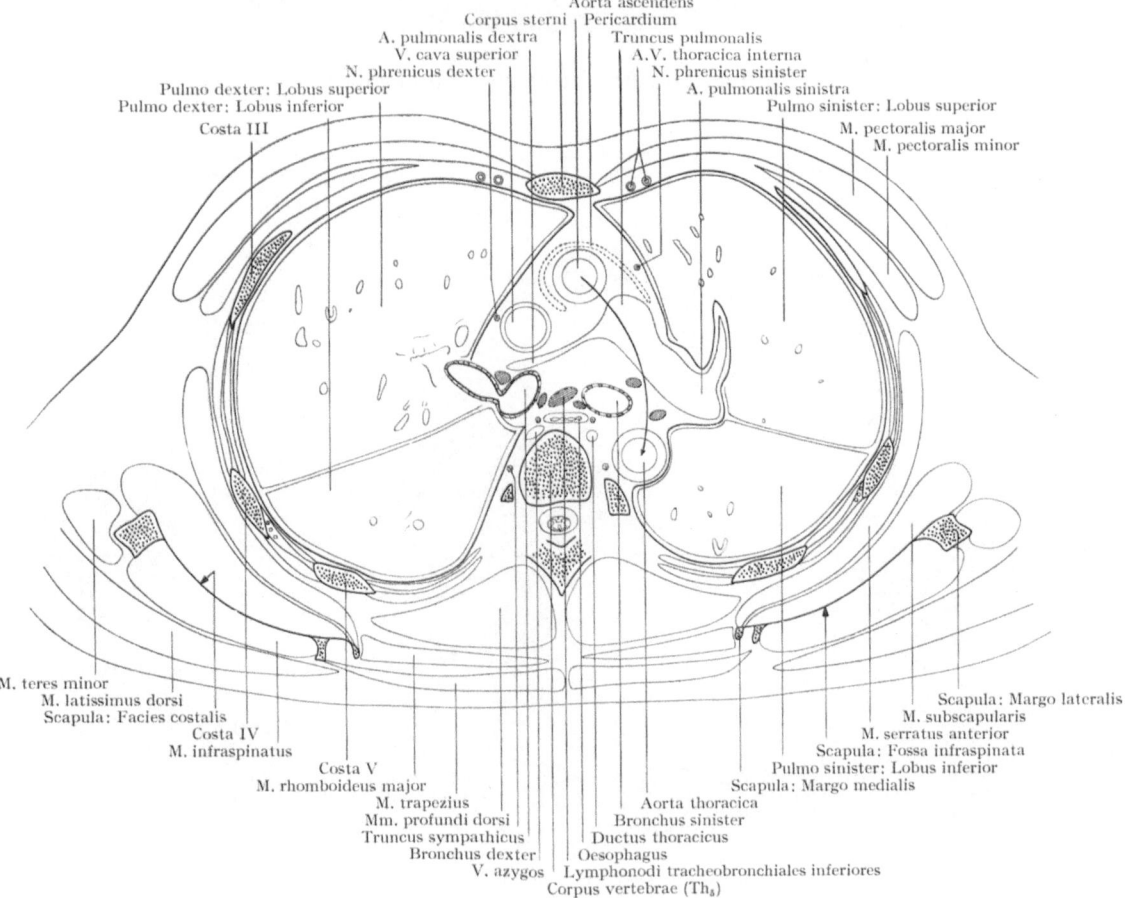

Fig. 217. Anatomical chart

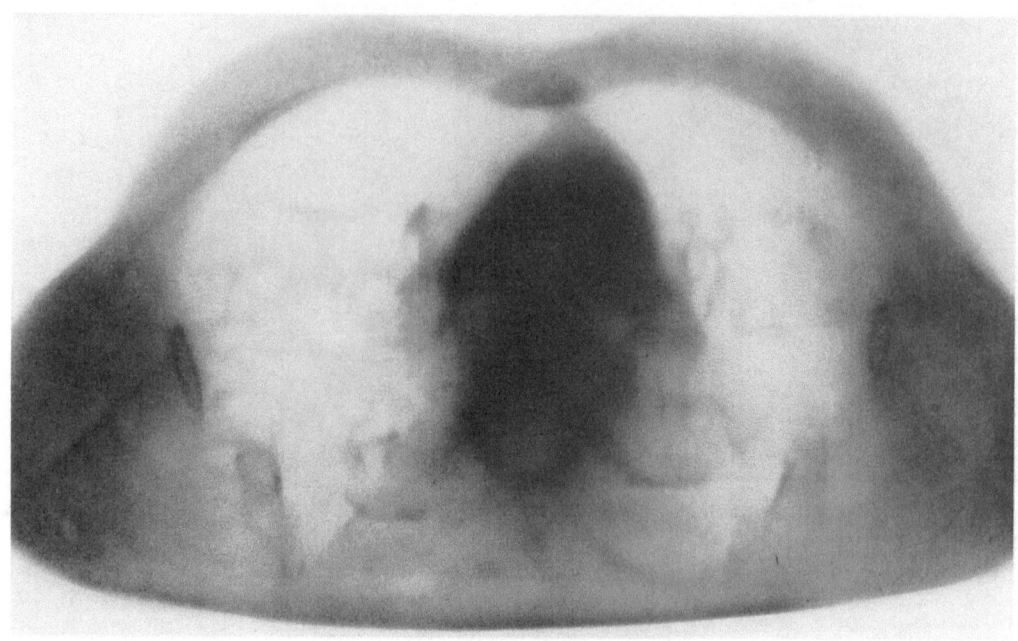

Fig. 218. Axial transverse tomogram

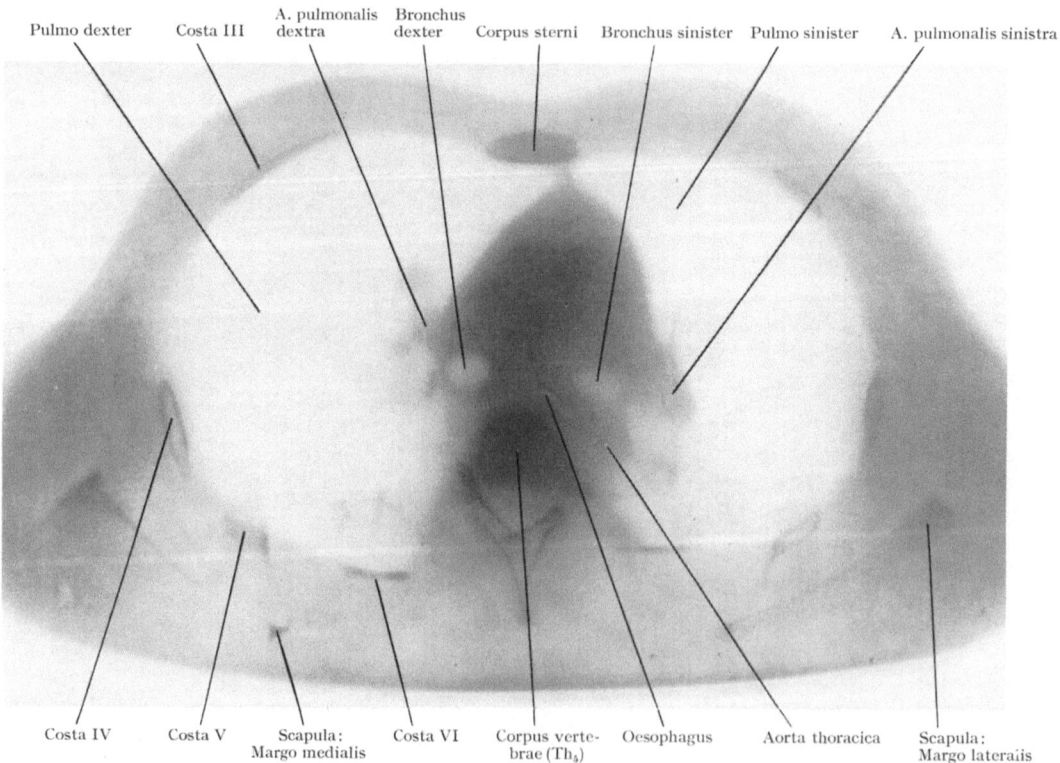

Pulmo dexter   Costa III   A. pulmonalis   Bronchus   Corpus sterni   Bronchus sinister   Pulmo sinister   A. pulmonalis sinistra
                              dextra   dexter

Costa IV   Costa V   Scapula: Costa VI   Corpus verte-   Oesophagus   Aorta thoracica   Scapula:
                       Margo medialis   brae (Th₅)   Margo lateralis

Fig. 219. Interpretation

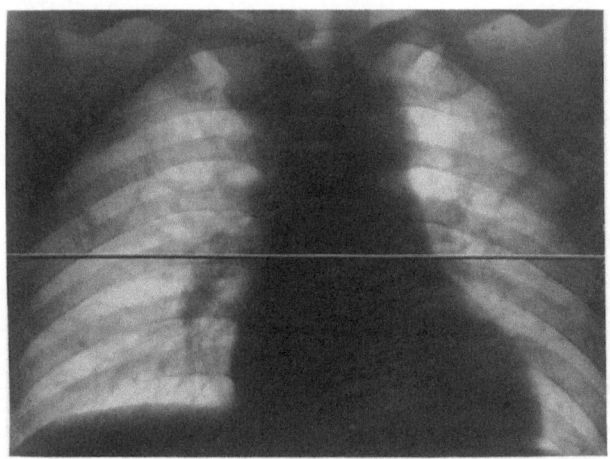

Fig. 220. Normal roentgenogram. Horizontal line showing the level tomographed

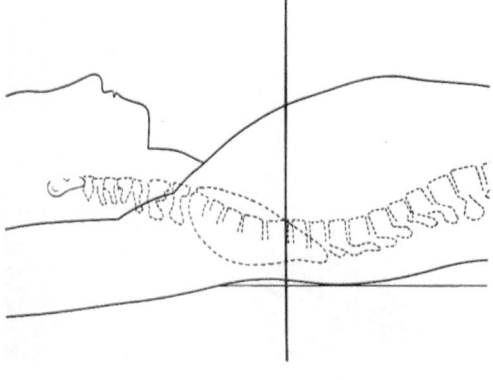

Fig. 221. Schematic drawing of the level tomographed. Subject supine with hands folded behind the head

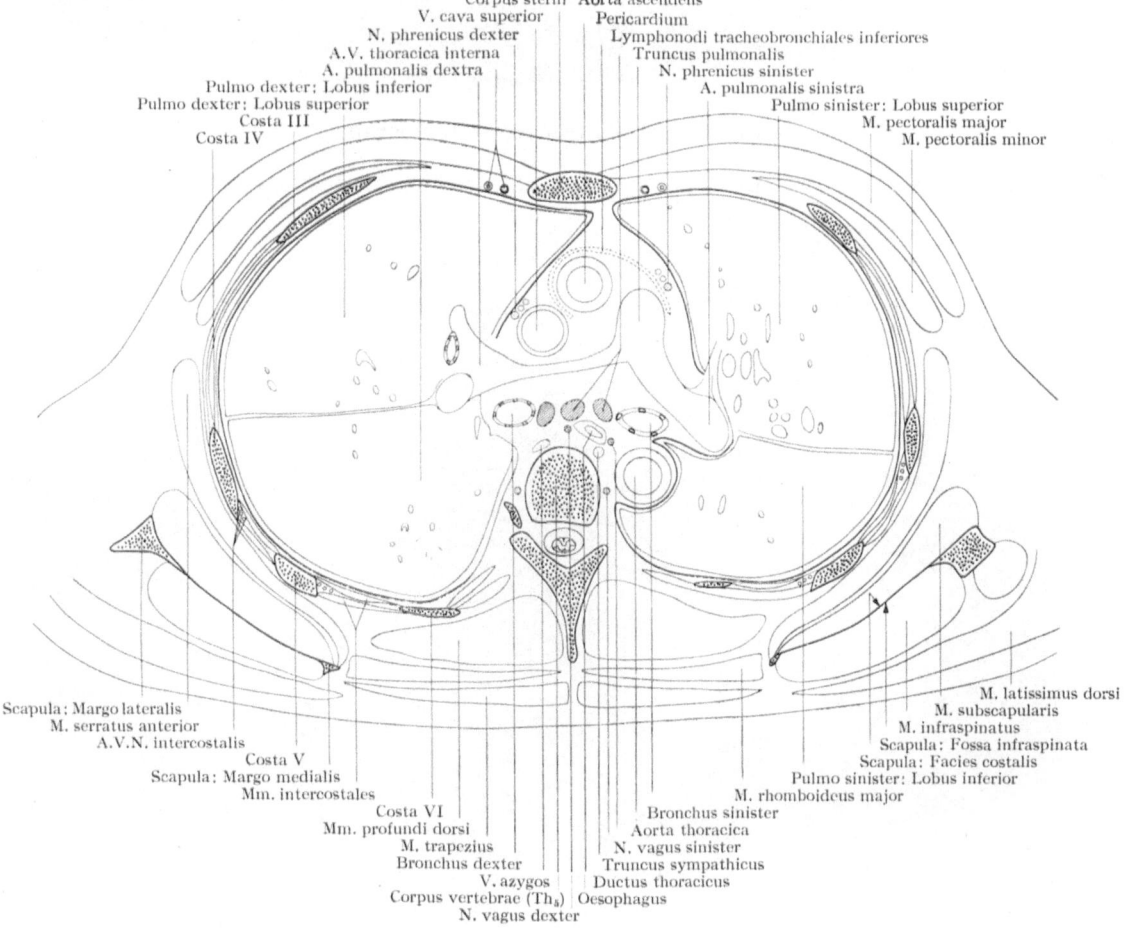

Corpus sterni Aorta ascendens
V. cava superior   Pericardium
N. phrenicus dexter   Lymphonodi tracheobronchiales inferiores
A.V. thoracica interna   Truncus pulmonalis
A. pulmonalis dextra   N. phrenicus sinister
Pulmo dexter; Lobus inferior   A. pulmonalis sinistra
Pulmo dexter; Lobus superior   Pulmo sinister: Lobus superior
Costa III   M. pectoralis major
Costa IV   M. pectoralis minor

M. latissimus dorsi
M. subscapularis
M. infraspinatus
Scapula: Fossa infraspinata
Scapula: Facies costalis
Pulmo sinister: Lobus inferior
M. rhomboideus major

Scapula; Margo lateralis
M. serratus anterior
A.V.N. intercostalis
Costa V
Scapula; Margo medialis
Mm. intercostales
Costa VI
Mm. profundi dorsi
M. trapezius
Bronchus dexter
V. azygos
Corpus vertebrae (Th₉)
N. vagus dexter

Bronchus sinister
Aorta thoracica
N. vagus sinister
Truncus sympathicus
Ductus thoracicus
Oesophagus

Fig. 222. Anatomical chart

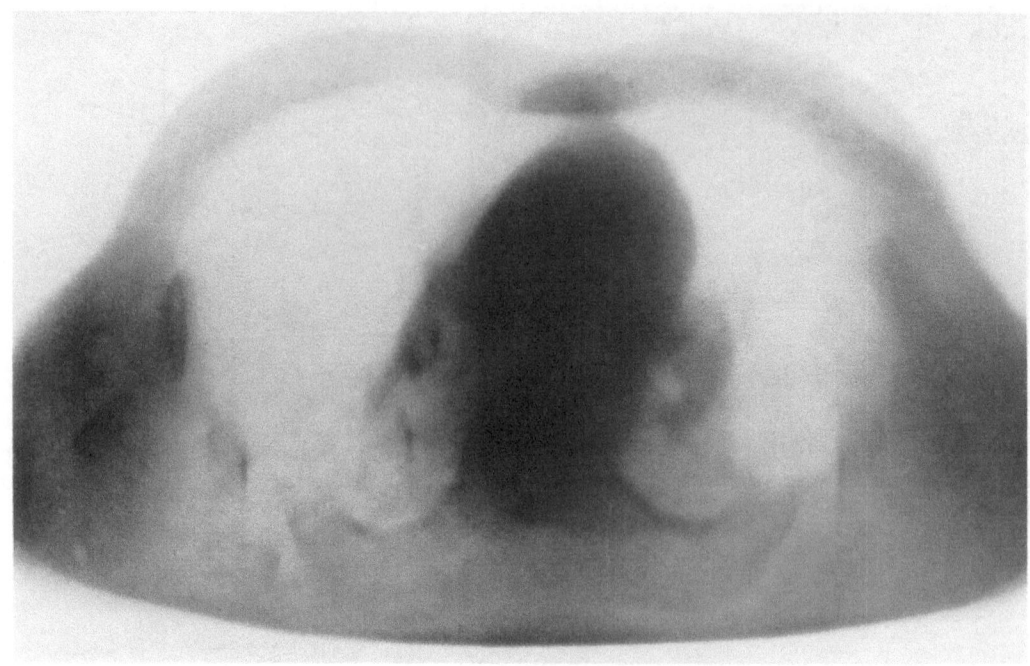

Fig. 223. Axial transverse tomogram

Costa IV Pulmo dexter Costa III Corpus sterni Cor A. pulmonalis sinistra Scapula: Margo lateralis

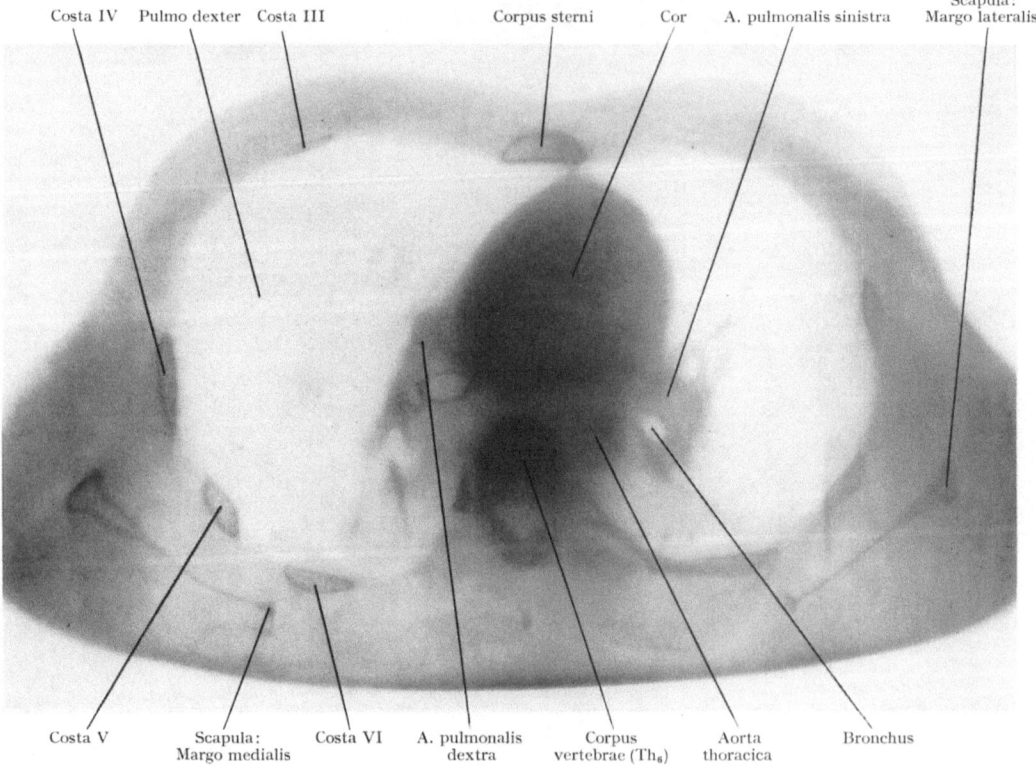

Costa V Scapula: Margo medialis Costa VI A. pulmonalis dextra Corpus vertebrae (Th$_6$) Aorta thoracica Bronchus

Fig. 224. Interpretation

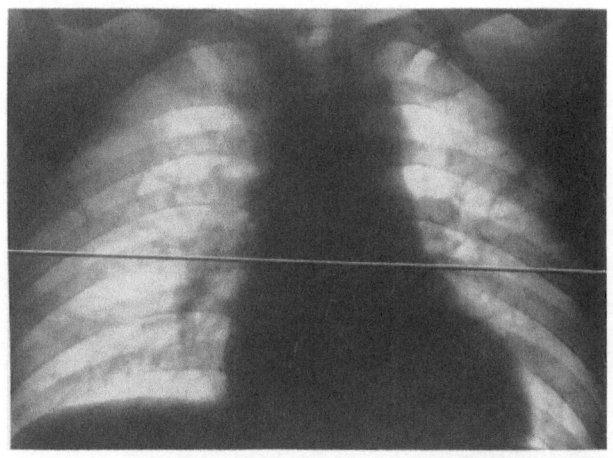

Fig. 225. Normal roentgenogram. Horizontal line showing the level tomographed

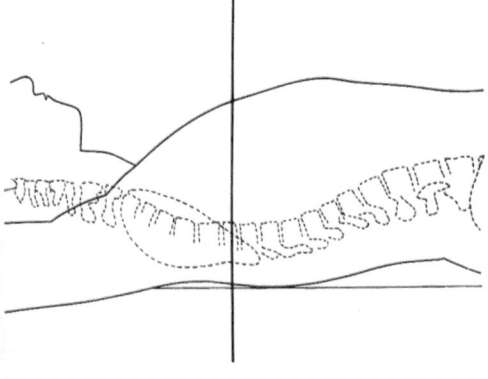

Fig. 226. Schematic drawing of the level tomographed. Subject supine with hands folded behind the head

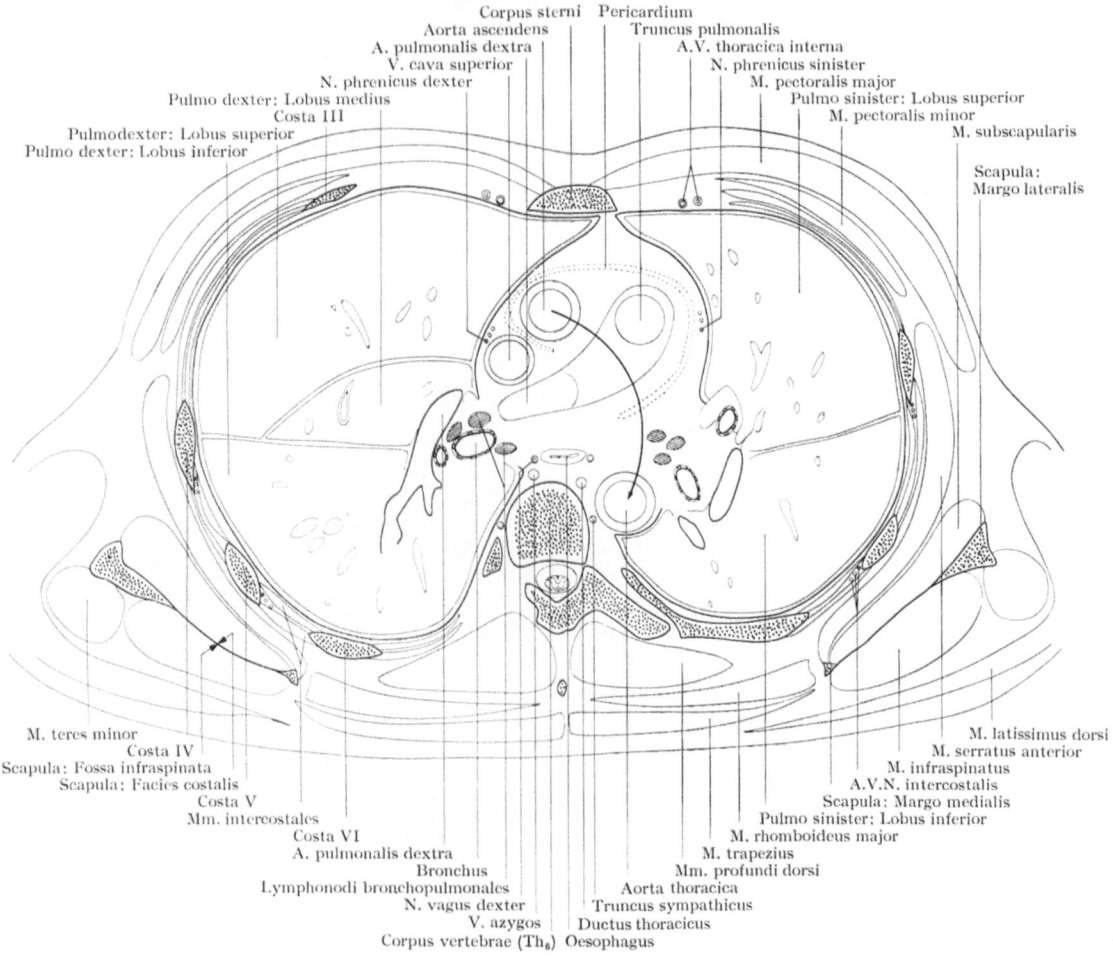

Corpus sterni Pericardium
Aorta ascendens Truncus pulmonalis
A. pulmonalis dextra A.V. thoracica interna
V. cava superior N. phrenicus sinister
N. phrenicus dexter M. pectoralis major
Pulmo dexter: Lobus medius Pulmo sinister: Lobus superior
Costa III M. pectoralis minor
Pulmodexter: Lobus superior M. subscapularis
Pulmo dexter: Lobus inferior Scapula: Margo lateralis

M. teres minor M. latissimus dorsi
Costa IV M. serratus anterior
Scapula: Fossa infraspinata M. infraspinatus
Scapula: Facies costalis A.V.N. intercostalis
Costa V Scapula: Margo medialis
Mm. intercostales Pulmo sinister: Lobus inferior
Costa VI M. rhomboideus major
A. pulmonalis dextra M. trapezius
Bronchus Mm. profundi dorsi
Lymphonodi bronchopulmonales Aorta thoracica
N. vagus dexter Truncus sympathicus
V. azygos Ductus thoracicus
Corpus vertebrae (Th₆) Oesophagus

Fig. 227. Anatomical chart

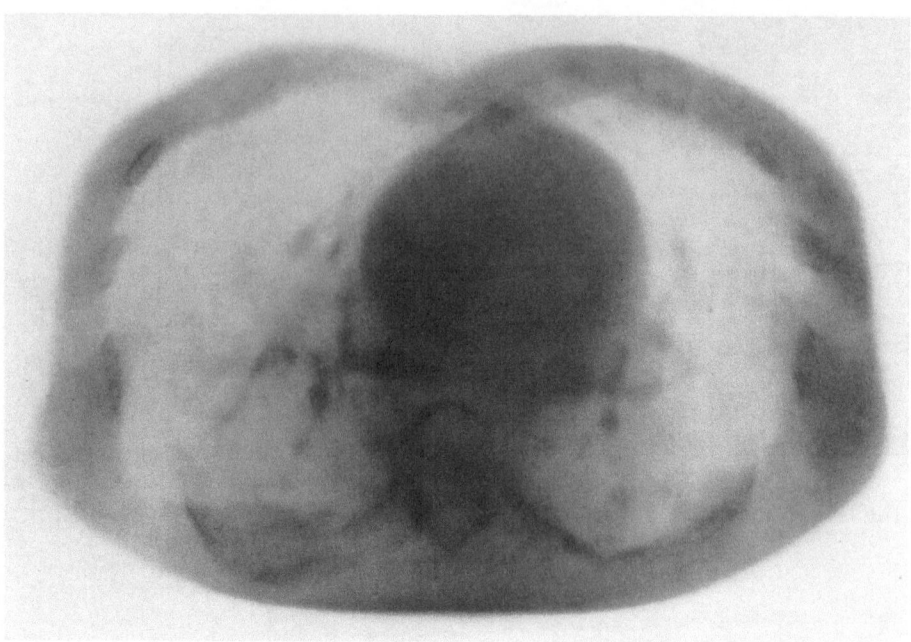

Fig. 228. Axial transverse tomogram

Costa VII Costa VI Costa V Corpus sterni Cor Pulmo sinister

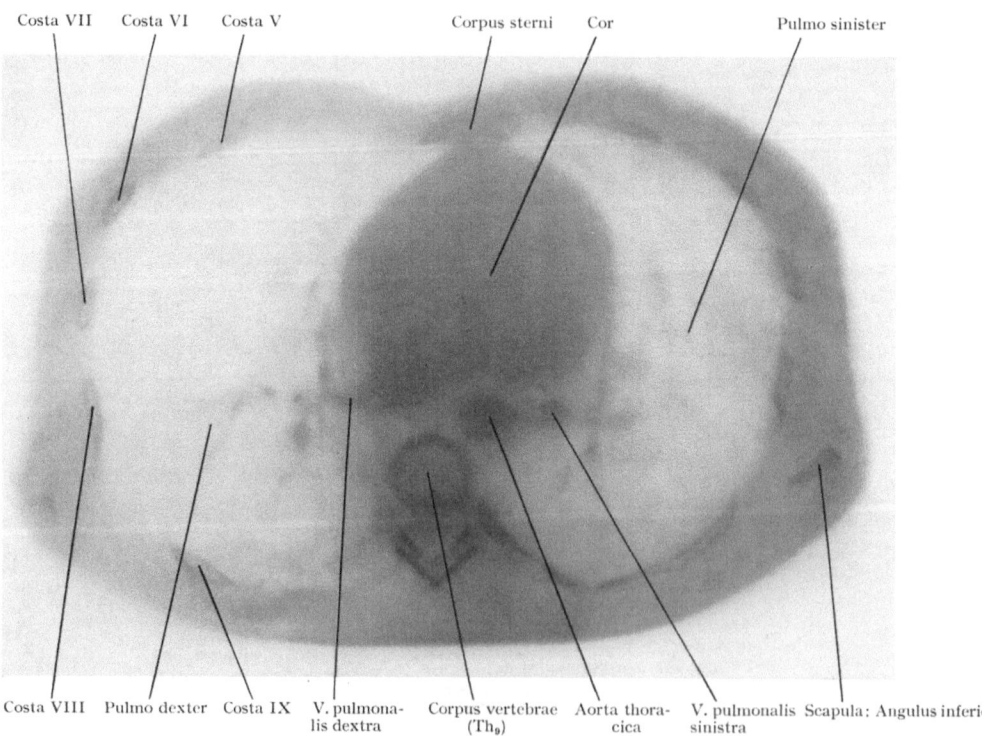

Costa VIII Pulmo dexter Costa IX V. pulmona- Corpus vertebrae Aorta thora- V. pulmonalis Scapula: Angulus inferior
                                     lis dextra (Th$_9$)   cica   sinistra

Fig. 229. Interpretation

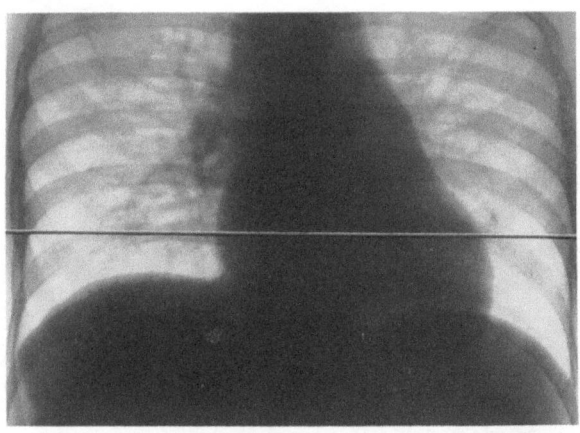

Fig. 230. Normal roentgenogram. Horizontal line showing the level tomographed

Fig. 231. Schematic drawing of the level tomographed. Subject supine with hands folded behind the head

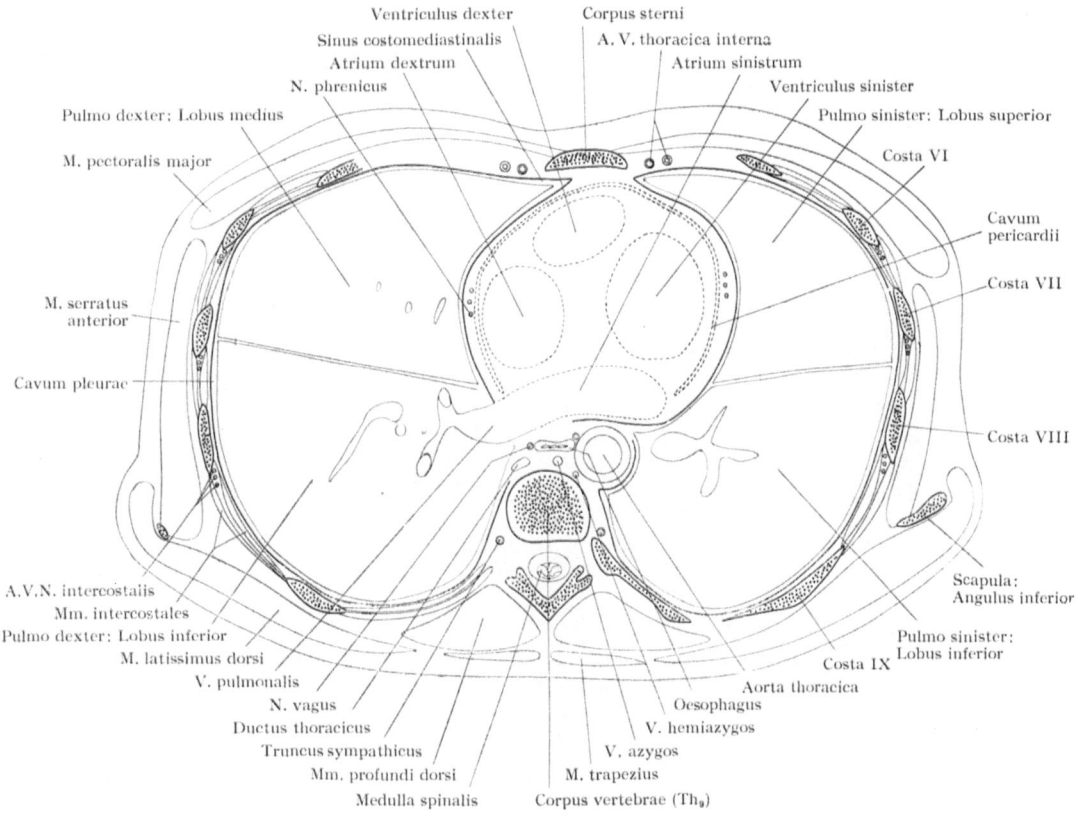

Ventriculus dexter
Sinus costomediastinalis
Atrium dextrum
N. phrenicus
Pulmo dexter; Lobus medius
M. pectoralis major
Corpus sterni
A. V. thoracica interna
Atrium sinistrum
Ventriculus sinister
Pulmo sinister: Lobus superior
Costa VI
Cavum pericardii
Costa VII
M. serratus anterior
Cavum pleurae
Costa VIII
A.V.N. intercostalis
Mm. intercostales
Pulmo dexter: Lobus inferior
M. latissimus dorsi
V. pulmonalis
N. vagus
Ductus thoracicus
Truncus sympathicus
Mm. profundi dorsi
Medulla spinalis
Corpus vertebrae (Th₉)
M. trapezius
V. azygos
V. hemiazygos
Oesophagus
Aorta thoracica
Costa IX
Pulmo sinister: Lobus inferior
Scapula: Angulus inferior

Fig. 232. Anatomical chart

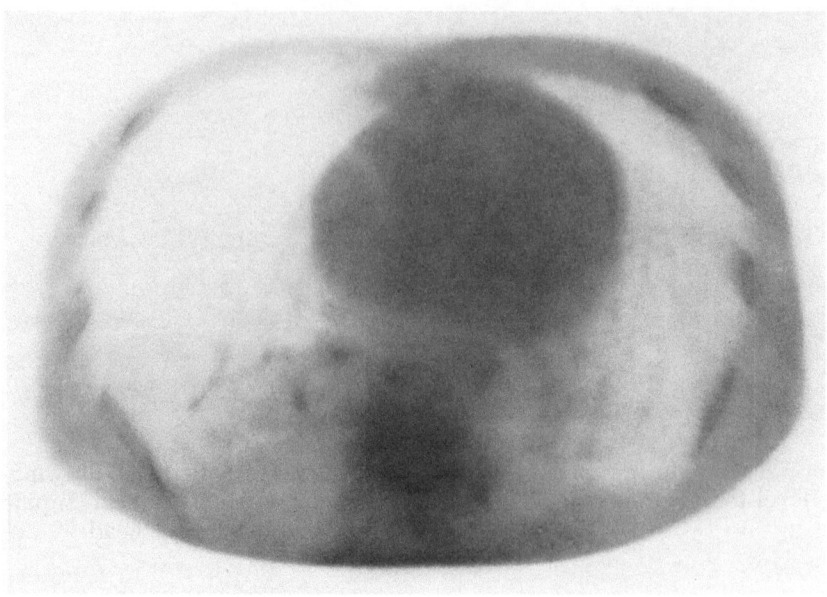

Fig. 233. Axial transverse tomogram

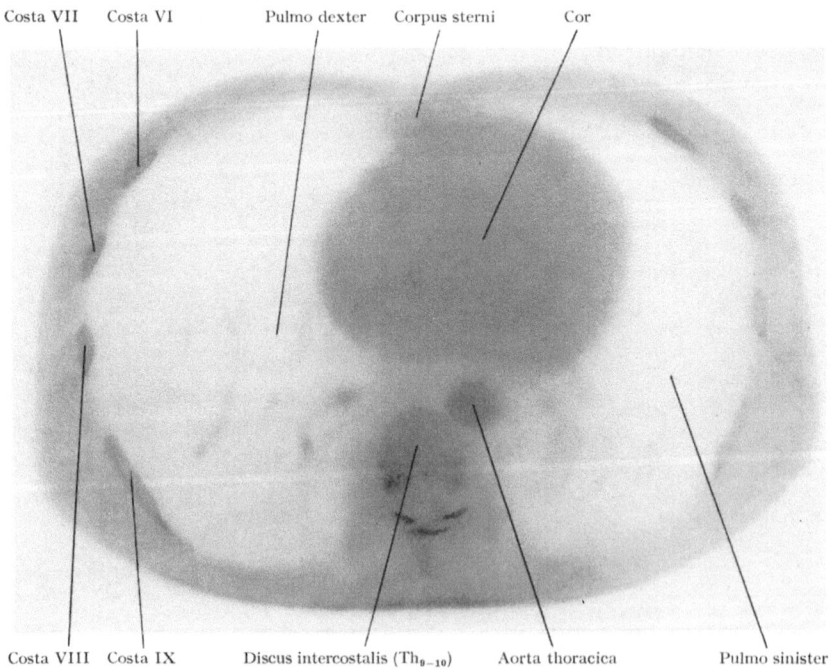

Costa VII   Costa VI   Pulmo dexter   Corpus sterni   Cor

Costa VIII   Costa IX   Discus intercostalis (Th$_{9-10}$)   Aorta thoracica   Pulmo sinister

Fig. 234. Interpretation

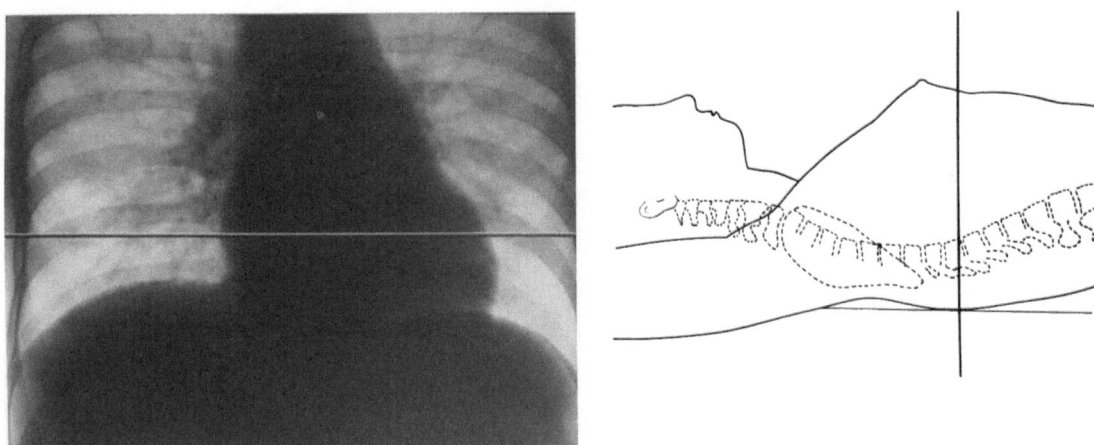

Fig. 235. Normal roentgenogram. Horizontal line showing the level tomographed

Fig. 236. Schematic drawing of the level tomographed. Subject supine with hands folded behind the head

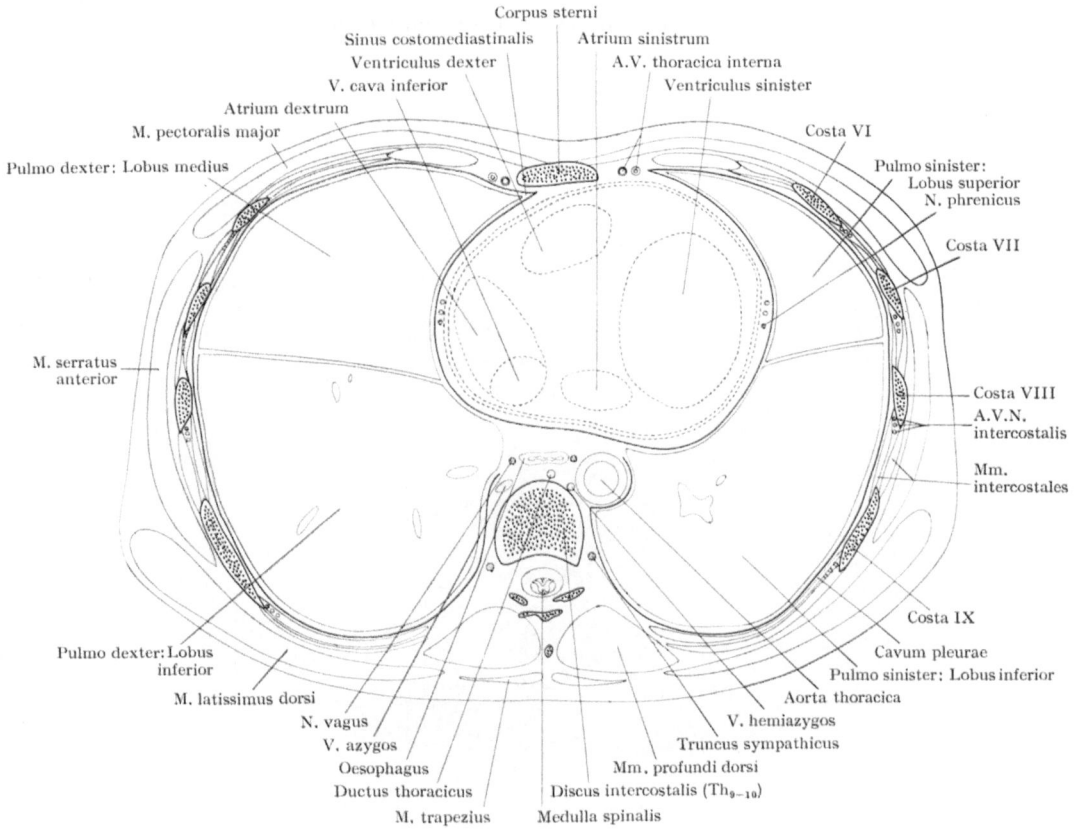

Corpus sterni
Sinus costomediastinalis
Atrium sinistrum
Ventriculus dexter
A.V. thoracica interna
V. cava inferior
Ventriculus sinister
Atrium dextrum
M. pectoralis major
Costa VI
Pulmo dexter: Lobus medius
Pulmo sinister: Lobus superior
N. phrenicus
Costa VII
M. serratus anterior
Costa VIII
A.V.N. intercostalis
Mm. intercostales
Costa IX
Cavum pleurae
Pulmo sinister: Lobus inferior
Pulmo dexter: Lobus inferior
Aorta thoracica
M. latissimus dorsi
V. hemiazygos
N. vagus
Truncus sympathicus
V. azygos
Mm. profundi dorsi
Oesophagus
Discus intercostalis (Th$_{9-10}$)
Ductus thoracicus
Medulla spinalis
M. trapezius

Fig. 237. Anatomical chart

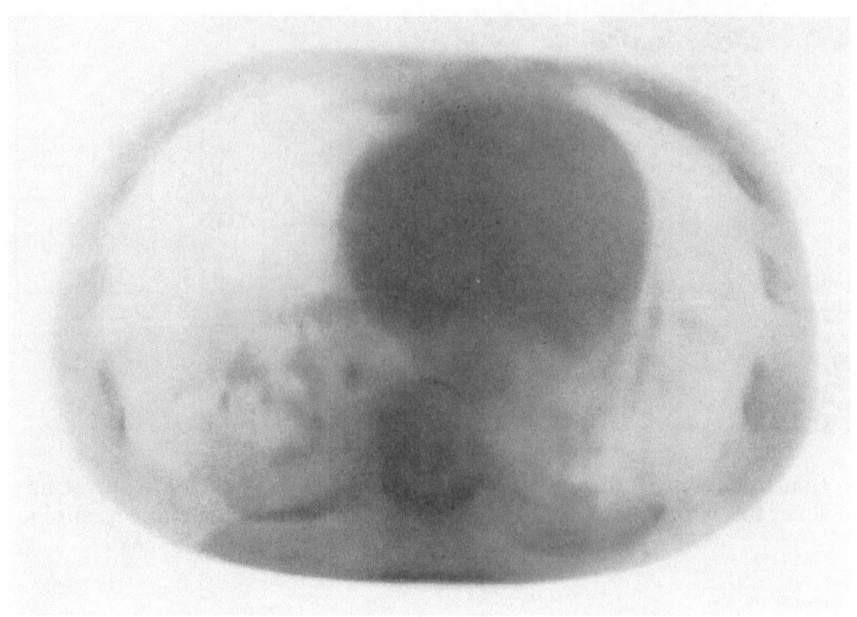

Fig. 238. Axial transverse tomogram

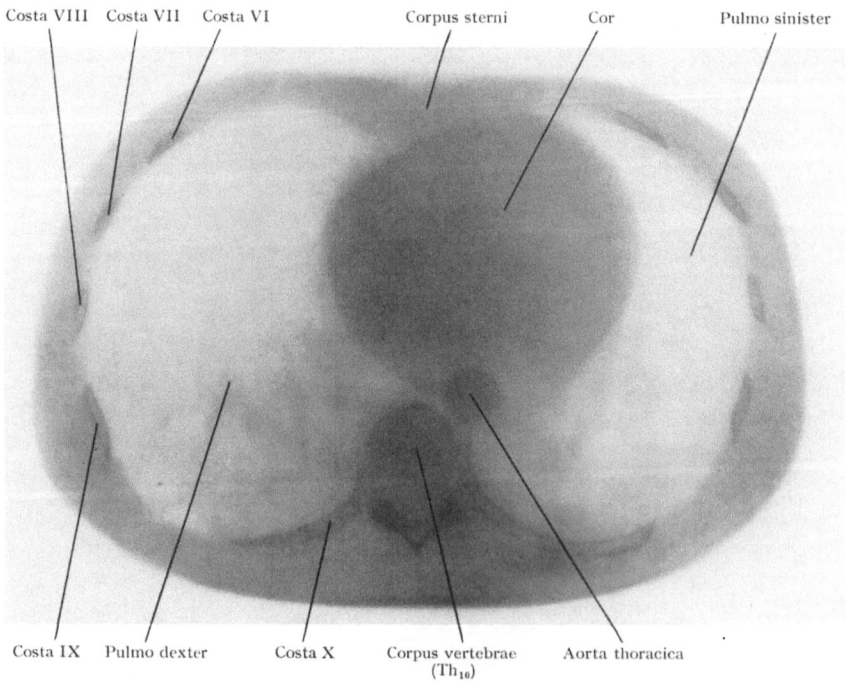

Costa VIII   Costa VII   Costa VI   Corpus sterni   Cor   Pulmo sinister

Costa IX   Pulmo dexter   Costa X   Corpus vertebrae   Aorta thoracica
(Th$_{10}$)

Fig. 239. Interpretation

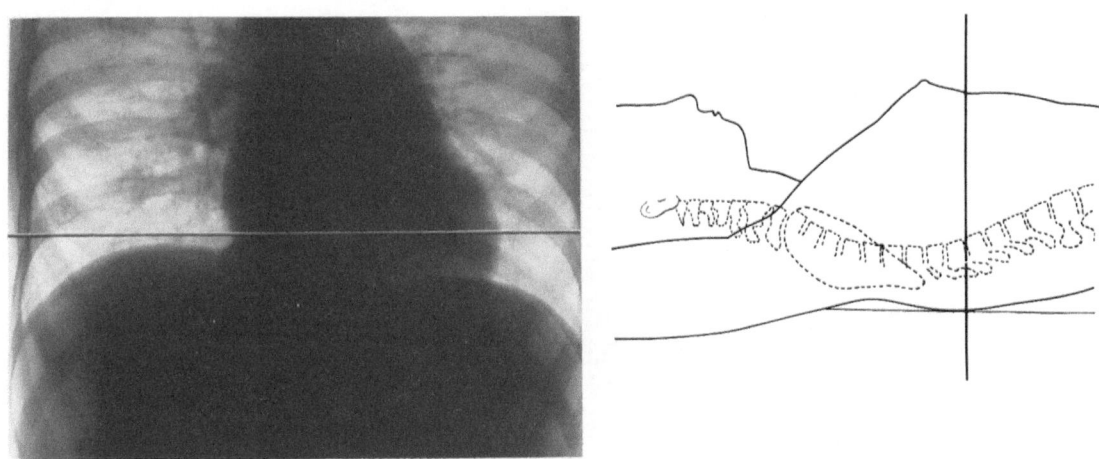

Fig. 240. Normal roentgenogram. Horizontal line showing the level tomographed

Fig. 241. Schematic drawing of the level tomographed. Subject supine with hands folded behind the head

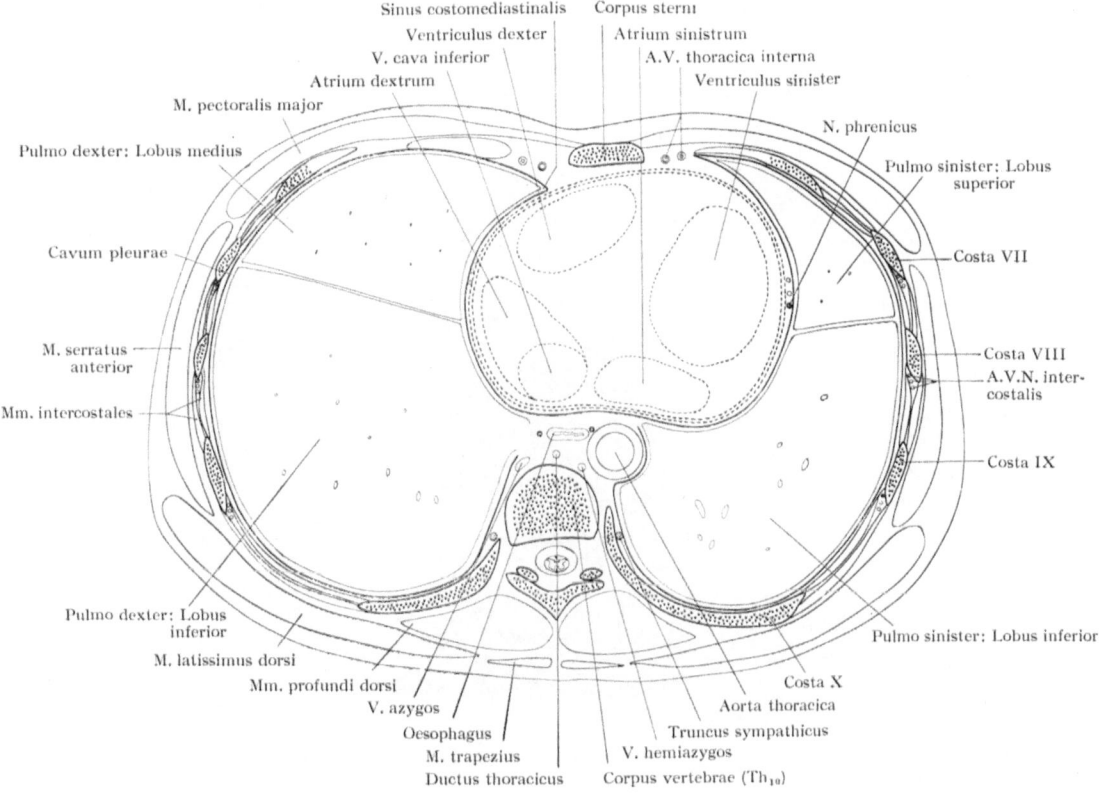

Fig. 242. Anatomical chart

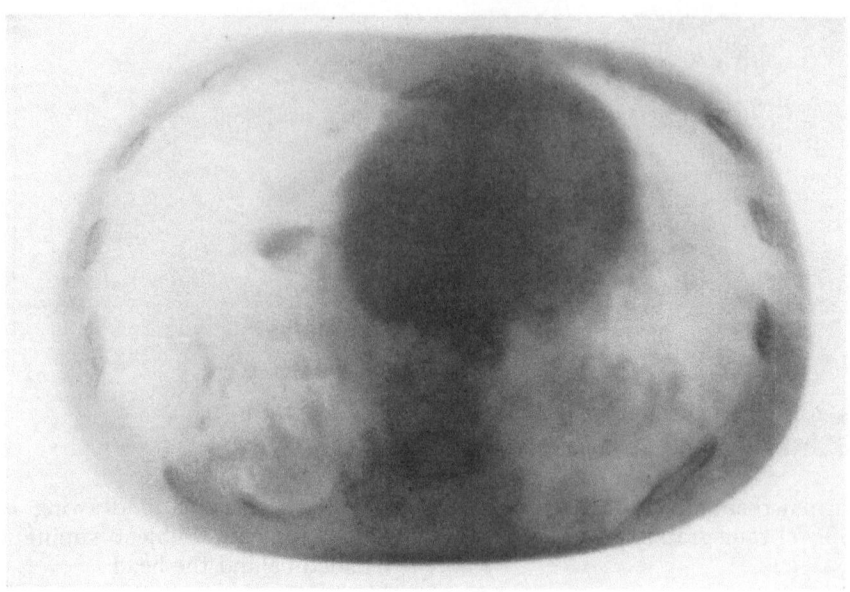

Fig. 243. Axial transverse tomogram

Costa VIII   Costa VII   Costa VI   Diaphragma   Corpus sterni   Cor   Pulmo sinister

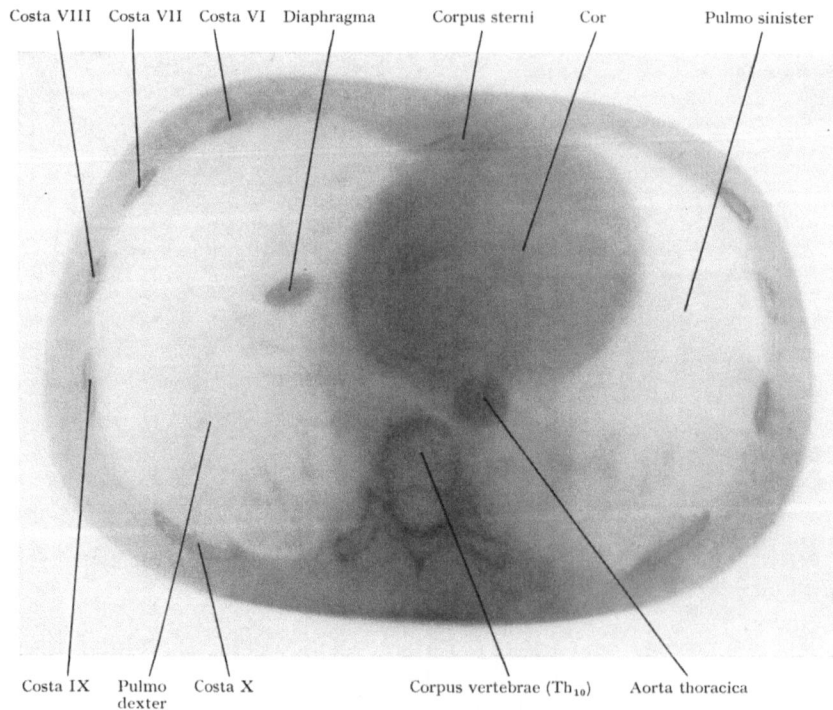

Costa IX   Pulmo   Costa X   Corpus vertebrae (Th$_{10}$)   Aorta thoracica
           dexter

Fig. 244. Interpretation

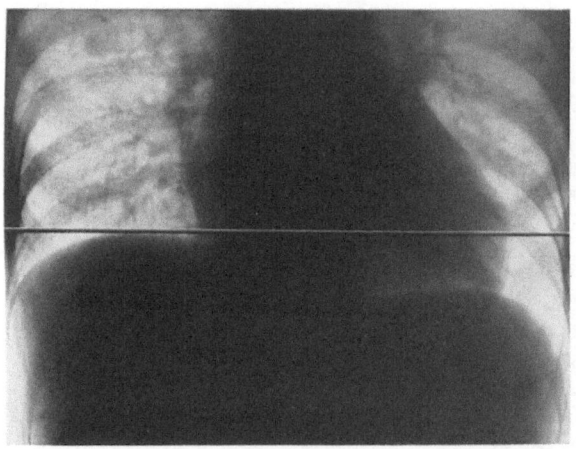

Fig. 245. Normal roentgenogram. Horizontal line showing the level tomographed

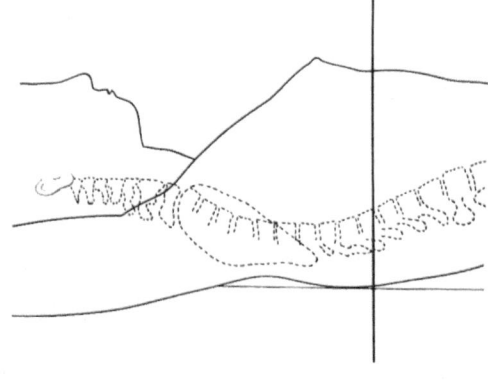

Fig. 246. Schematic drawing of the level tomographed. Subject supine with hands folded behind the head

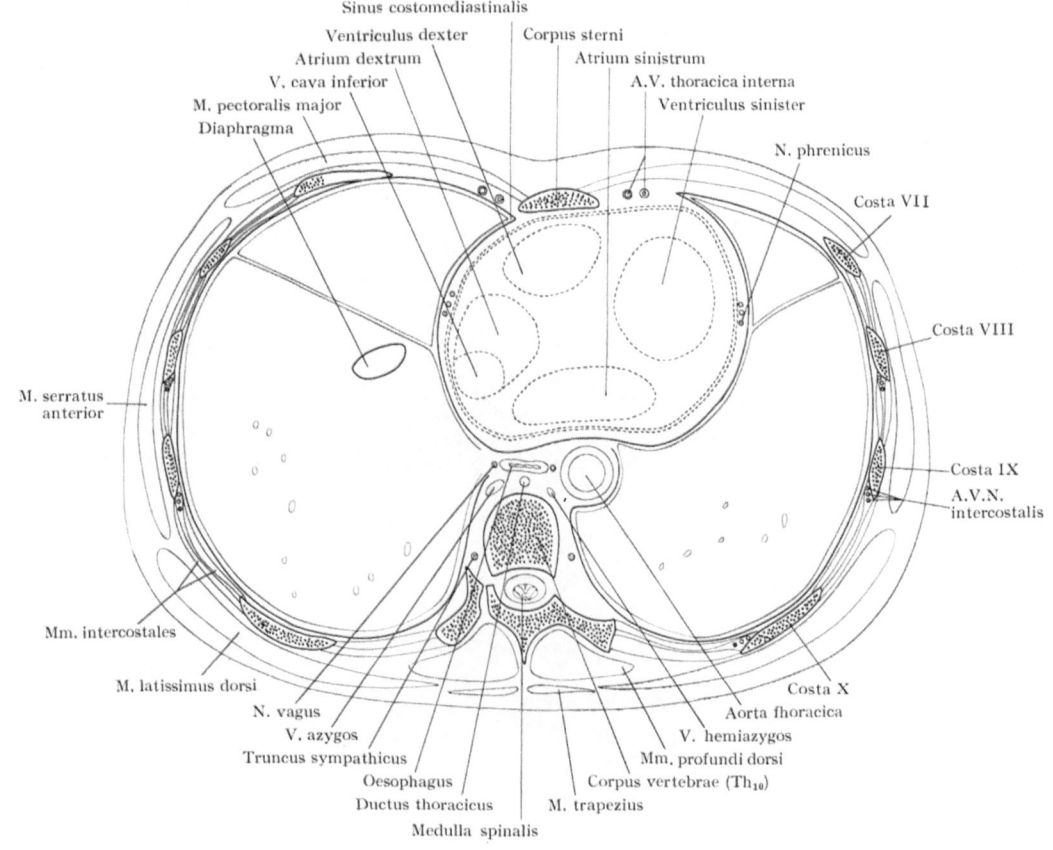

Fig. 247. Anatomical chart

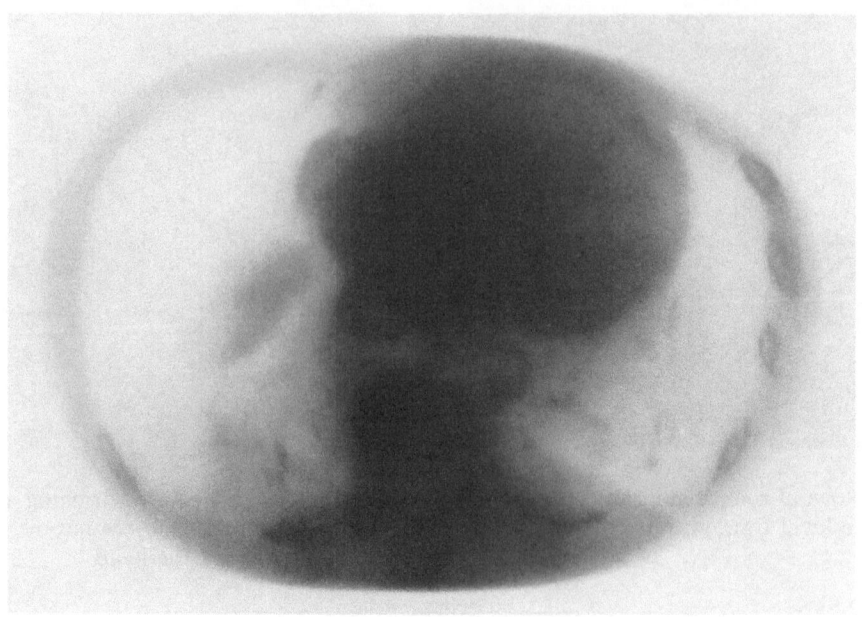

Fig. 248. Axial transverse tomogram

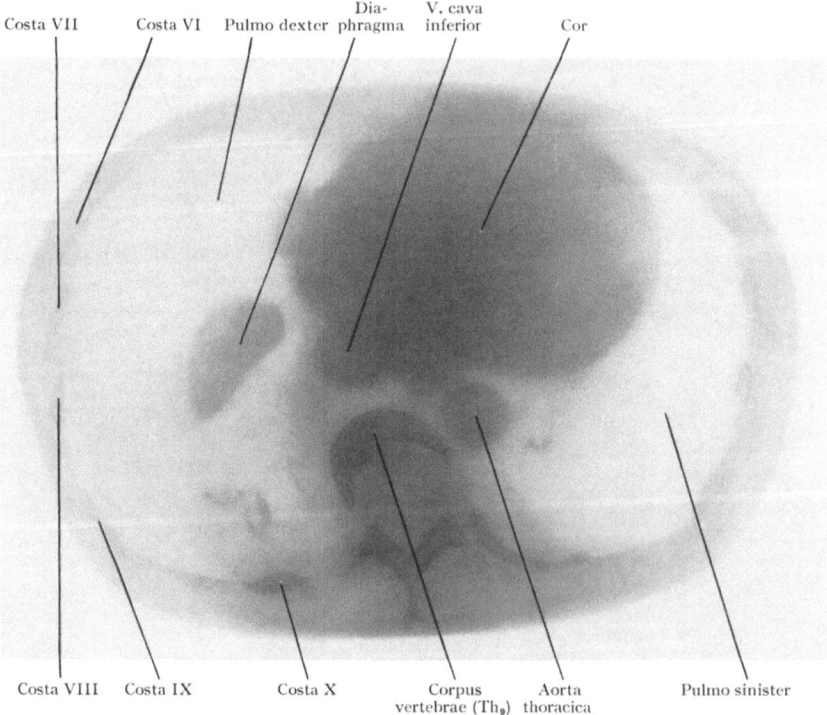

Fig. 249. Interpretation

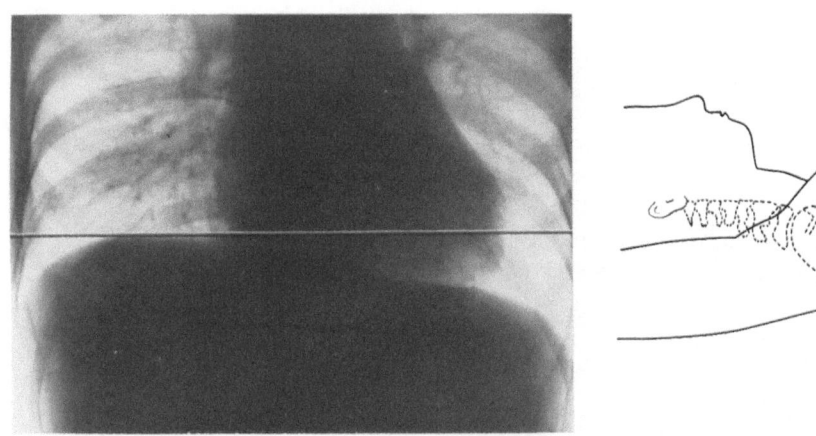

Fig. 250. Normal roentgenogram. Horizontal line showing the level tomographed

Fig. 251. Schematic drawing of the level tomographed. Subject supine with hands folded behind the head

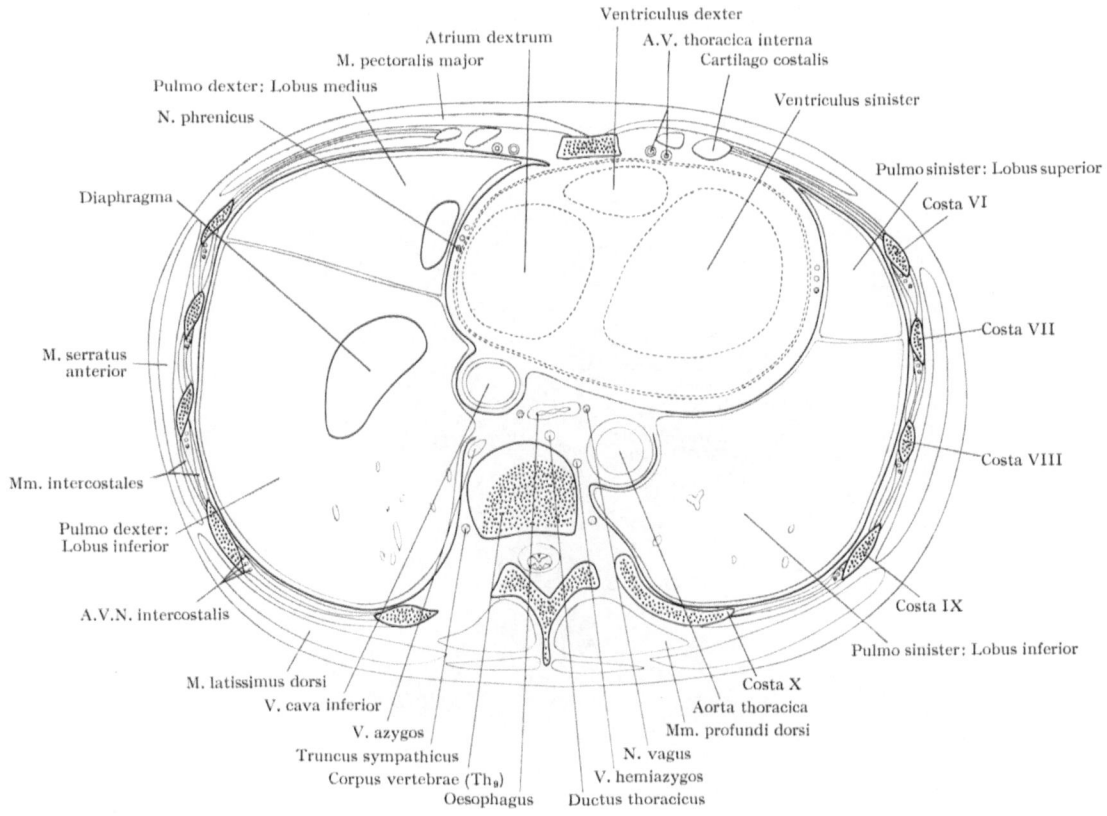

Fig. 252. Anatomical chart

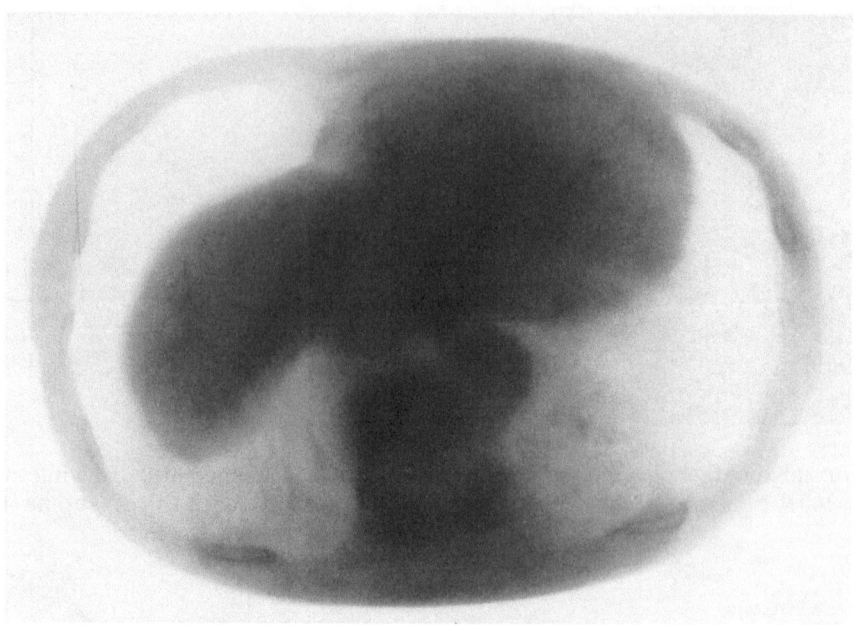

Fig. 253. Axial transverse tomogram

Costa VII   Costa VI   Pulmo dexter   Diaphragma   V. cava inferior   Cor

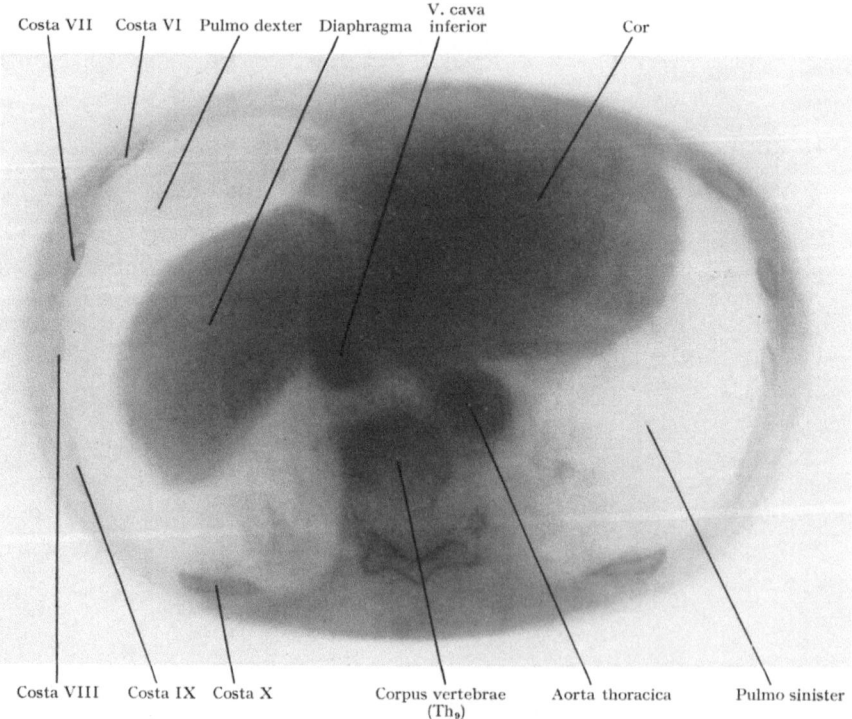

Costa VIII   Costa IX   Costa X   Corpus vertebrae (Th$_9$)   Aorta thoracica   Pulmo sinister

Fig. 254. Interpretation

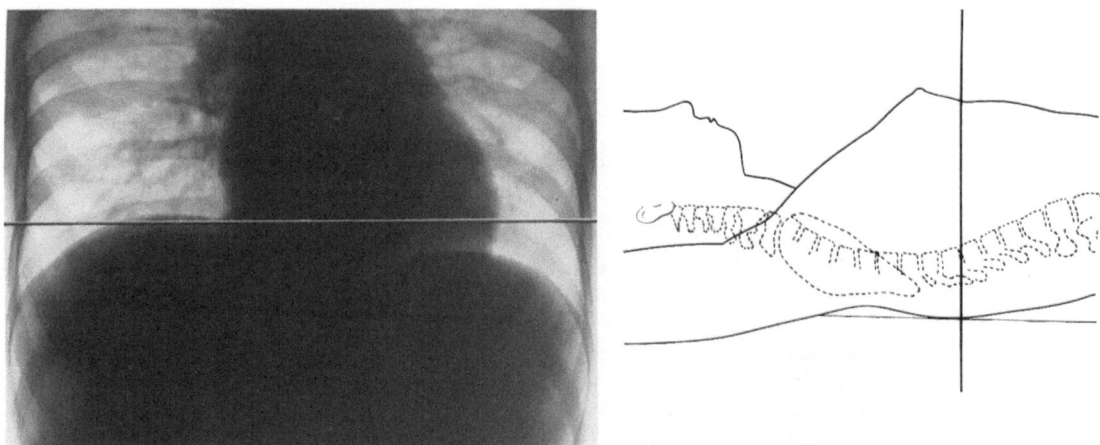

Fig. 255. Normal roentgenogram. Horizontal line showing the level tomographed

Fig. 256. Schematic drawing of the level tomographed. Subject supine with hands folded behind the head

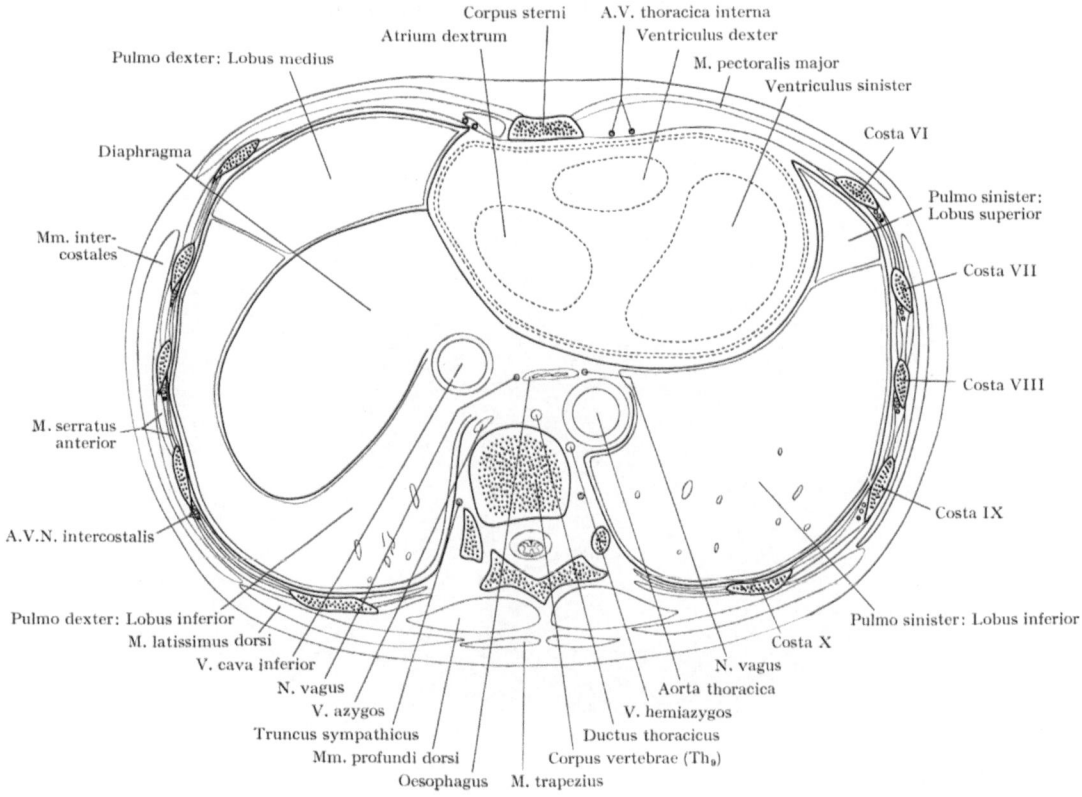

Fig. 257. Anatomical chart

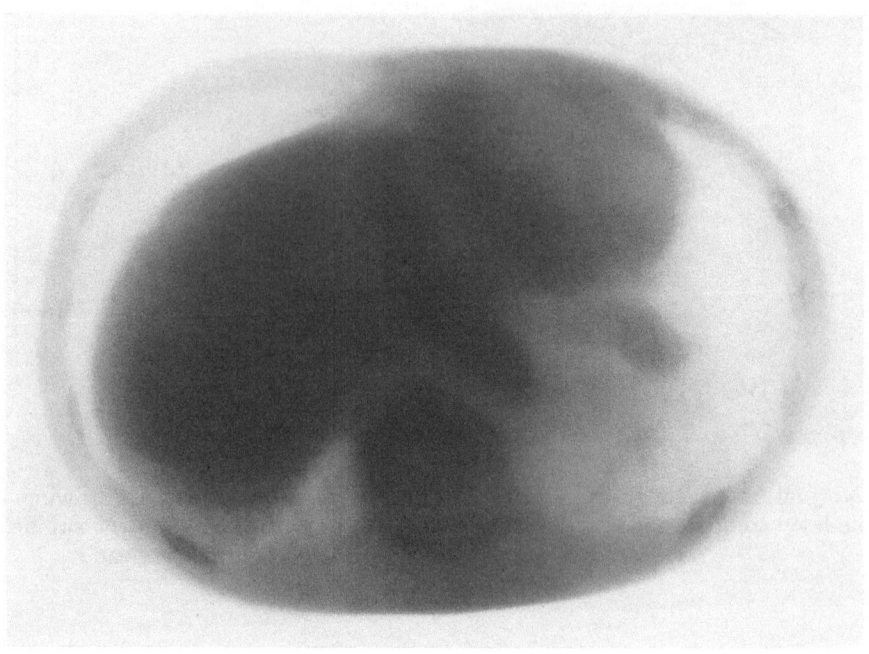

Fig. 258. Axial transverse tomogram

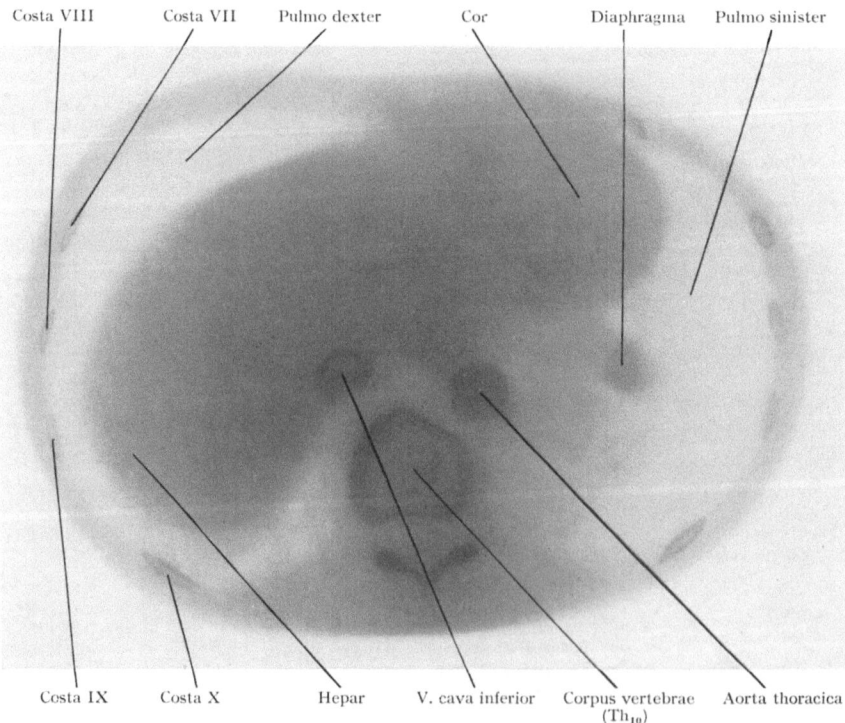

Costa VIII   Costa VII   Pulmo dexter   Cor   Diaphragma   Pulmo sinister

Costa IX   Costa X   Hepar   V. cava inferior   Corpus vertebrae (Th$_{10}$)   Aorta thoracica

Fig. 259. Interpretation

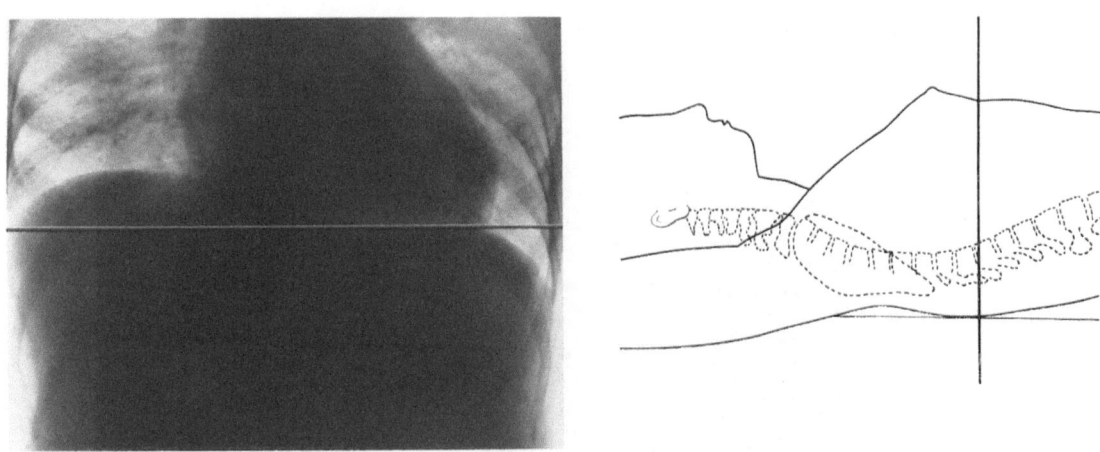

Fig. 260. Normal roentgenogram. Horizontal line showing the level tomographed

Fig. 261. Schematic drawing of the level tomographed. Subject supine with hands folded behind the head

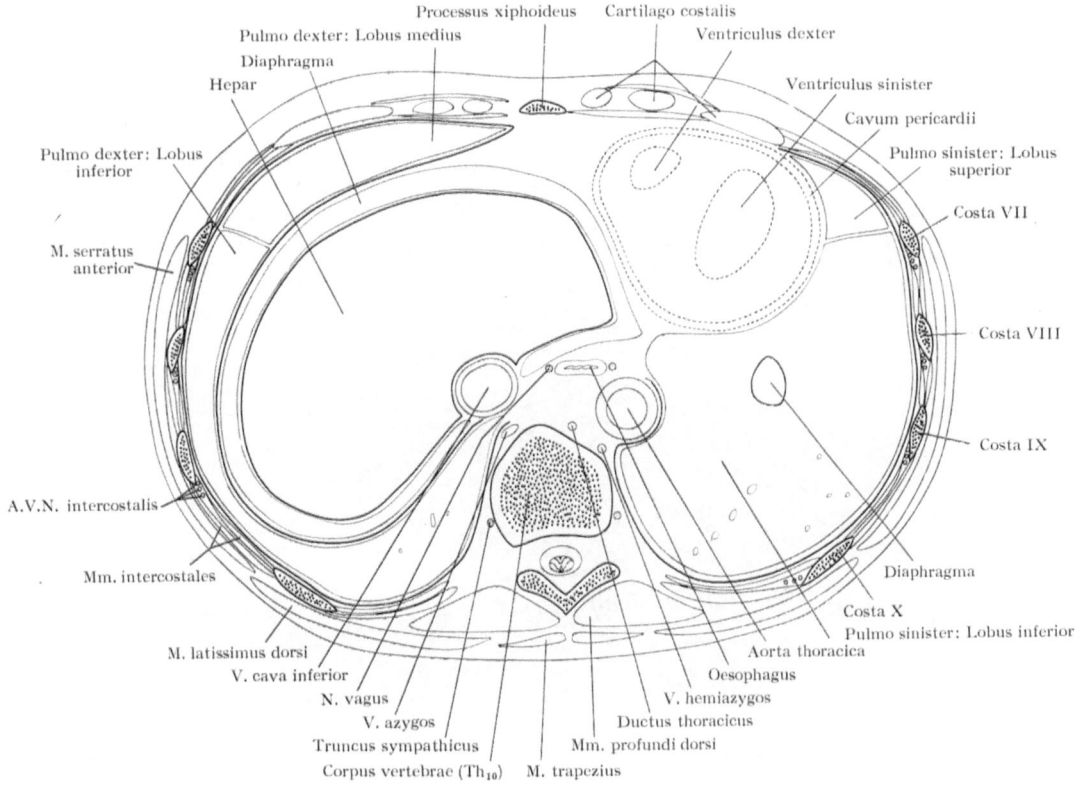

Fig. 262. Anatomical chart

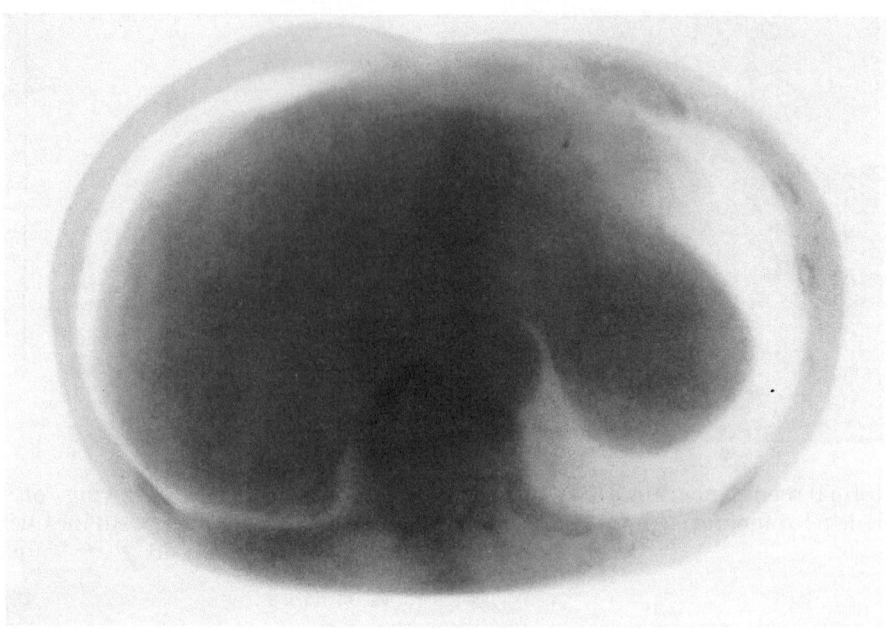

Fig. 263. Axial transverse tomogram

Costa VIII Costa VII Pulmo dexter Cor Pulmo sinister

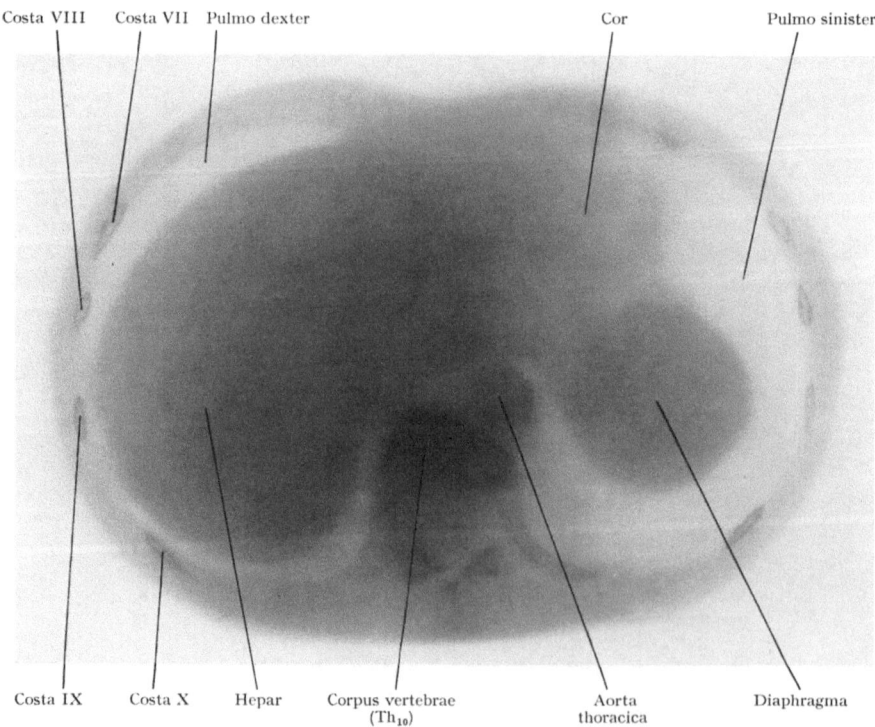

Costa IX Costa X Hepar Corpus vertebrae (Th$_{10}$) Aorta thoracica Diaphragma

Fig. 264. Interpretation

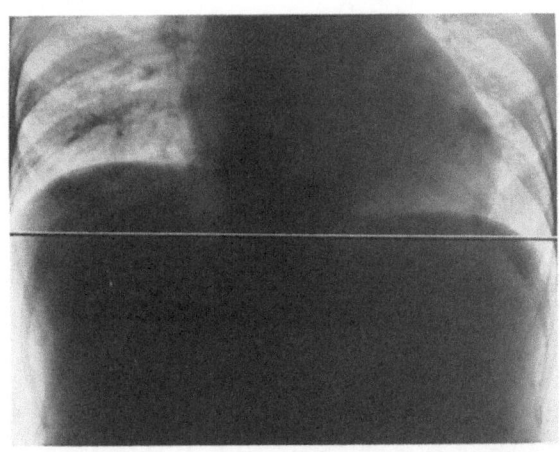

Fig. 265. Normal roentgenogram. Horizontal line showing the level tomographed

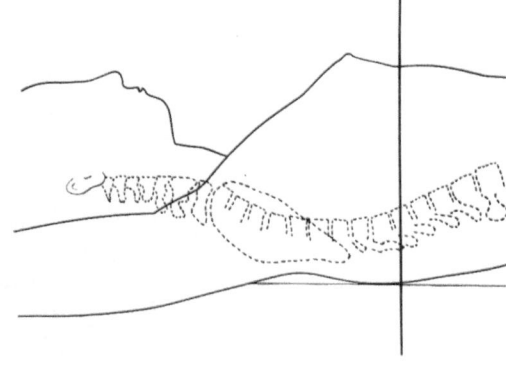

Fig. 266. Schematic drawing of the level tomographed. Subject supine with hands folded behind the head

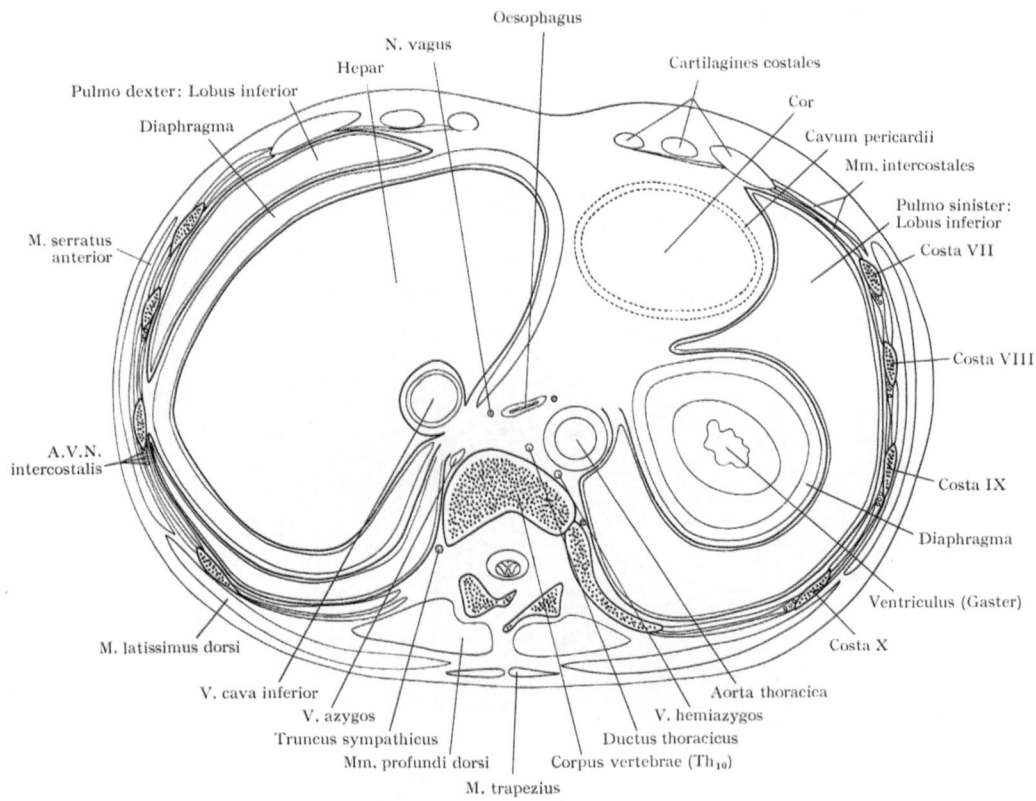

Fig. 267. Anatomical chart

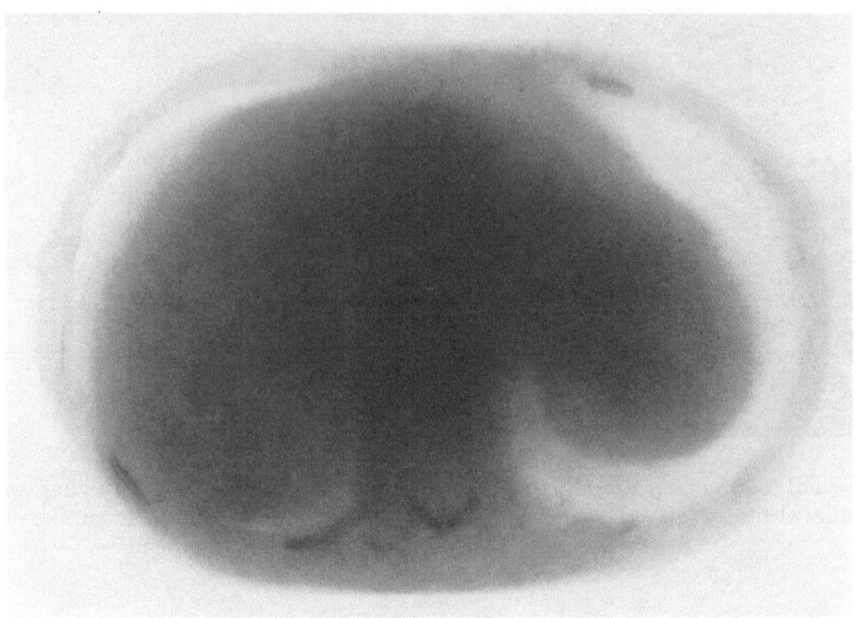

Fig. 268. Axial transverse tomogram

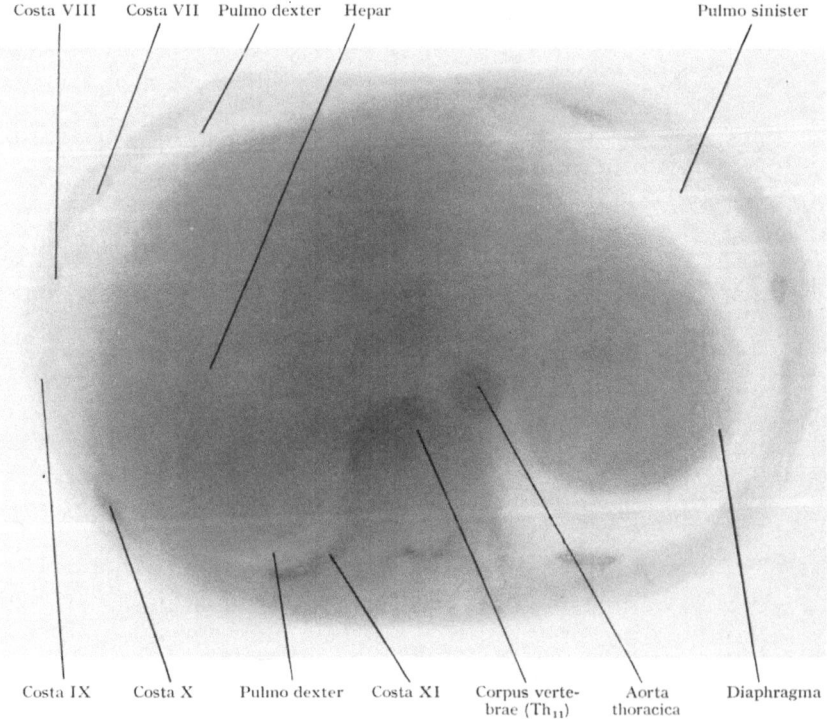

Costa VIII   Costa VII   Pulmo dexter   Hepar   Pulmo sinister

Costa IX   Costa X   Pulmo dexter   Costa XI   Corpus verte-   Aorta   Diaphragma
                                                    brae (Th$_{11}$)   thoracica

Fig. 269. Interpretation

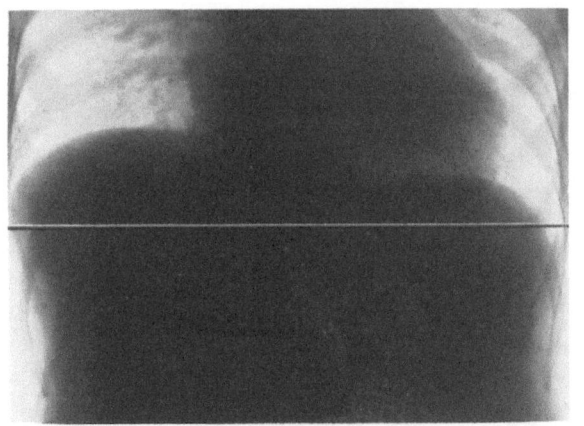

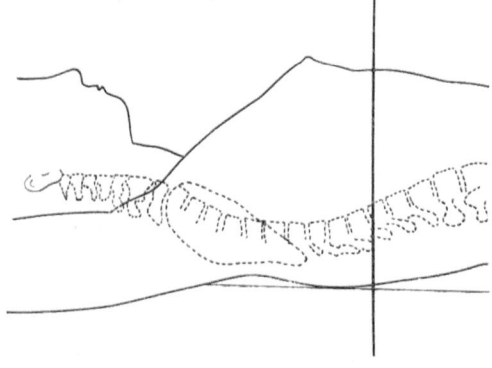

Fig. 270. Normal roentgenogram. Horizontal line showing the level tomographed

Fig. 271. Schematic drawing of the level tomographed. Subject supine with hands folded behind the head

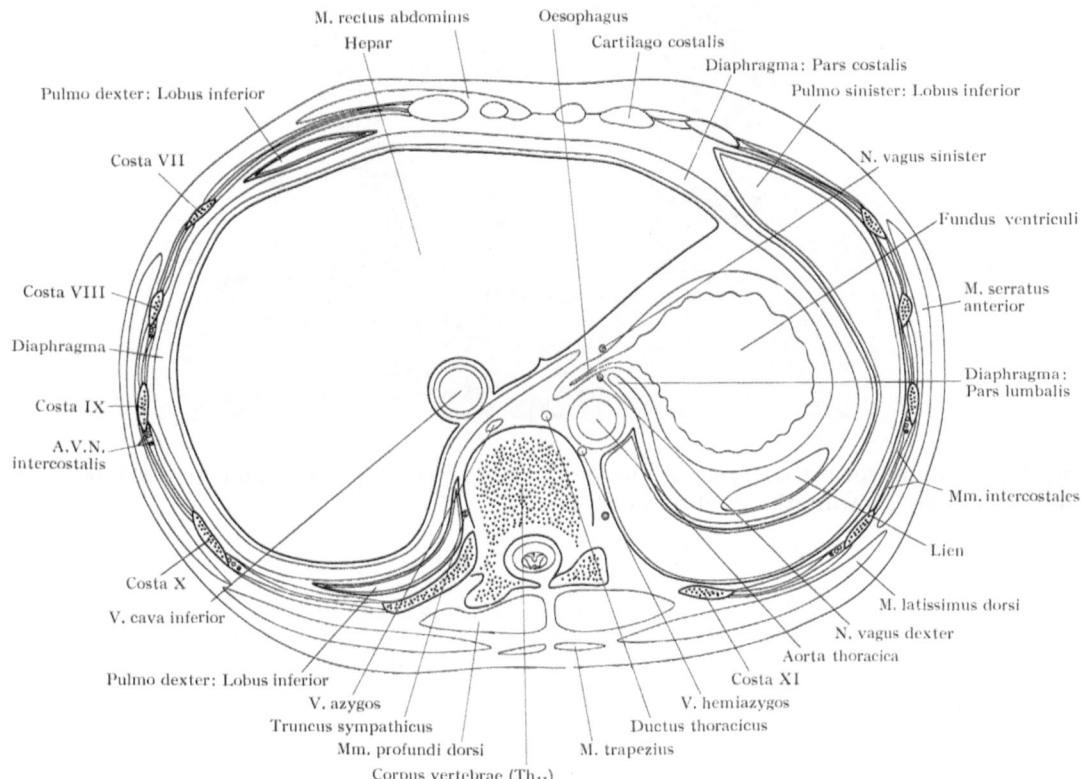

Fig. 272. Anatomical chart

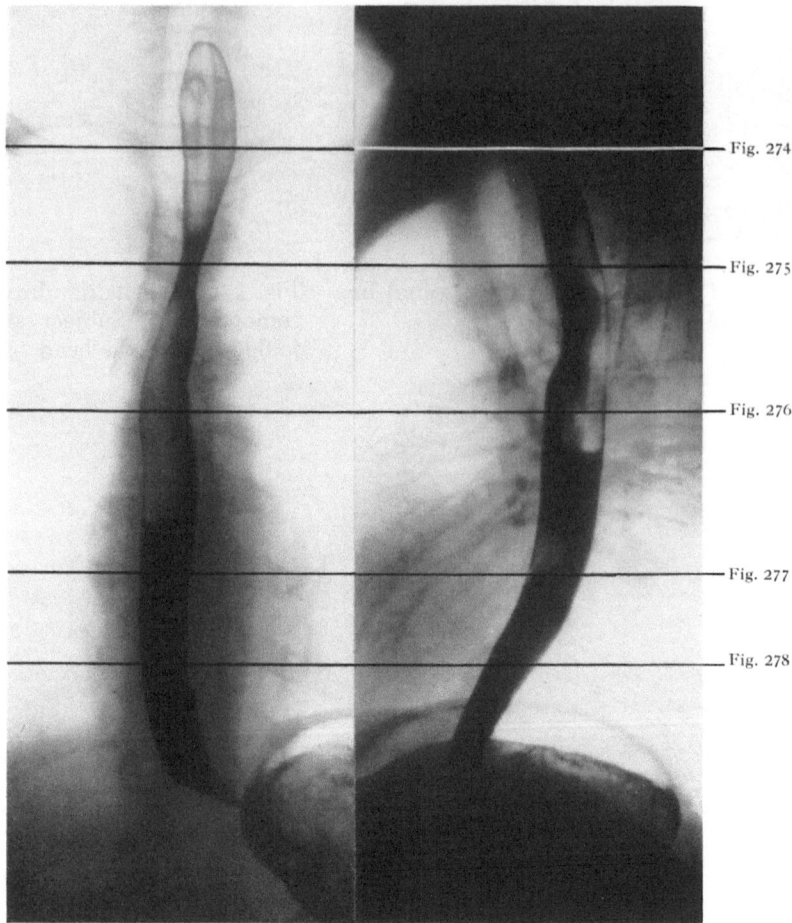

Fig. 274

Fig. 275

Fig. 276

Fig. 277

Fig. 278

Fig. 273. Normal roentgenograms of the esophagus in the a.p. view and in the lateral view. Horizontal lines showing the level tomographed

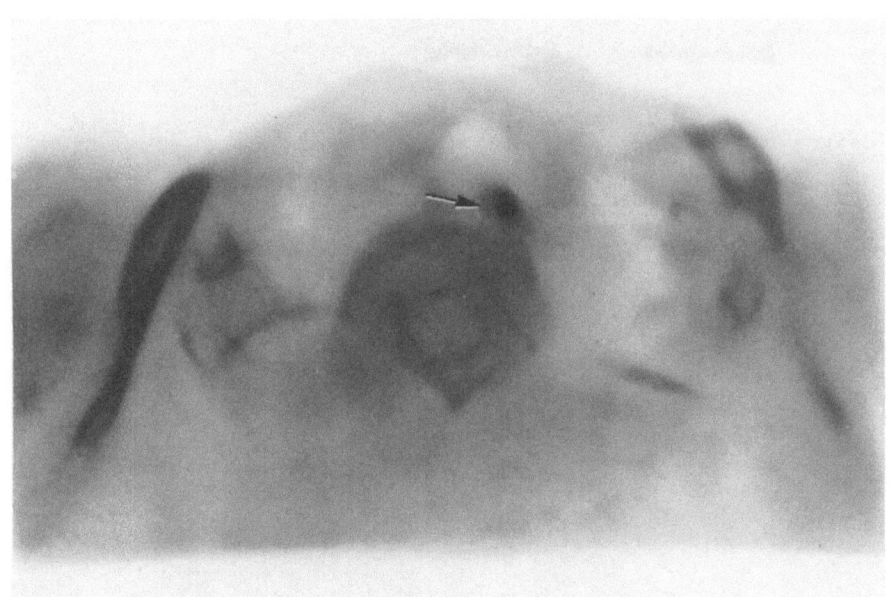

Fig. 274. Axial transverse tomogram of the esophagus (↗) (see Figs. 158—162)

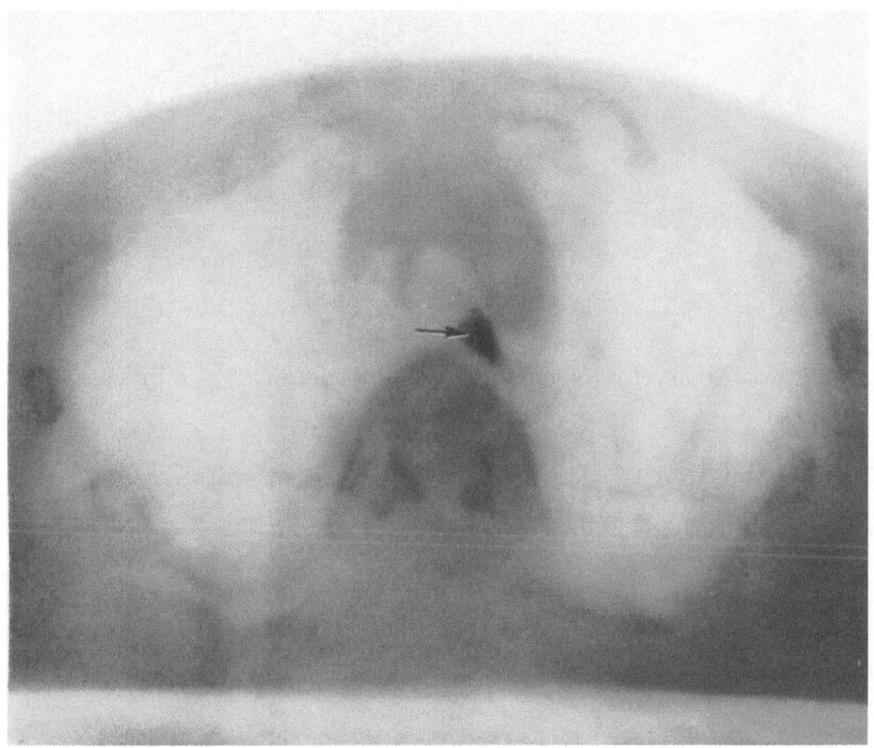

Fig. 275. Axial transverse tomogram of the esophagus (↗) (see Figs. 178—182)

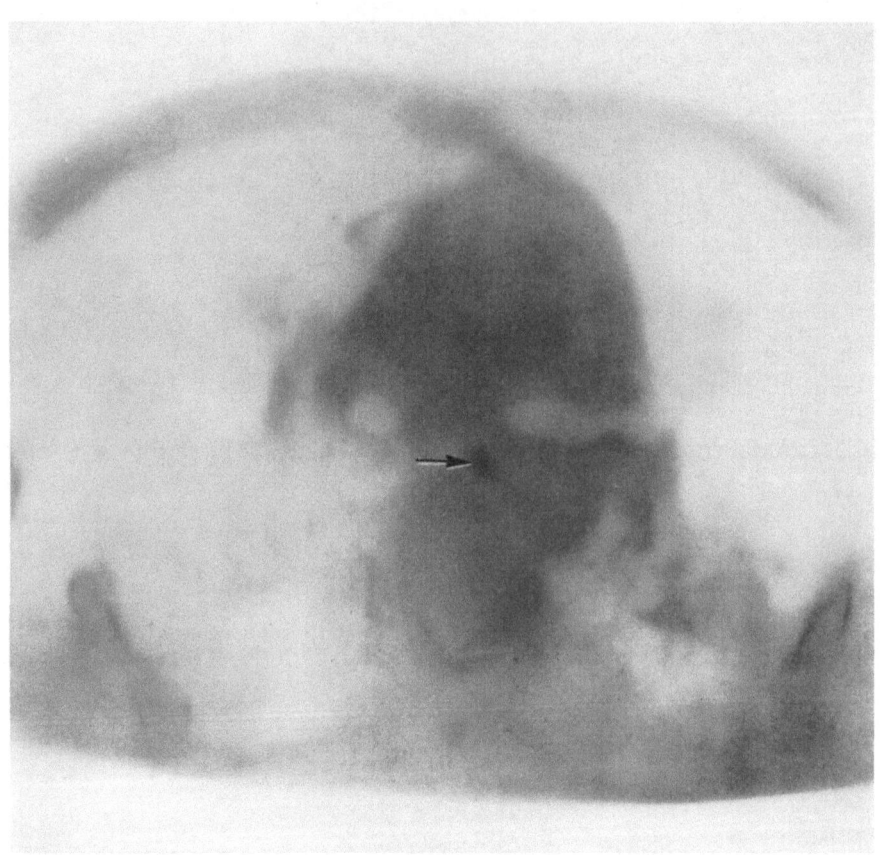

Fig. 276. Axial transverse tomogram of the esophagus (↗) (see Figs. 218—222)

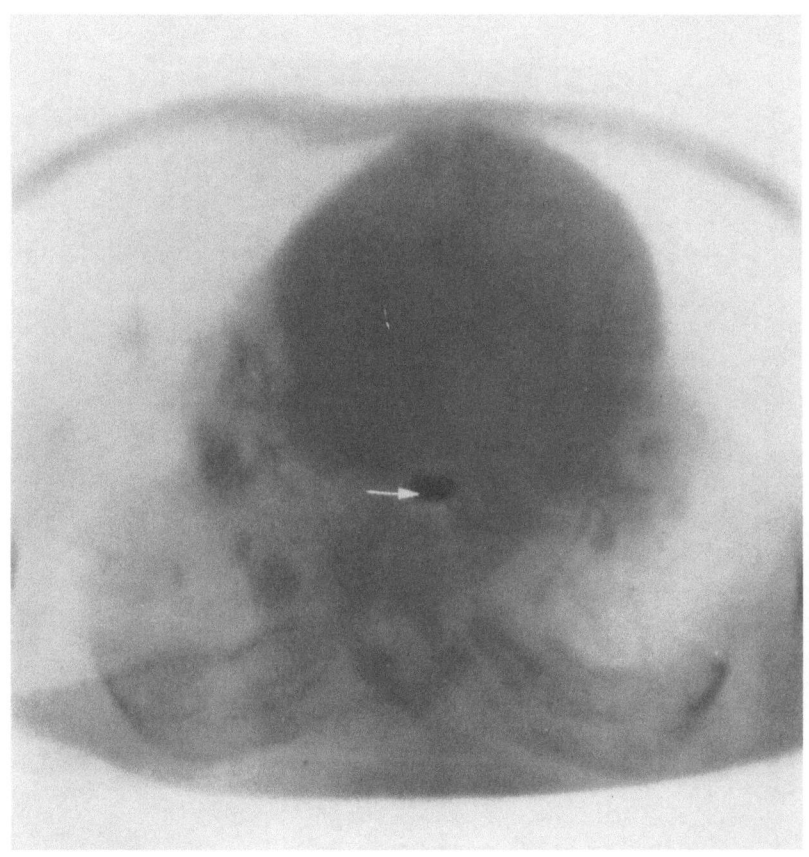

Fig. 277. Axial transverse tomogram of the esophagus (↗) (see Figs. 228—232)

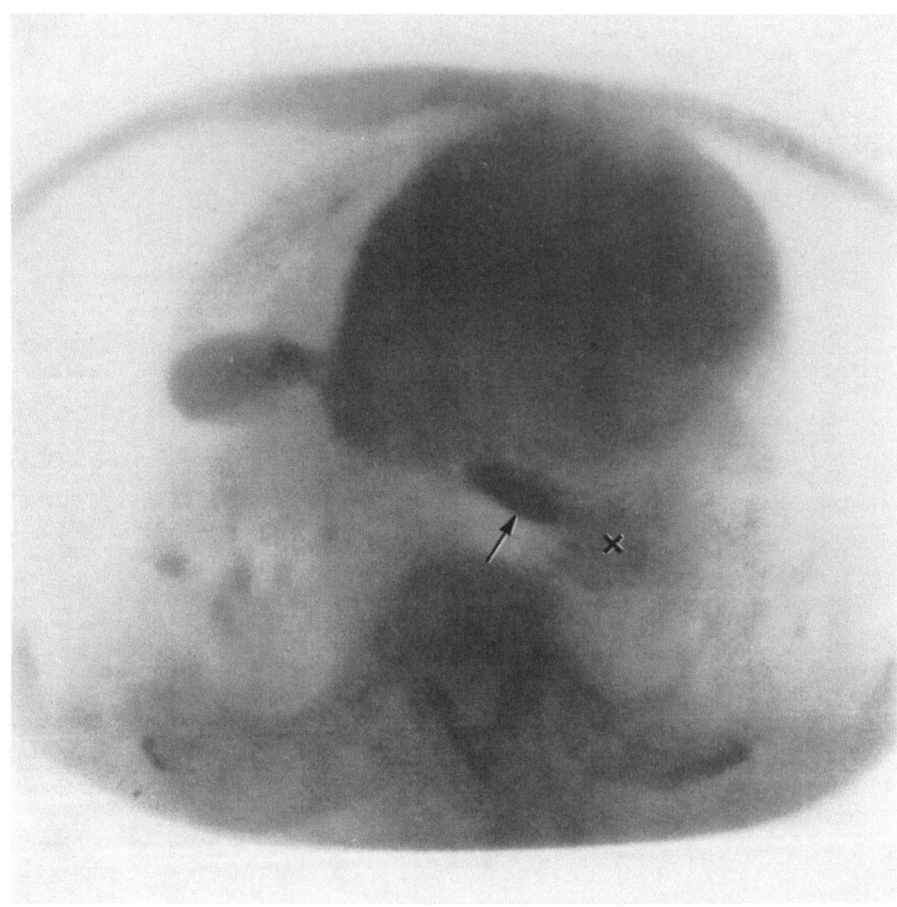

Fig. 278. Axial transverse tomogram of the esophagus (╱) (see Figs. 243—247). Thoracic aorta (✕)

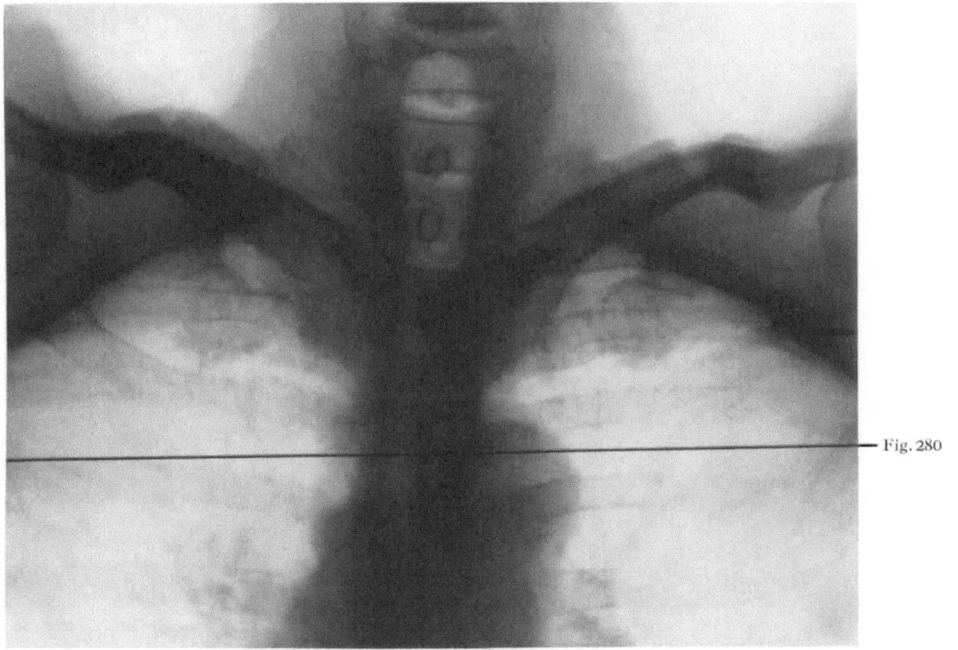

Fig. 280

Fig. 279. Normal roentgenogram of the thoracic duct. Horizontal line showing the level tomographed

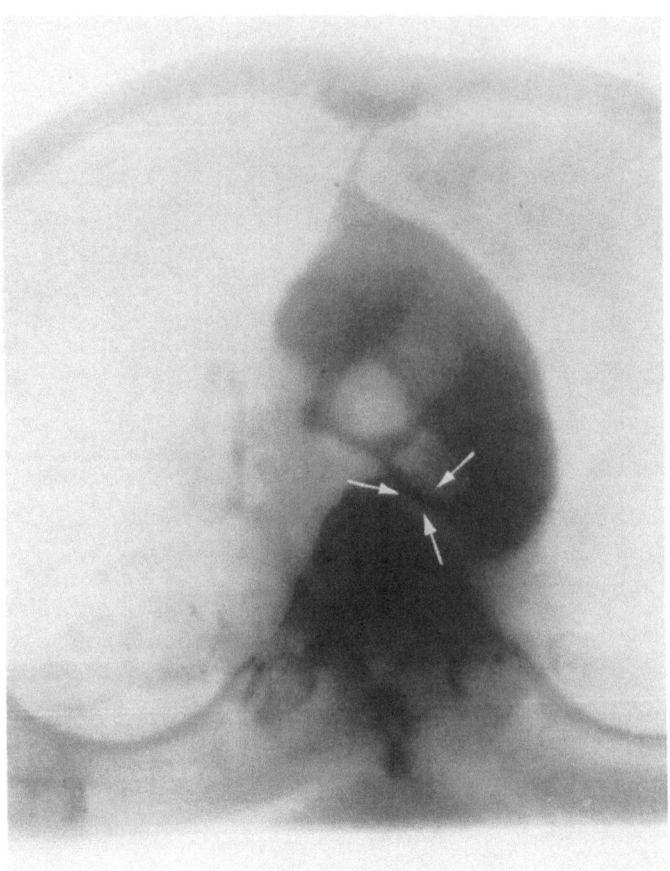

Fig. 280. Axial transverse tomogram of the thoracic duct (↗) (see Figs. 188—192)

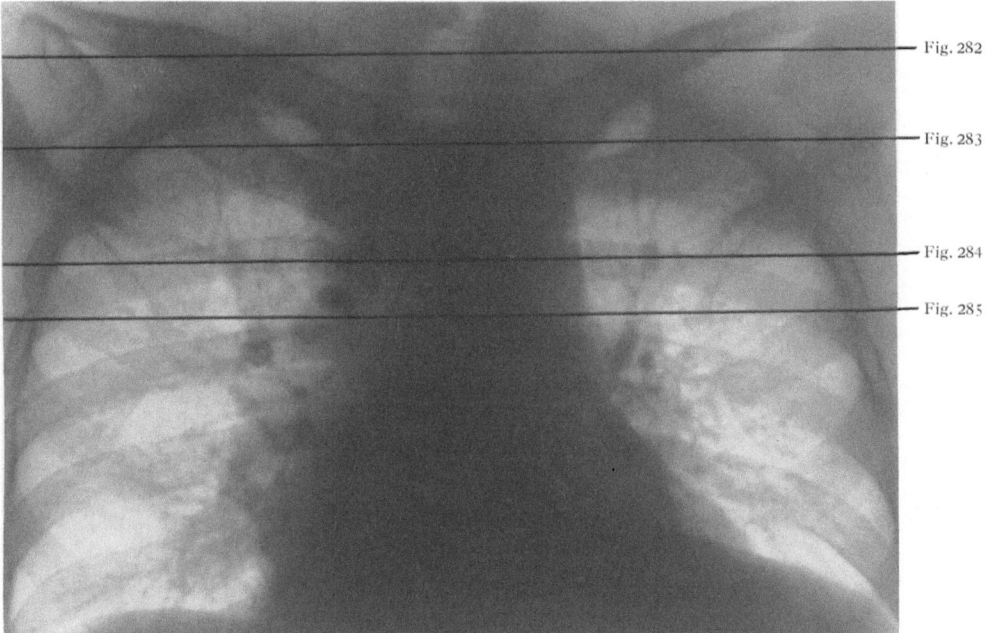

Fig. 282

Fig. 283

Fig. 284

Fig. 285

Fig. 281. Normal roentgenogram of the intrathoracic lymph nodes. Horizontal lines showing the level tomographed

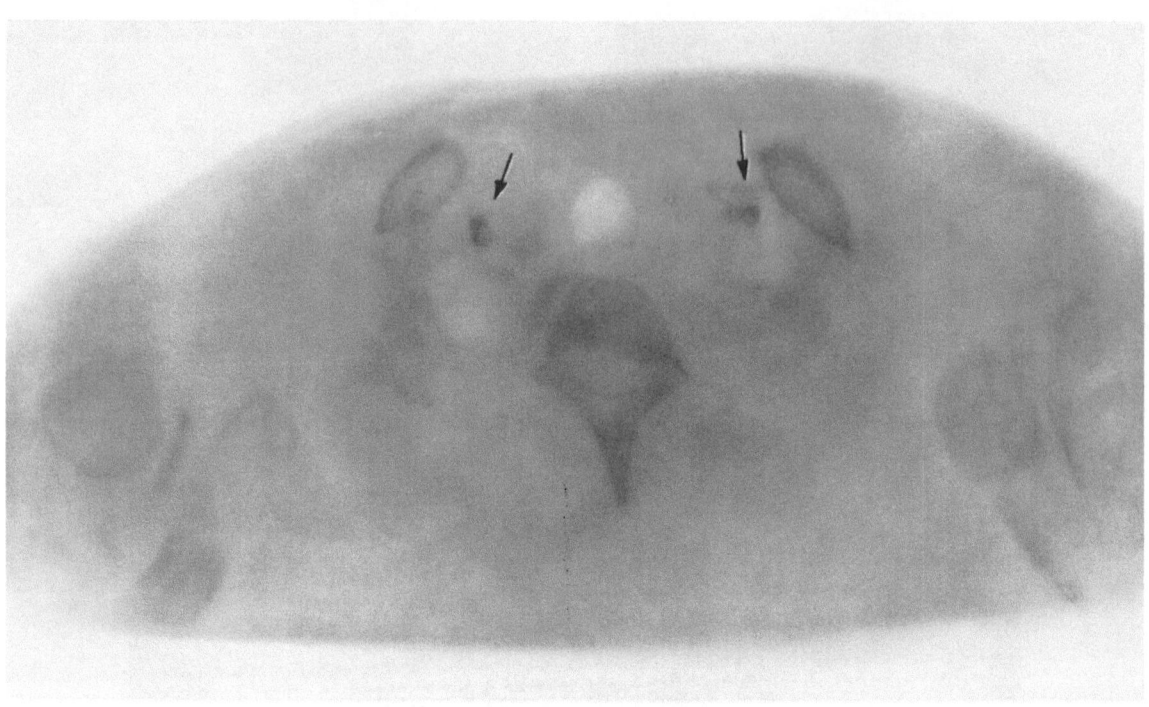

Fig. 282. Axial transverse tomogram of the infraclavicular lymph nodes (⟋) (see Figs. 158—162)

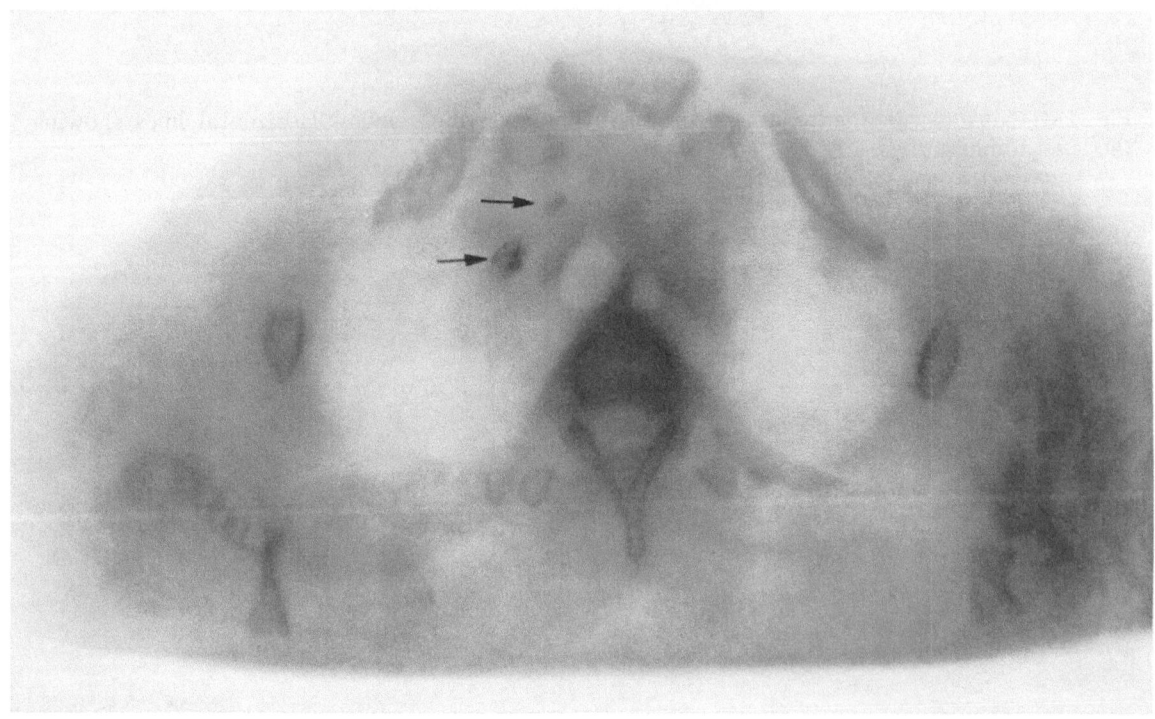

Fig. 283. Axial transverse tomogram of the tracheal lymph nodes (⟋) (see Figs. 173—177)

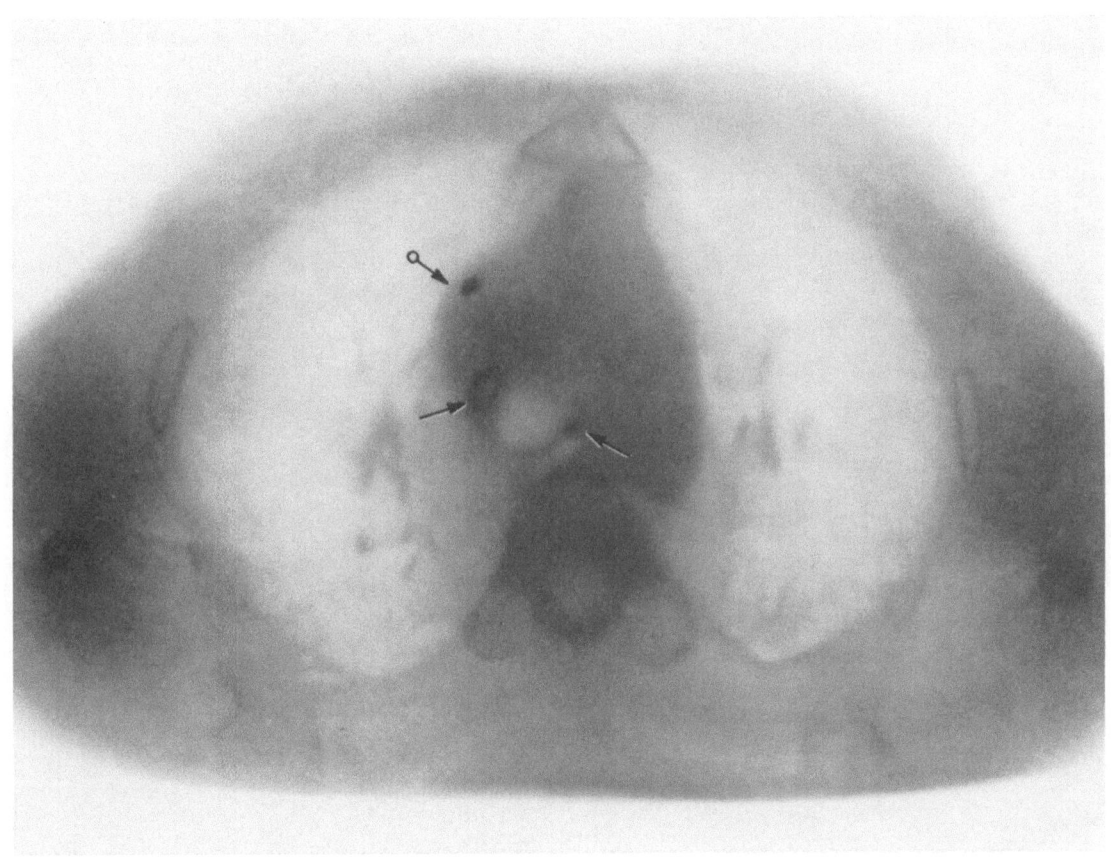

Fig. 284. Axial transverse tomogram of the tracheal lymph nodes (⟋) and anterior mediastinal lymph nodes (⟋) (see Figs. 193—222)

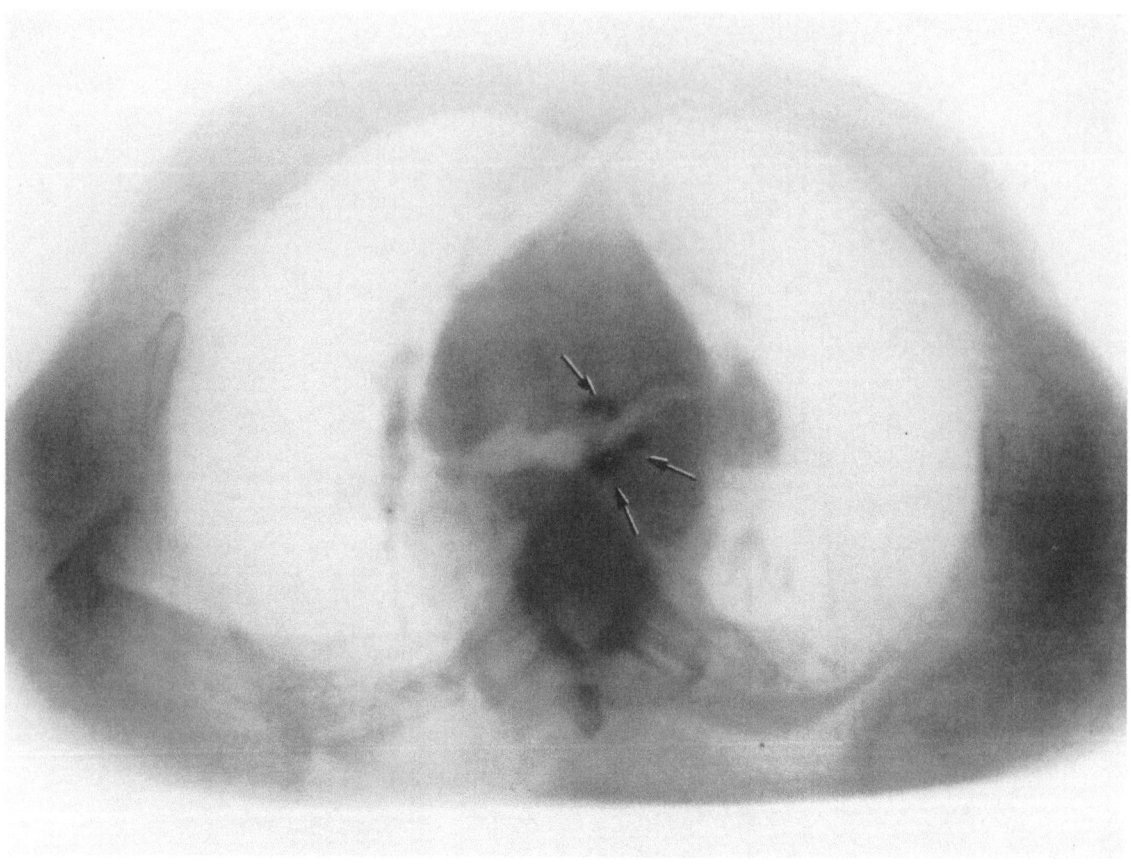

Fig. 285. Axial transverse tomogram of the superior tracheobronchial lymph nodes (↗) (see Figs. 213—217)

Upper Abdomen

Seventeen axial transverse tomograms of the subject with air insufflated into the retroperitoneal space.

Appendices:
1. Axial transverse tomograms of the duodenal loop with duodenal tube introduced.
2. Axial transverse tomogram of the stomach, the duodenum, the gall bladder and the renal pelvis.

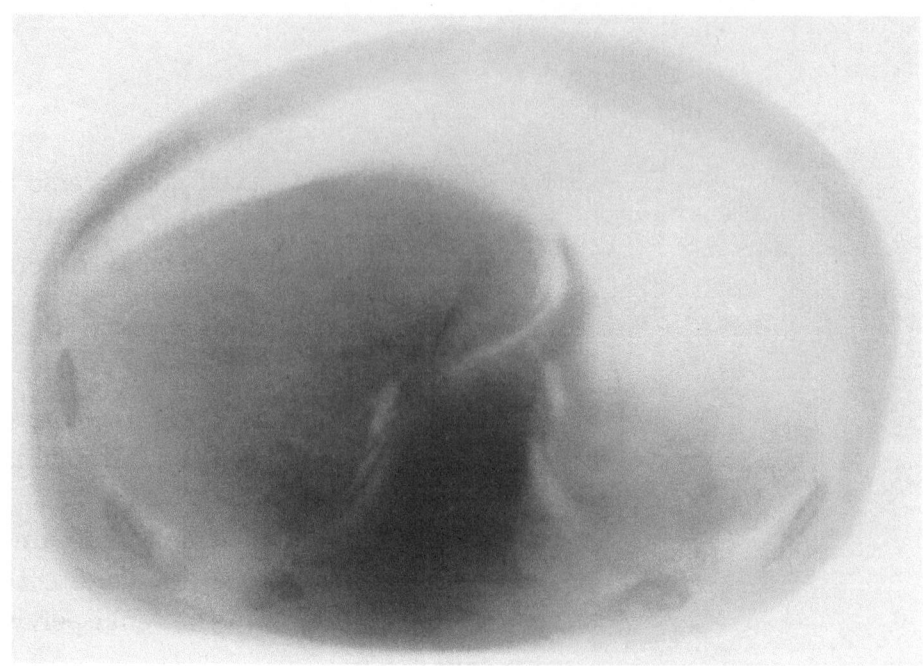

Fig. 286. Axial transverse tomogram

Costa   Hepar   Aer   Aorta thoracica   Ventriculus   Flexura coli sinistra

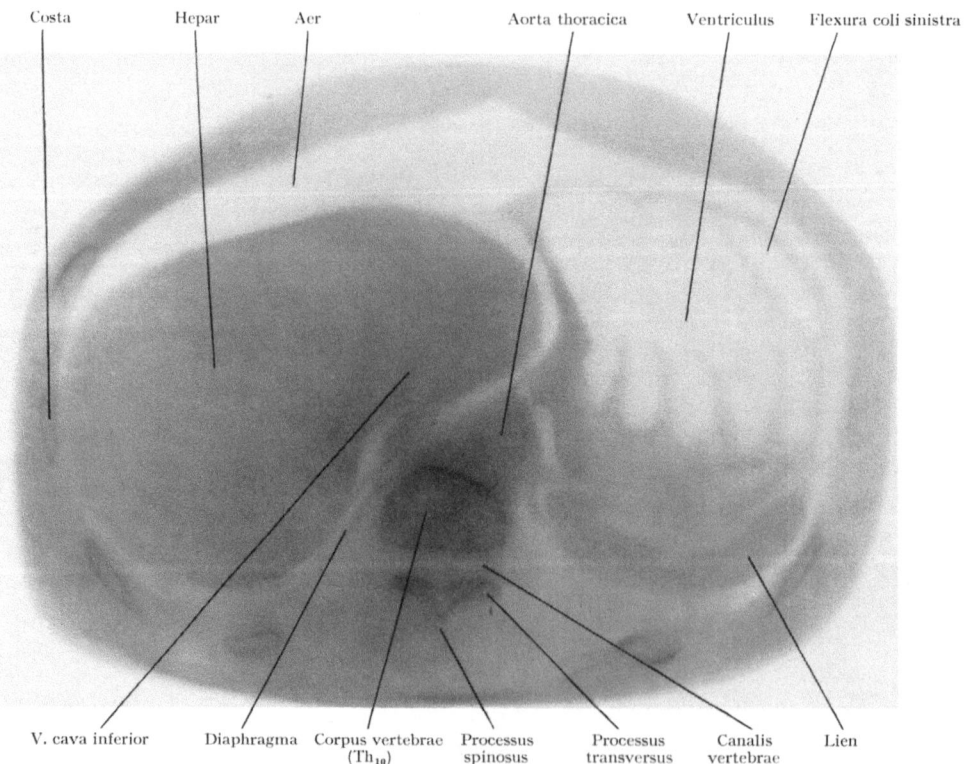

V. cava inferior   Diaphragma   Corpus vertebrae   Processus   Processus   Canalis   Lien
                                     (Th₁₀)   spinosus   transversus   vertebrae

Fig. 287. Interpretation

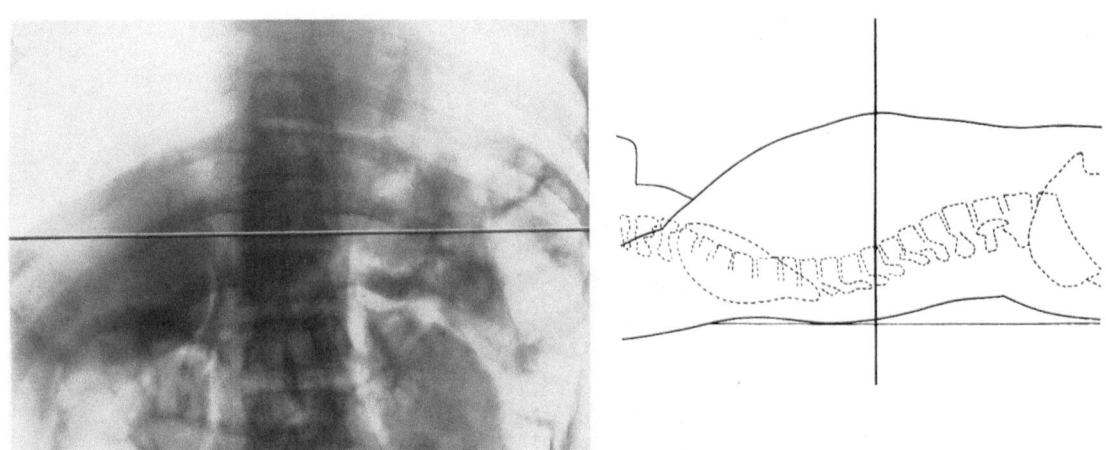

Fig. 288. Normal roentgenogram. Horizontal line showing the level tomographed

Fig. 289. Schematic drawing of the level tomographed

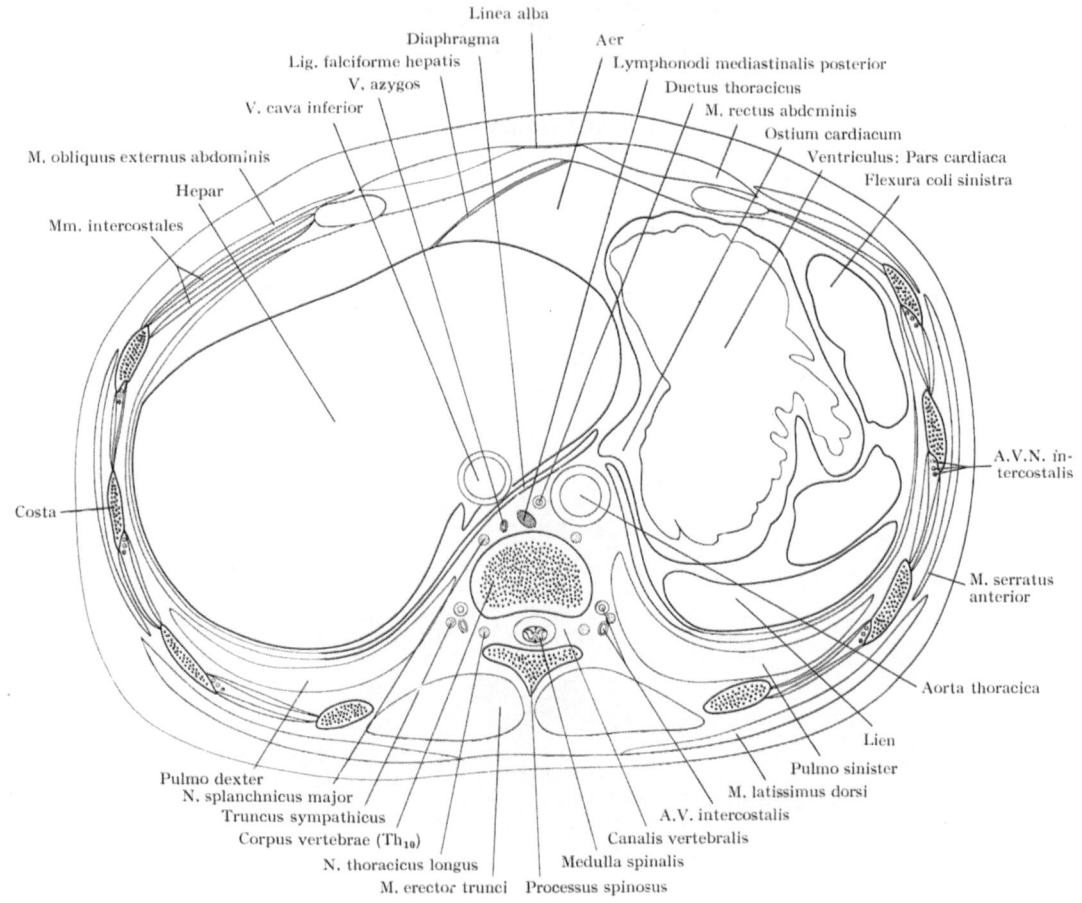

Linea alba
Diaphragma
Lig. falciforme hepatis
V. azygos
V. cava inferior
Aer
Lymphonodi mediastinalis posterior
Ductus thoracicus
M. rectus abdominis
Ostium cardiacum
M. obliquus externus abdominis
Ventriculus: Pars cardiaca
Flexura coli sinistra
Hepar
Mm. intercostales
A.V.N. intercostalis
Costa
M. serratus anterior
Aorta thoracica
Lien
Pulmo sinister
Pulmo dexter
M. latissimus dorsi
N. splanchnicus major
A.V. intercostalis
Truncus sympathicus
Canalis vertebralis
Corpus vertebrae (Th$_{10}$)
Medulla spinalis
N. thoracicus longus
Processus spinosus
M. erector trunci

Fig. 290. Anatomical chart

141

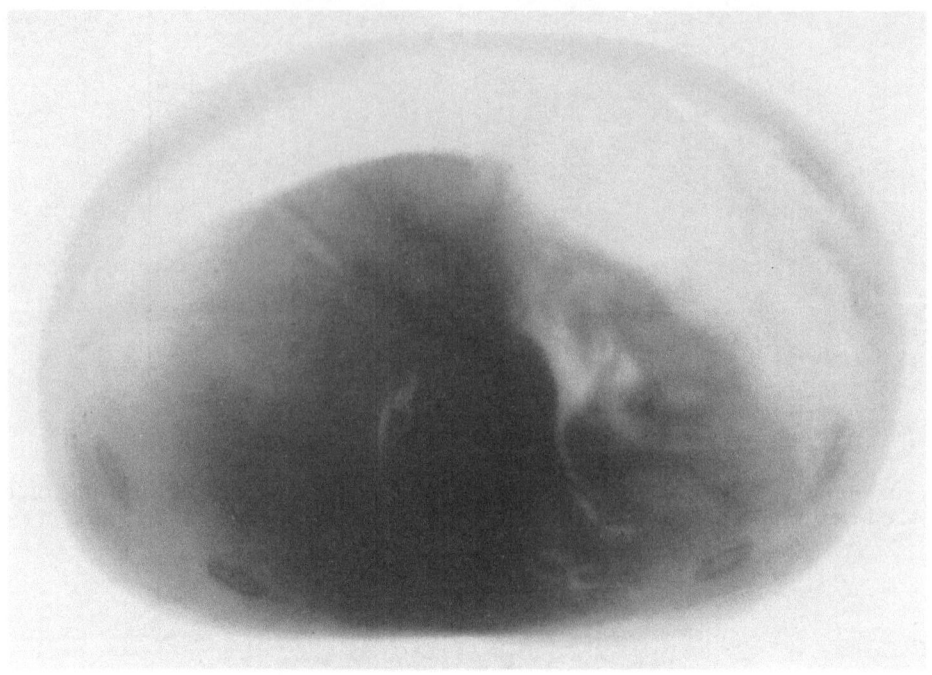

Fig. 291. Axial transverse tomogram

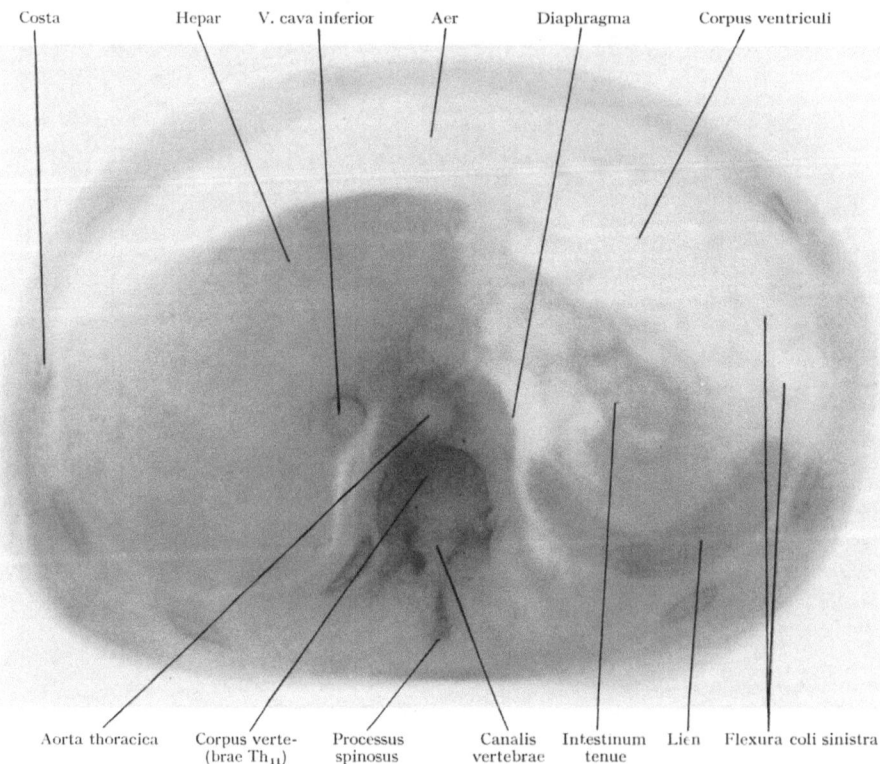

Costa   Hepar   V. cava inferior   Aer   Diaphragma   Corpus ventriculi

Aorta thoracica   Corpus verte-   Processus   Canalis   Intestinum   Lien   Flexura coli sinistra
              (brae Th$_{11}$)   spinosus   vertebrae   tenue

Fig. 292. Interpretation

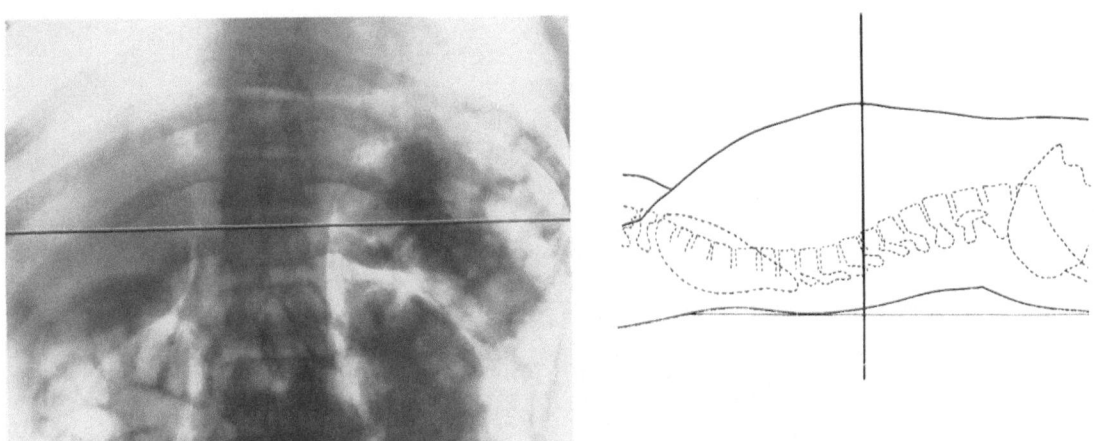

Fig. 293. Normal roentgenogram. Horizontal line showing the level tomographed

Fig. 294. Schematic drawing of the level tomographed

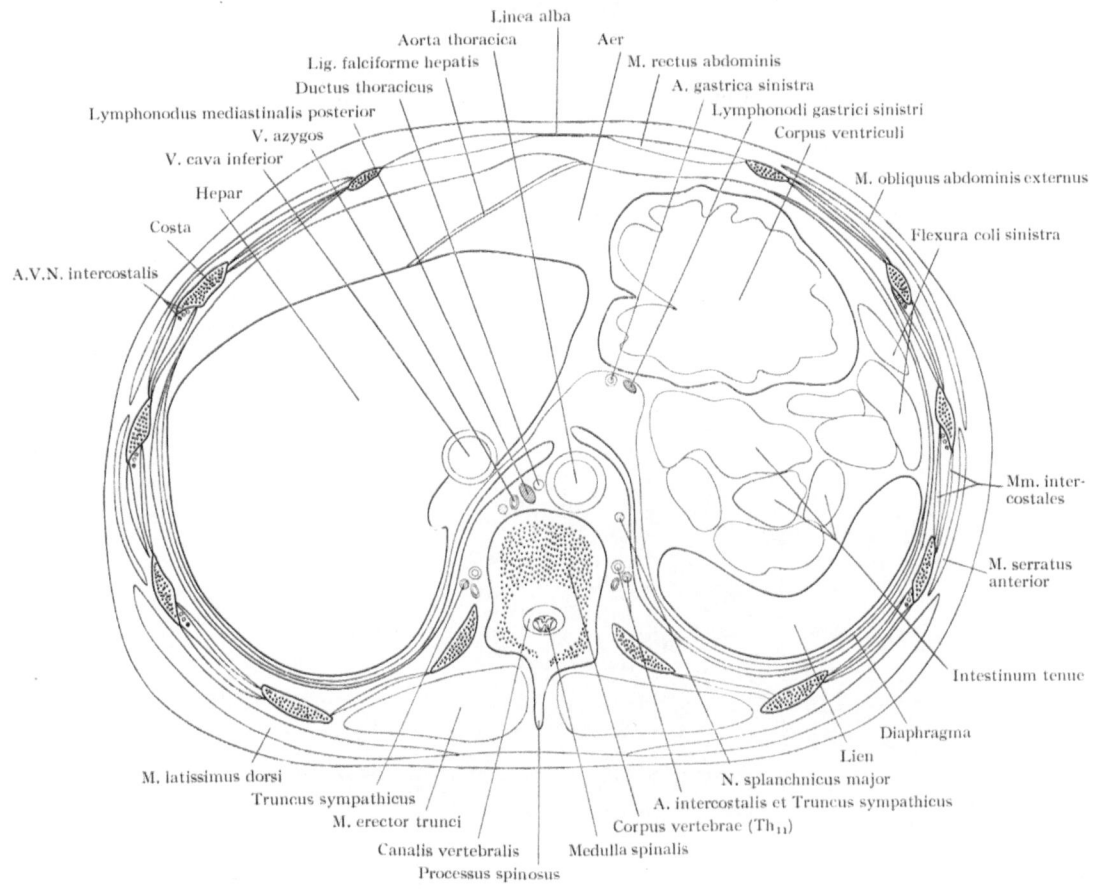

Fig. 295. Anatomical chart

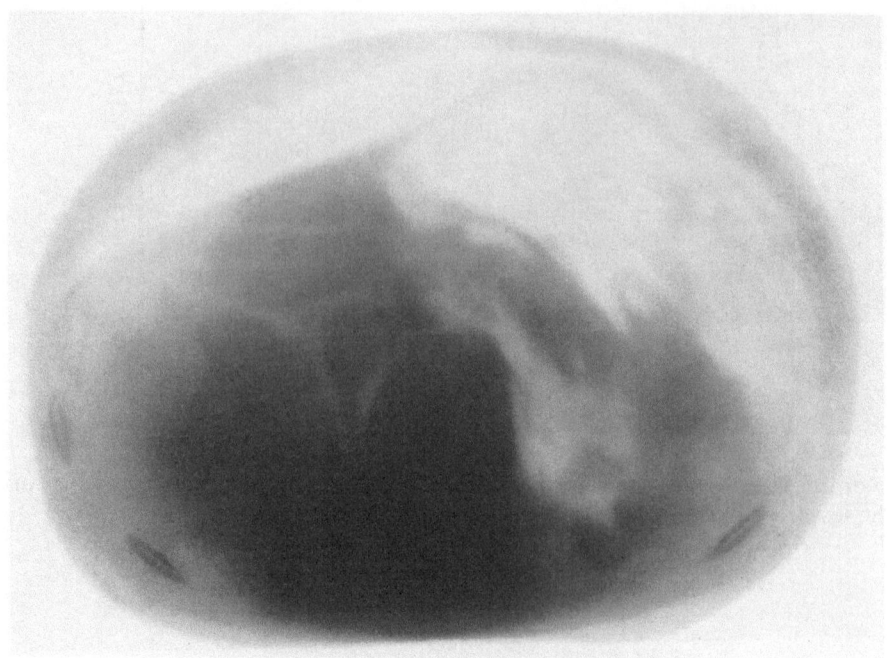

Fig. 296. Axial transverse tomogram

Hepar V. cava inferior Pancreas Aer Corpus ventriculi Flexura coli sinistra

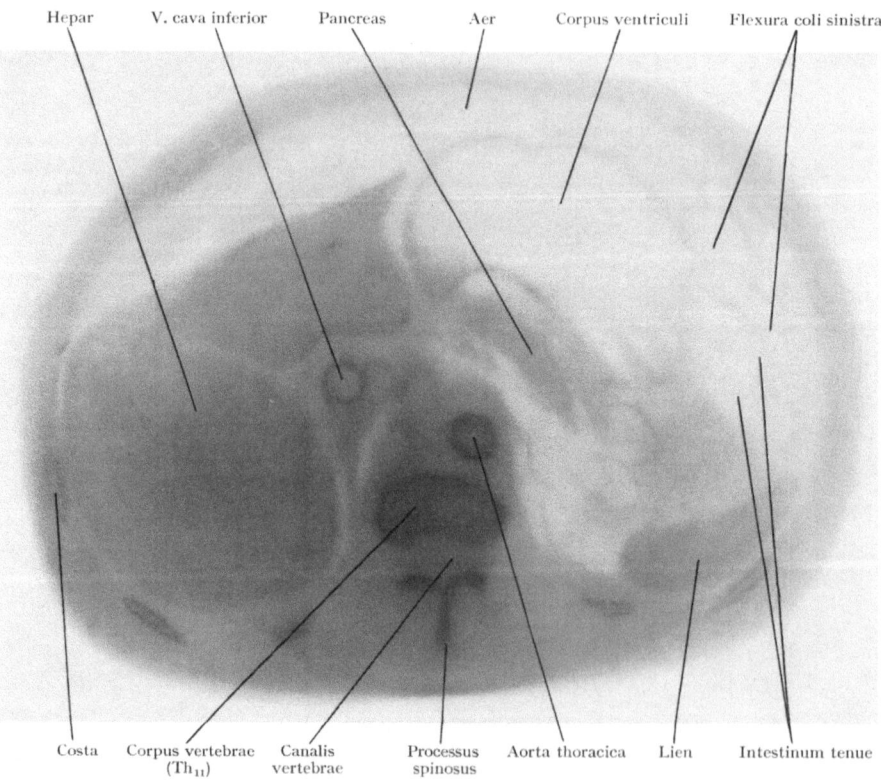

Costa Corpus vertebrae (Th₁₁) Canalis vertebrae Processus spinosus Aorta thoracica Lien Intestinum tenue

Fig. 297. Interpretation

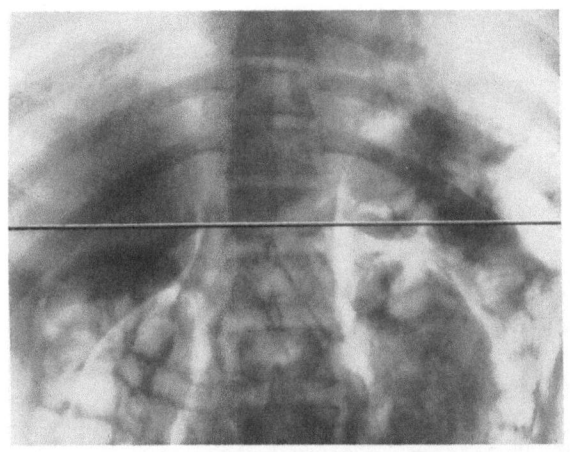

Fig. 298. Normal roentgenogram. Horizontal line showing the level tomographed

Fig. 299. Schematic drawing of the level tomographed

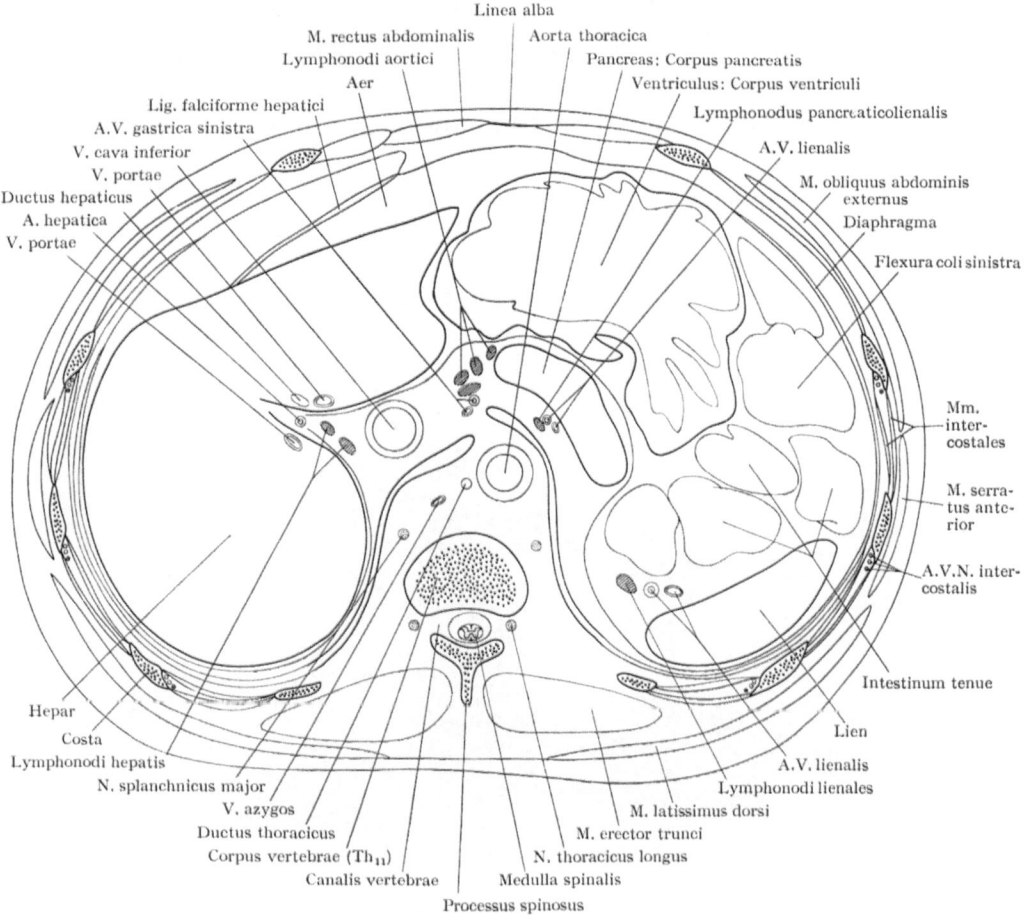

Fig. 300. Anatomical chart

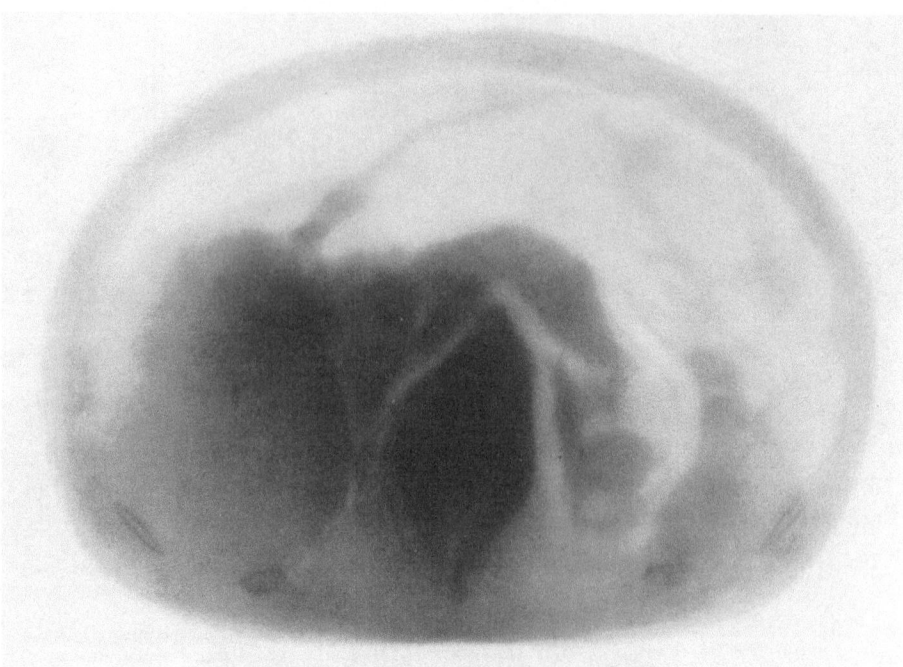

Fig. 301. Axial transverse tomogram

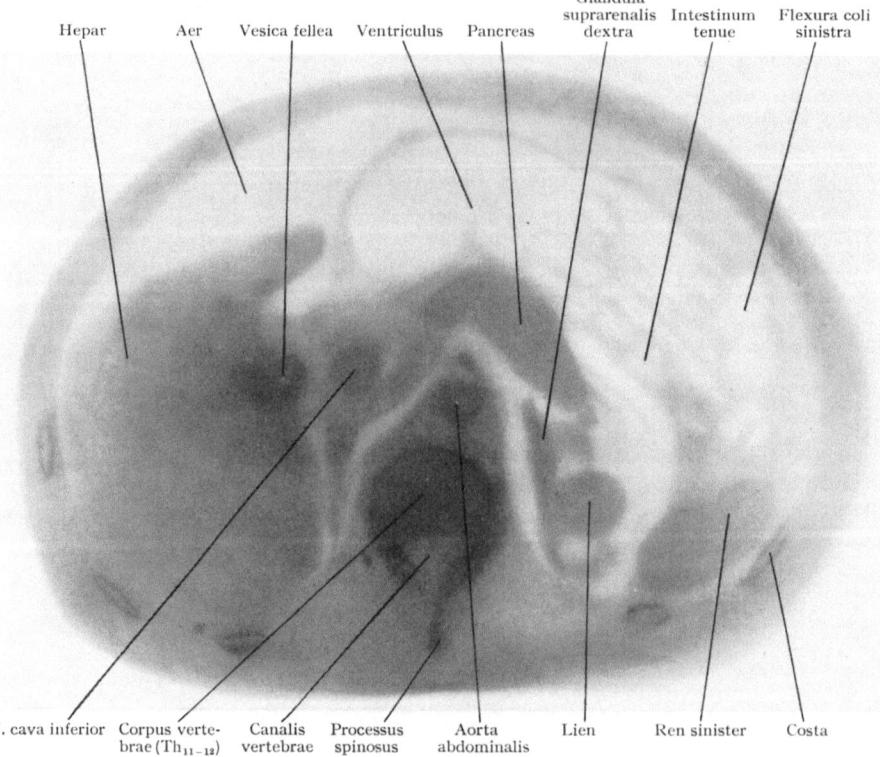

Fig. 302. Interpretation

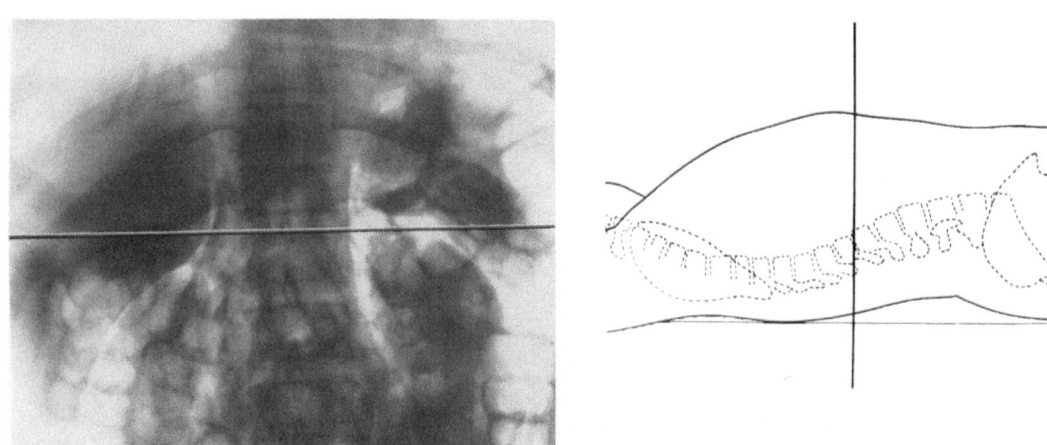

Fig. 303. Normal roentgenogram. Horizontal line showing the level tomographed

Fig. 304. Schematic drawing of the level tomographed

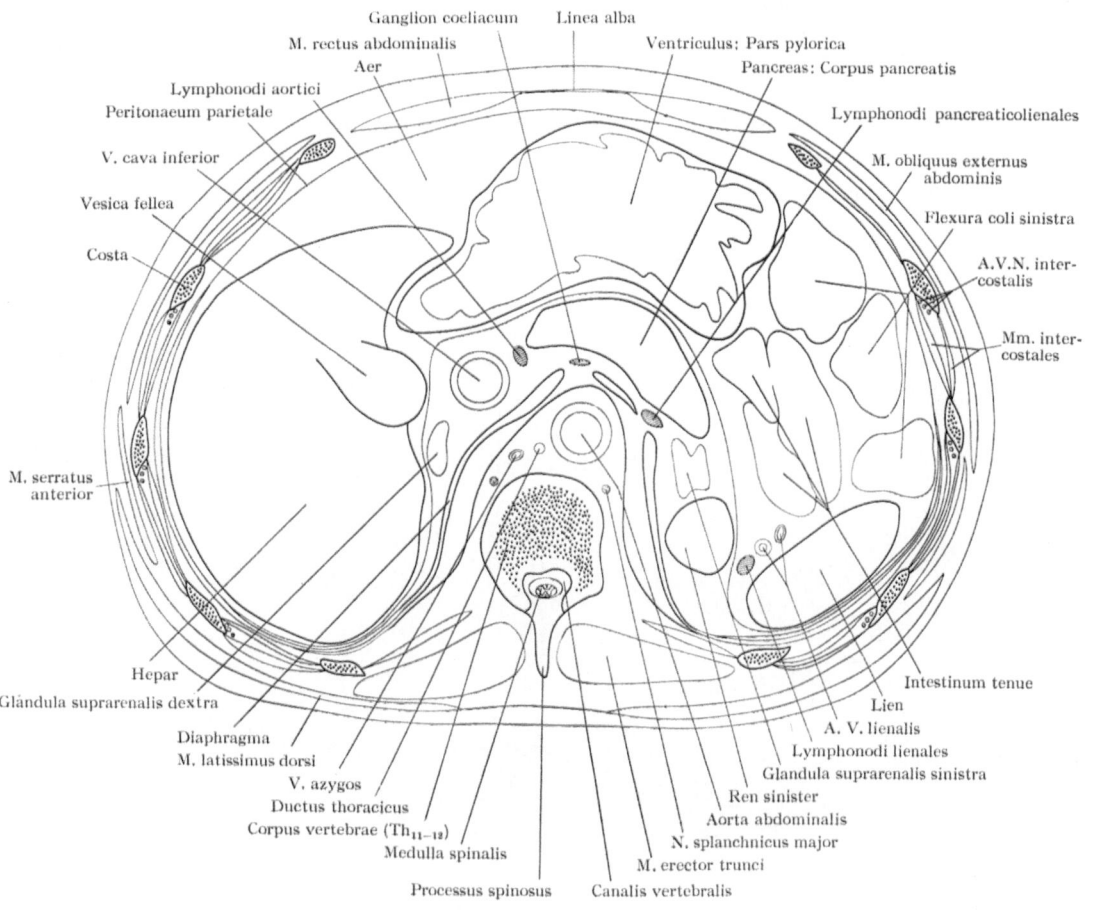

Ganglion coeliacum

Linea alba

M. rectus abdominalis

Aer

Ventriculus: Pars pylorica

Pancreas: Corpus pancreatis

Lymphonodi aortici

Peritonaeum parietale

Lymphonodi pancreaticolienales

V. cava inferior

M. obliquus externus abdominis

Vesica fellea

Flexura coli sinistra

Costa

A.V.N. inter-costalis

Mm. inter-costales

M. serratus anterior

Hepar

Intestinum tenue

Glandula suprarenalis dextra

Lien

Diaphragma

A. V. lienalis

M. latissimus dorsi

Lymphonodi lienales

V. azygos

Glandula suprarenalis sinistra

Ductus thoracicus

Ren sinister

Corpus vertebrae (Th₁₁₋₁₂)

Aorta abdominalis

Medulla spinalis

N. splanchnicus major

M. erector trunci

Processus spinosus

Canalis vertebralis

Fig. 305. Anatomical chart

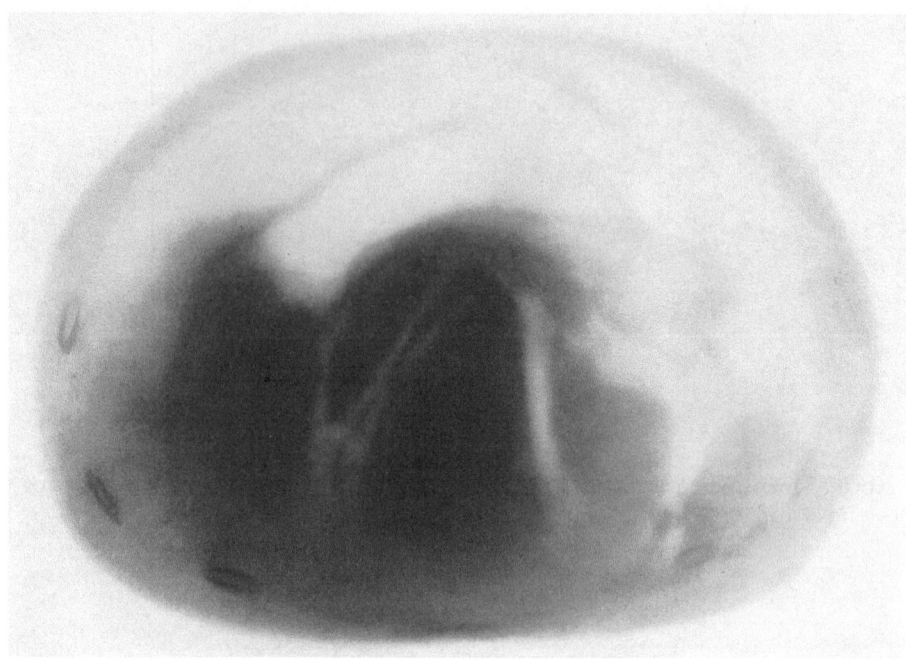

Fig. 306. Axial transverse tomogram

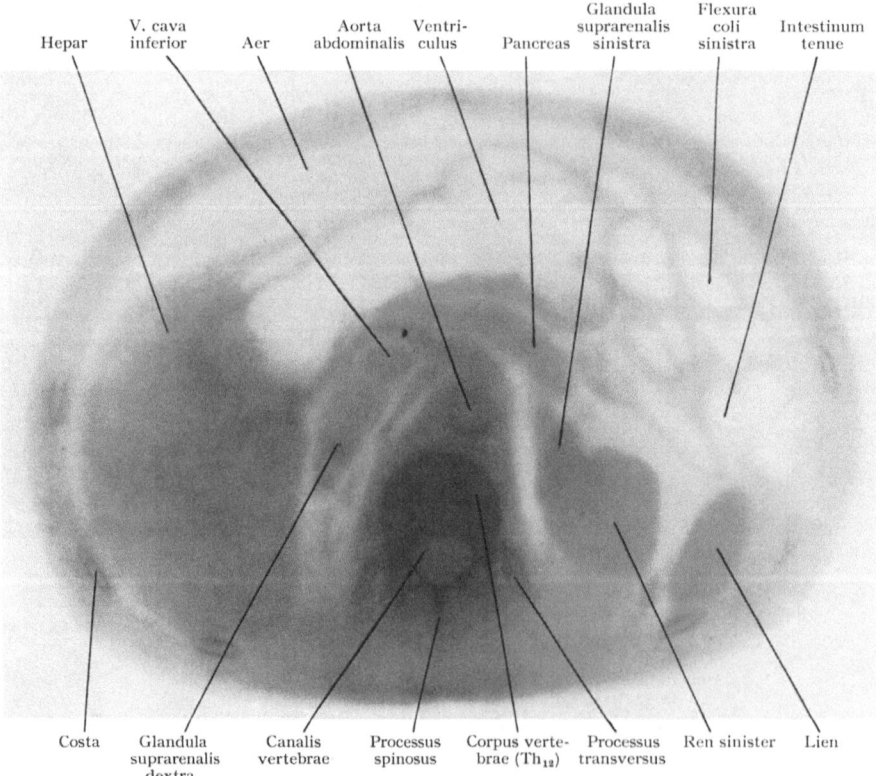

Fig. 307. Interpretation

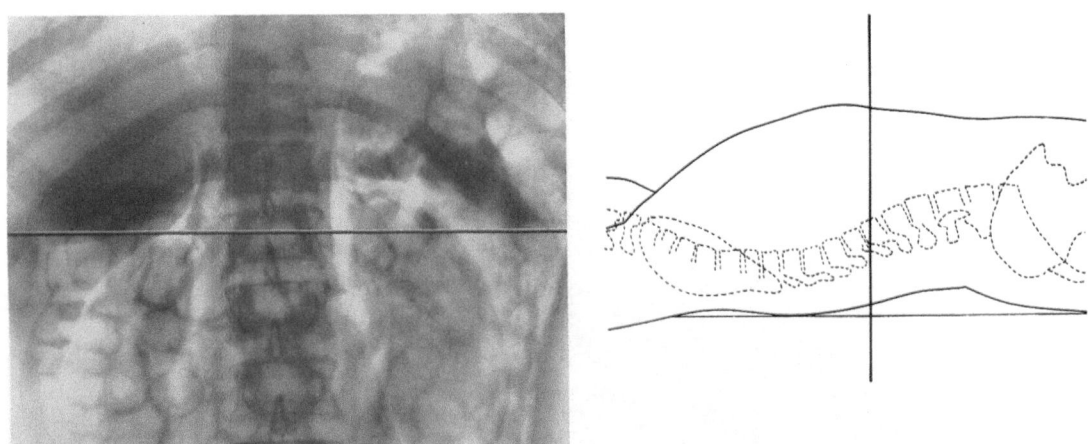

Fig. 308. Normal roentgenogram. Horizontal line showing the level tomographed

Fig. 309. Schematic drawing of the level tomographed

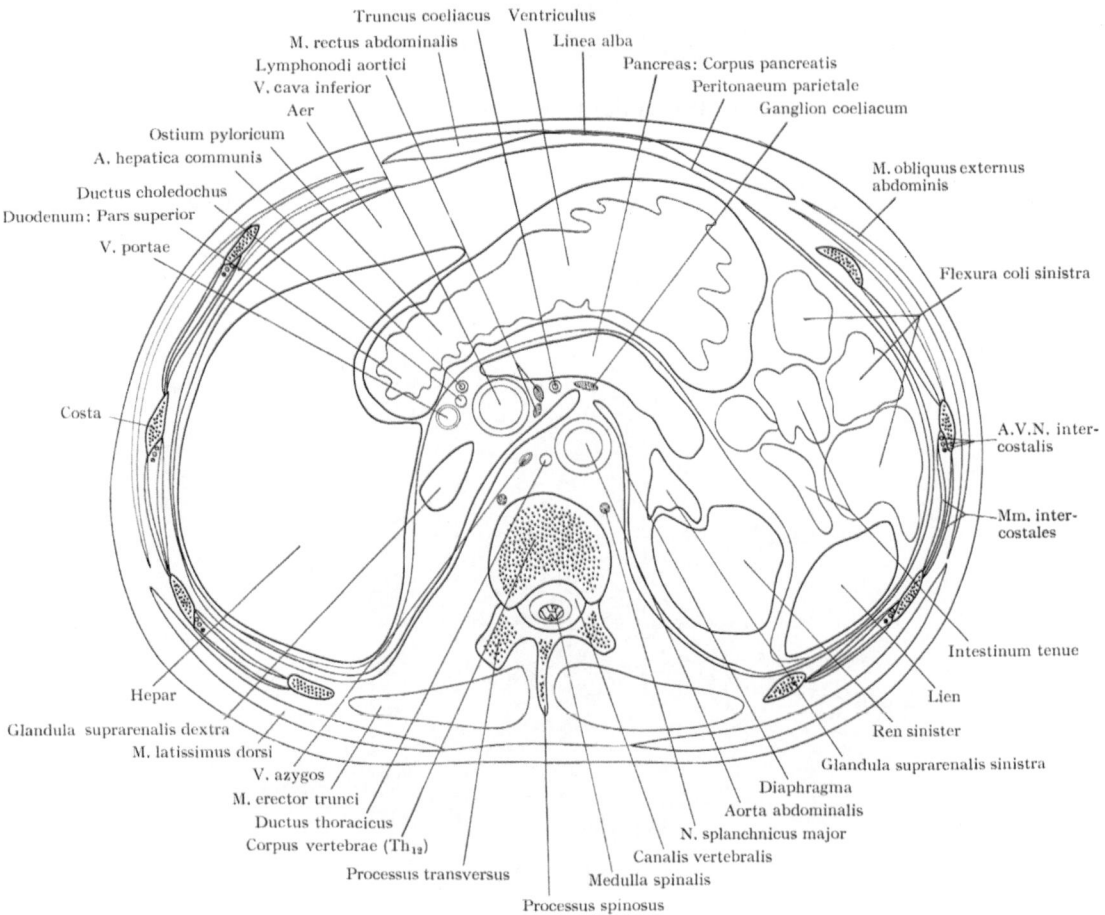

Fig. 310. Anatomical chart

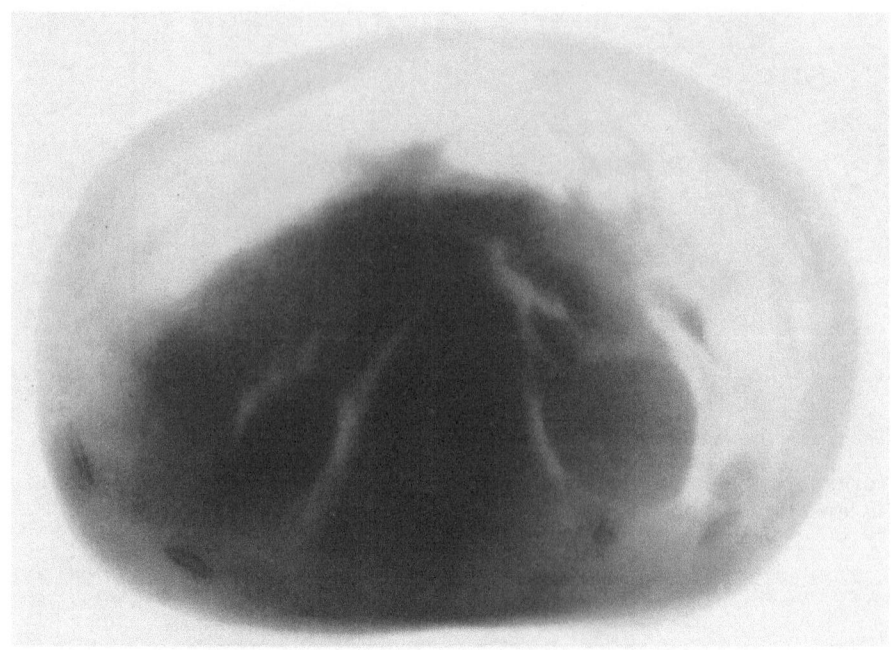

Fig. 311. Axial transverse tomogram

Colon transversum   Duodenum   Pancreas   V. cava inferior   Aorta abdominalis   Dia-phragma   Glandula suprarenalis sinistra   Intestinum tenue   Colon transversum

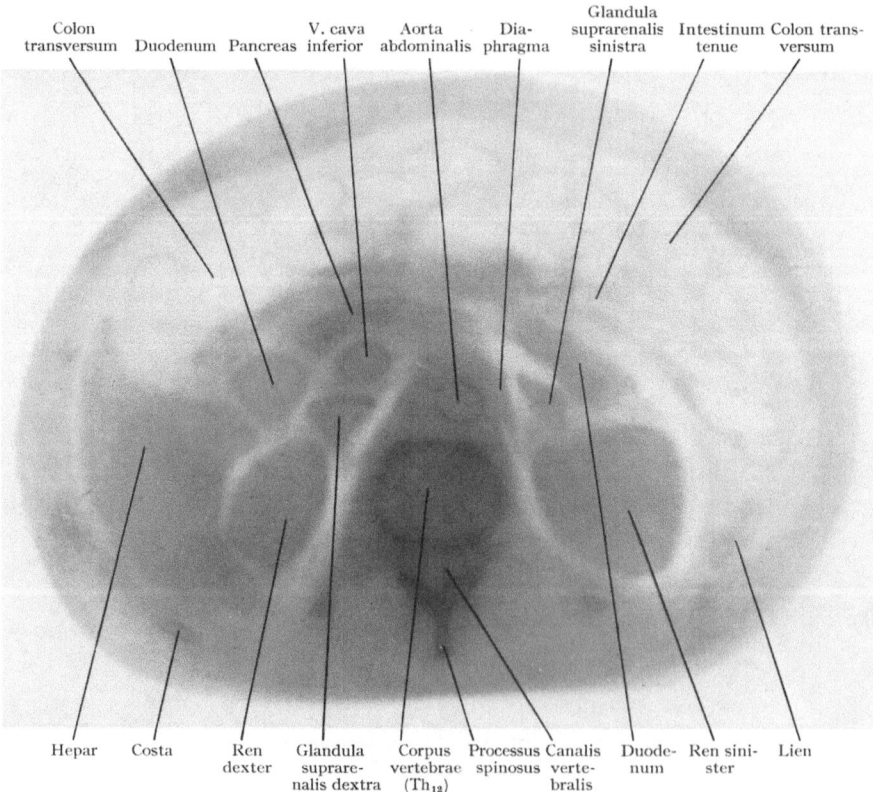

Hepar   Costa   Ren dexter   Glandula suprarenalis dextra   Corpus vertebrae (Th$_{12}$)   Processus spinosus   Canalis vertebralis   Duodenum   Ren sinister   Lien

Fig. 312. Interpretation

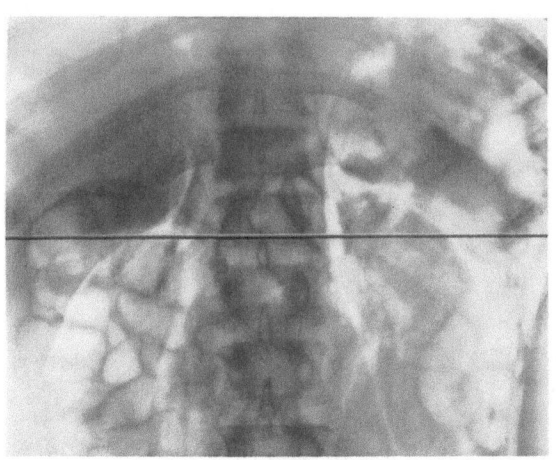

Fig. 313. Normal roentgenogram. Horizontal line showing the level tomographed

Fig. 314. Schematic drawing of the level tomographed

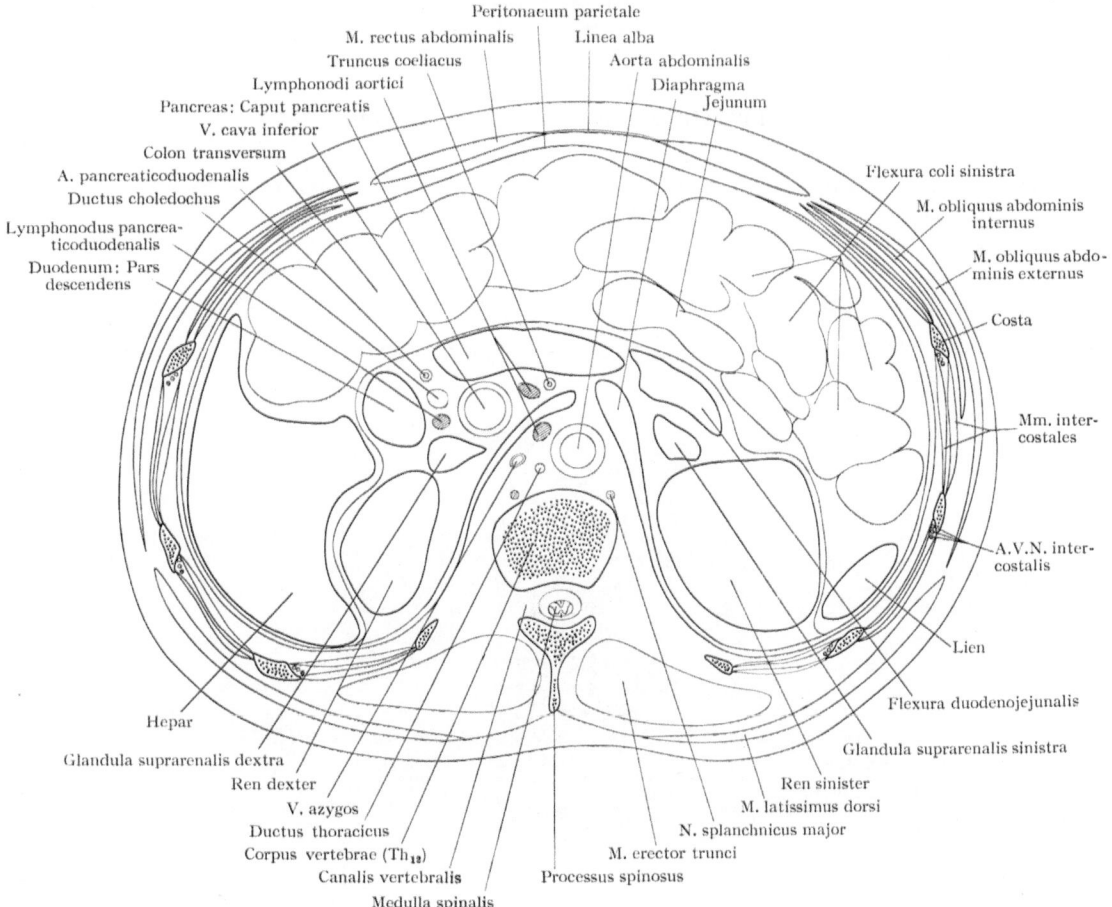

Peritonaeum parietale
M. rectus abdominalis
Truncus coeliacus
Lymphonodi aortici
Pancreas: Caput pancreatis
V. cava inferior
Colon transversum
A. pancreaticoduodenalis
Ductus choledochus
Lymphonodus pancrea-
ticoduodenalis
Duodenum: Pars
descendens

Linea alba
Aorta abdominalis
Diaphragma
Jejunum

Flexura coli sinistra
M. obliquus abdominis
internus
M. obliquus abdo-
minis externus
Costa
Mm. inter-
costales
A.V.N. inter-
costalis
Lien
Flexura duodenojejunalis
Glandula suprarenalis sinistra

Hepar
Glandula suprarenalis dextra
Ren dexter
V. azygos
Ductus thoracicus
Corpus vertebrae (Th$_{12}$)
Canalis vertebralis
Medulla spinalis

Ren sinister
M. latissimus dorsi
N. splanchnicus major
M. erector trunci
Processus spinosus

Fig. 315. Anatomical chart

151

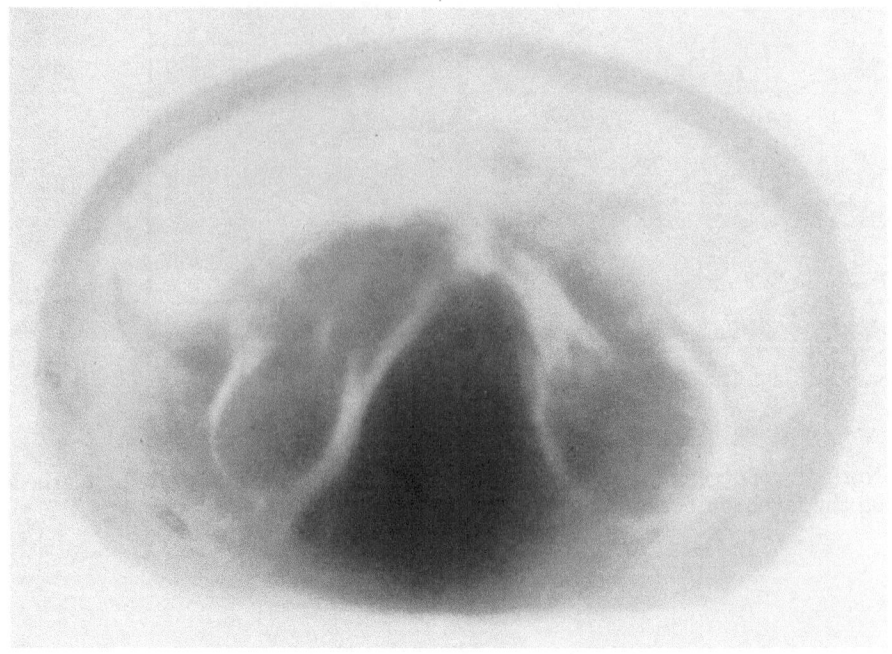

Fig. 316. Axial transverse tomogram

Flexura coli dextra   Pancreas   Colon transversum   V. cava inferior!   Aer   Duodenum   Aorta abdominalis   Intestinum tenue

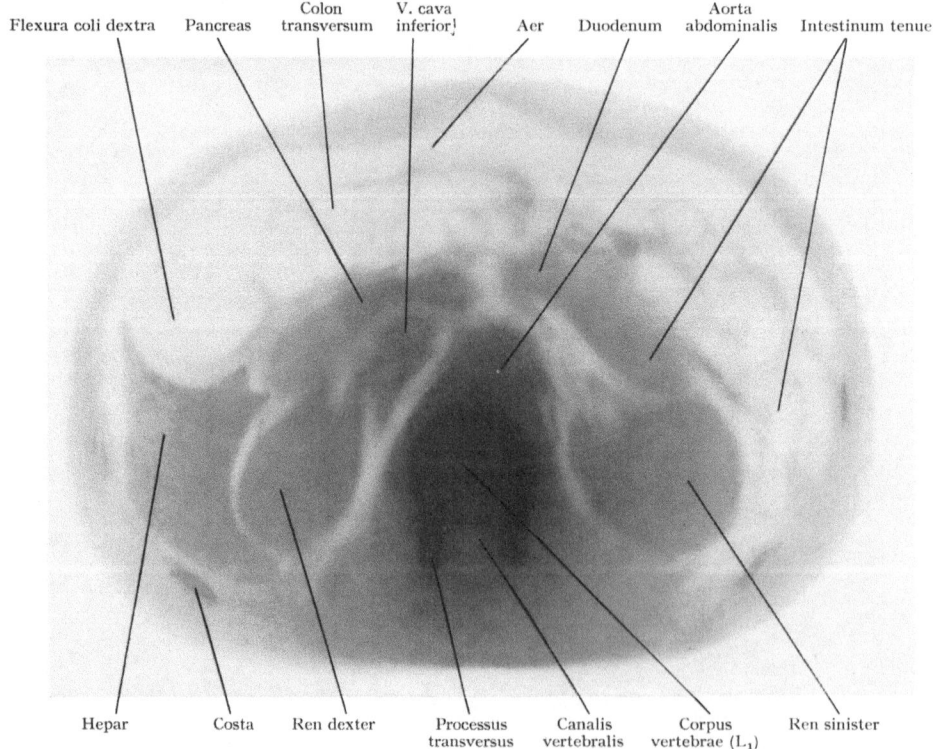

Hepar   Costa   Ren dexter   Processus transversus   Canalis vertebralis   Corpus vertebrae (L₁)   Ren sinister

Fig. 317. Interpretation

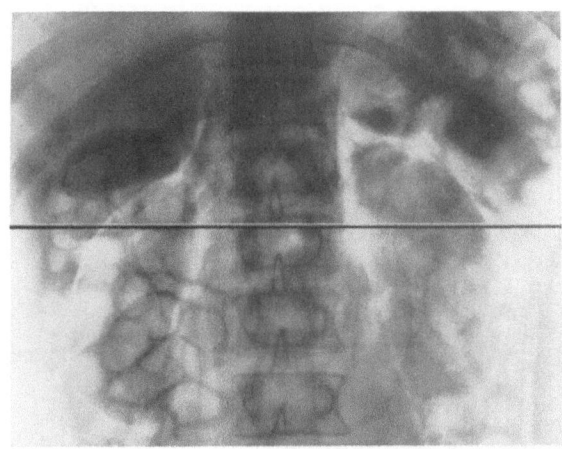

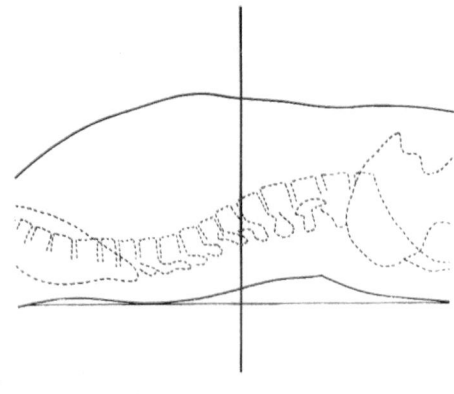

Fig. 318. Normal roentgenogram. Horizontal line showing the level tomographed

Fig. 319. Schematic drawing of the level tomographed

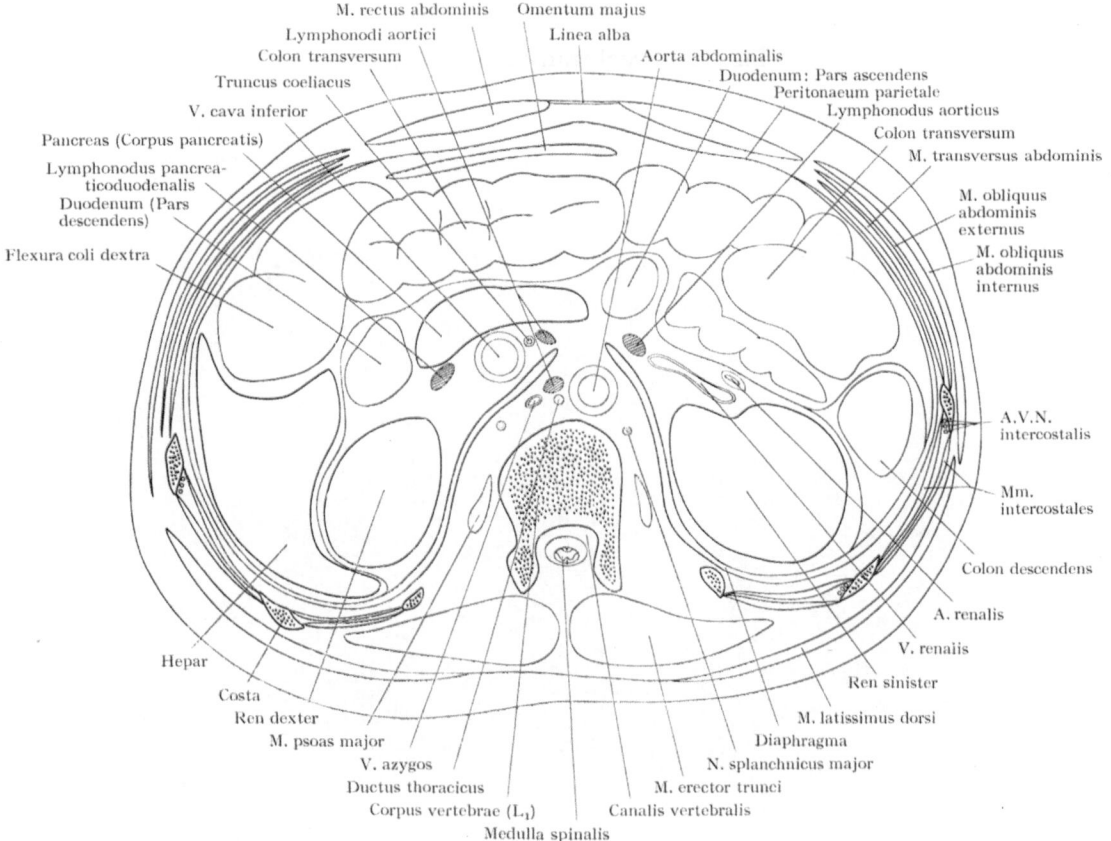

Fig. 320. Anatomical chart

153

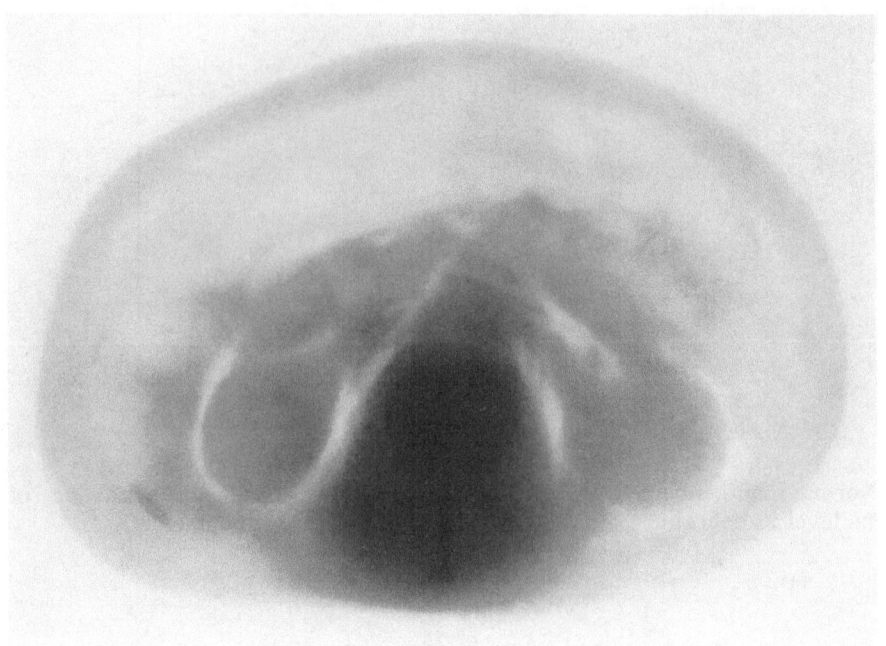

Fig. 321. Axial transverse tomogram

Duodenum (Pars ascendens)   Colon transversum   Aer   V. cava inferior   Pancreas   Aorta abdominalis   Duodenum   Intestinum tenue

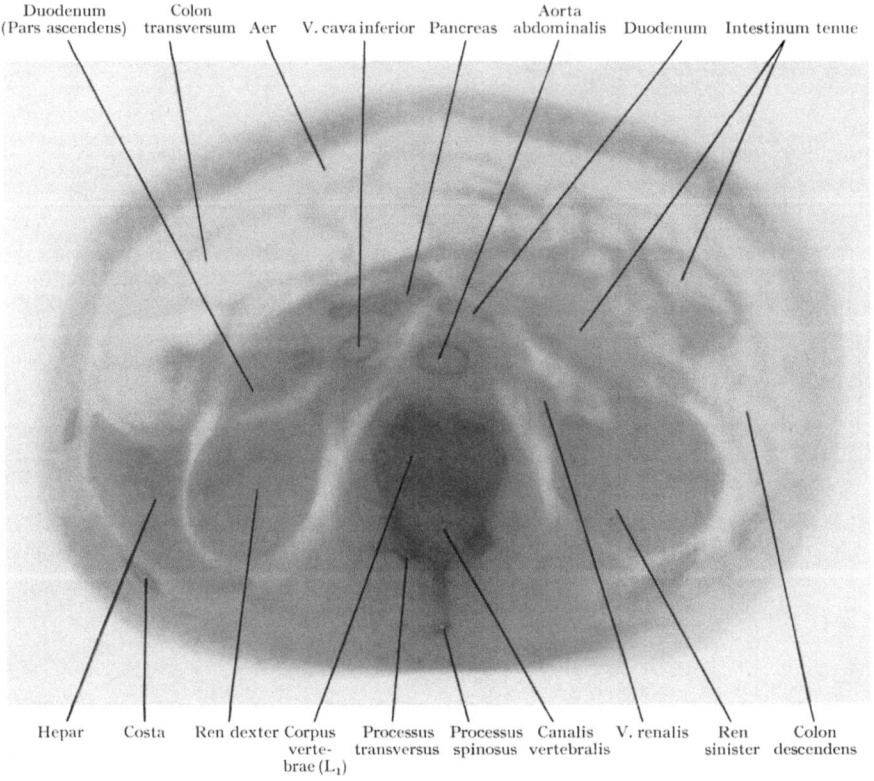

Hepar   Costa   Ren dexter   Corpus vertebrae (L₁)   Processus transversus   Processus spinosus   Canalis vertebralis   V. renalis   Ren sinister   Colon descendens

Fig. 322. Interpretation

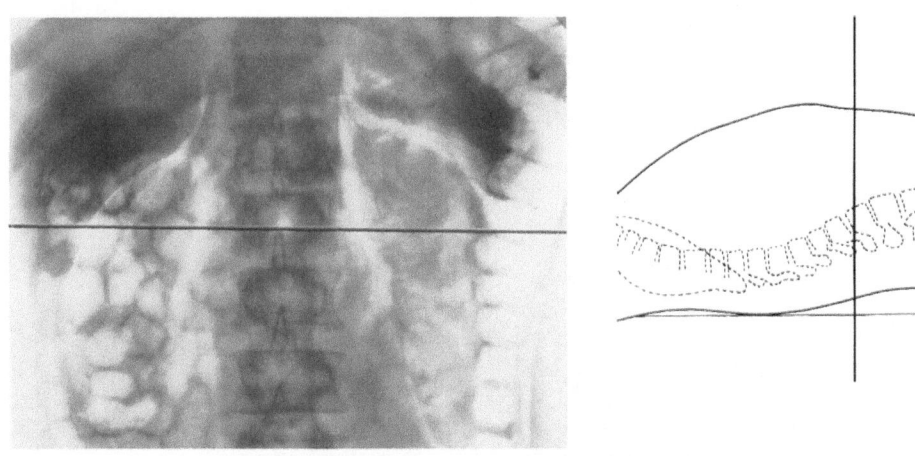

Fig. 323. Normal roentgenogram. Horizontal line showing the level tomographed

Fig. 324. Schematic drawing of the level tomographed

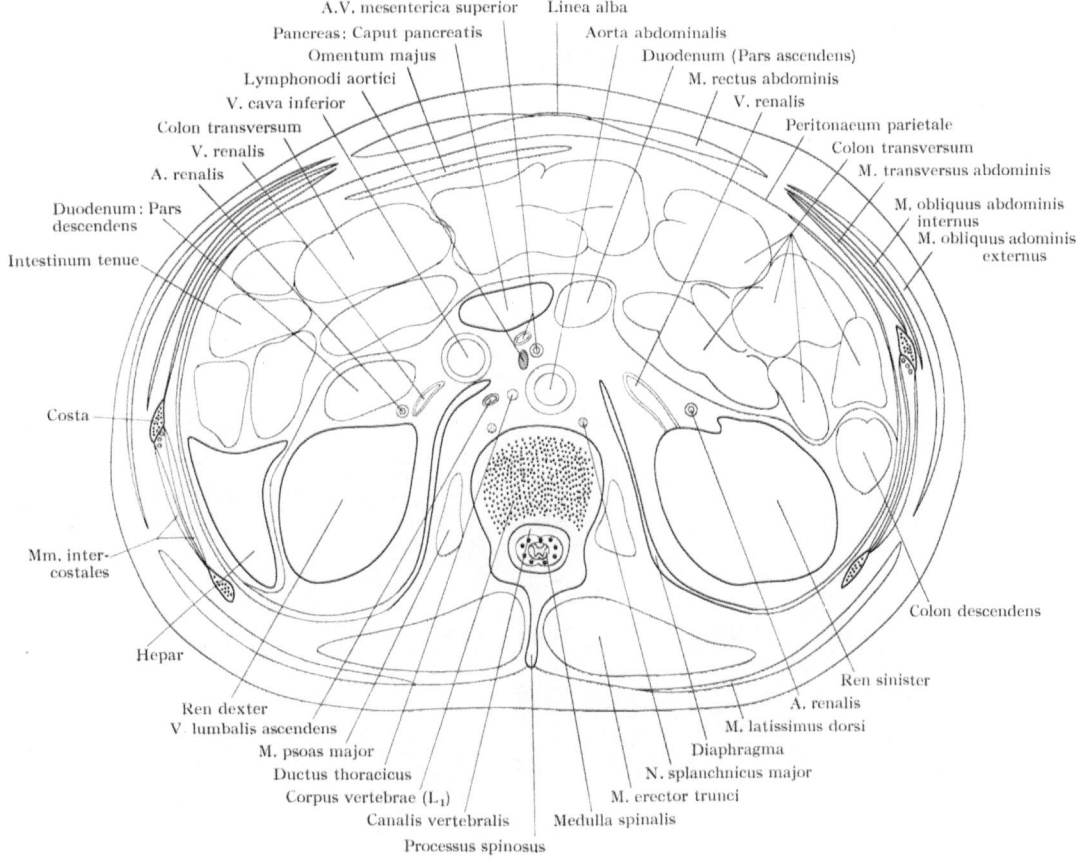

A.V. mesenterica superior
Pancreas: Caput pancreatis
Omentum majus
Lymphonodi aortici
V. cava inferior
Colon transversum
V. renalis
A. renalis
Duodenum: Pars descendens
Intestinum tenue
Costa
Mm. intercostales
Hepar
Ren dexter
V. lumbalis ascendens
M. psoas major
Ductus thoracicus
Corpus vertebrae (L₁)
Canalis vertebralis
Processus spinosus

Linea alba
Aorta abdominalis
Duodenum (Pars ascendens)
M. rectus abdominis
V. renalis
Peritonaeum parietale
Colon transversum
M. transversus abdominis
M. obliquus abdominis internus
M. obliquus adominis externus
Colon descendens
Ren sinister
A. renalis
M. latissimus dorsi
Diaphragma
N. splanchnicus major
M. erector trunci
Medulla spinalis

Fig. 325. Anatomical chart

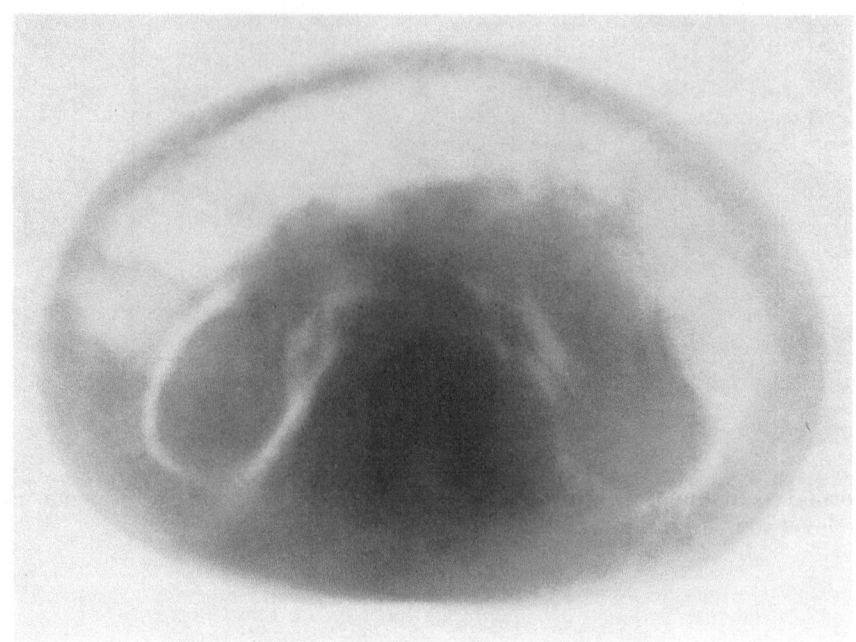

Fig. 326. Axial transverse tomogram

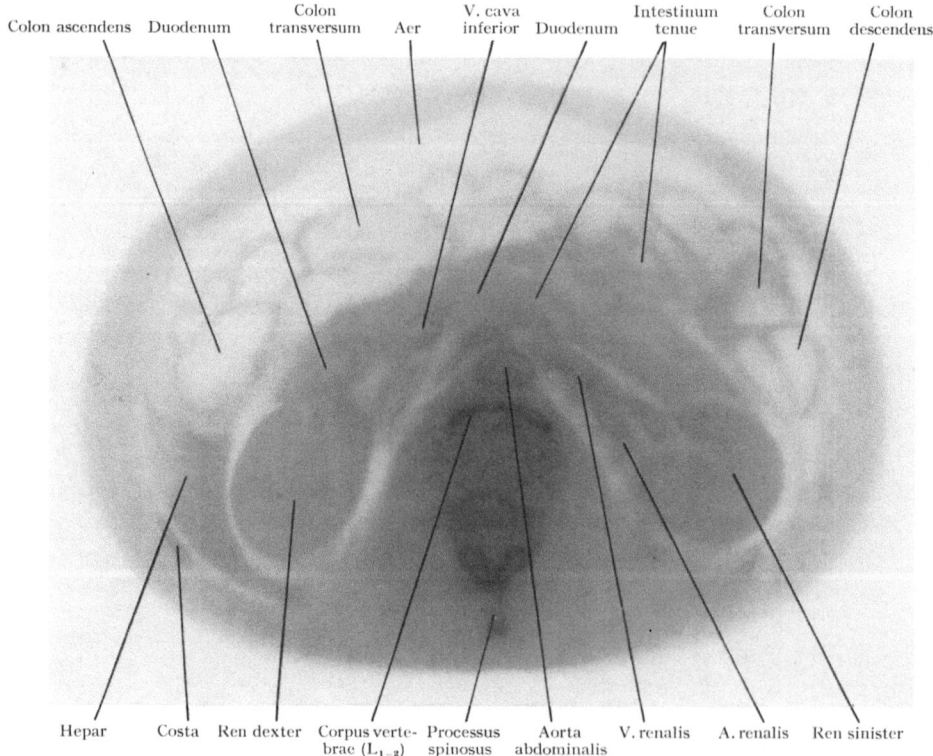

Fig. 327. Interpretation

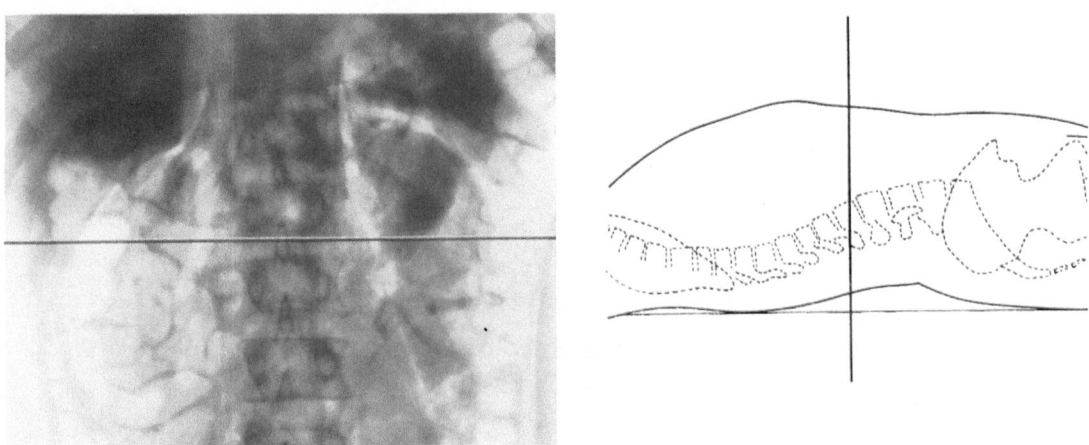

Fig. 328. Normal roentgenogram. Horizontal line showing the level tomographed

Fig. 329. Schematic drawing of the level tomographed

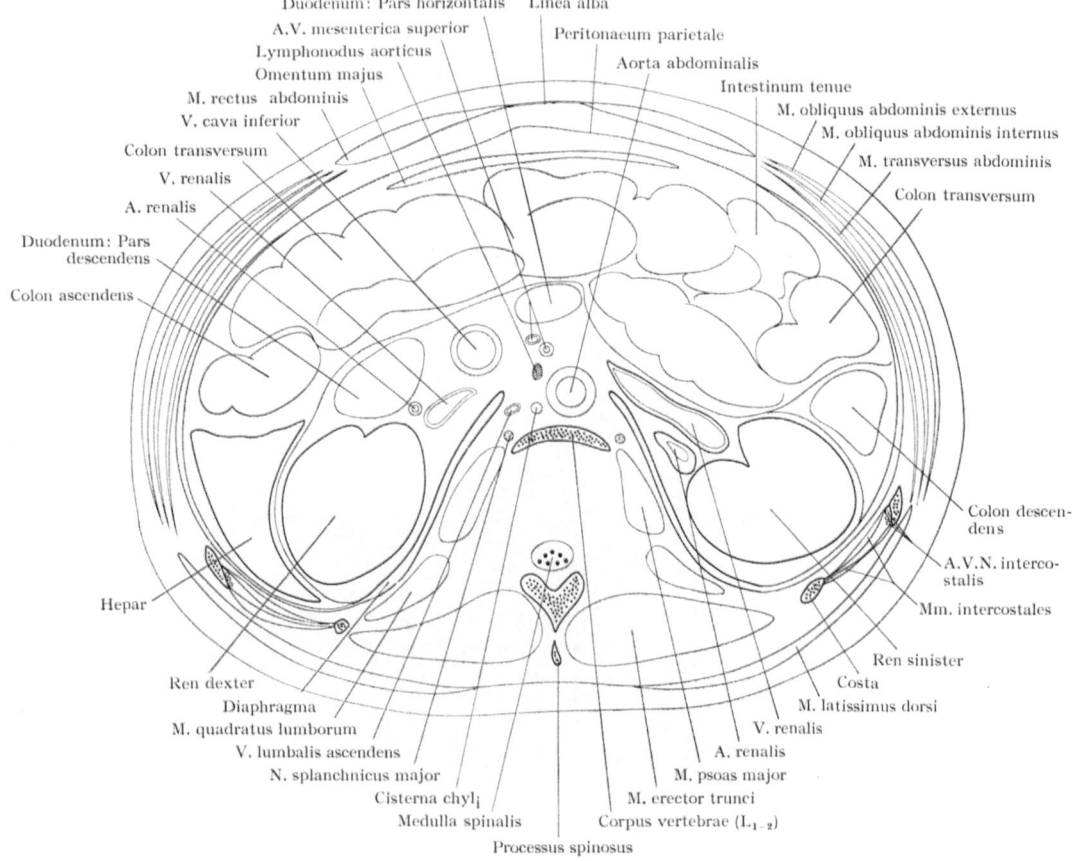

Duodenum: Pars horizontalis
A.V. mesenterica superior
Lymphonodus aorticus
Omentum majus
M. rectus abdominis
V. cava inferior
Colon transversum
V. renalis
A. renalis
Duodenum: Pars descendens
Colon ascendens
Hepar
Ren dexter
Diaphragma
M. quadratus lumborum
V. lumbalis ascendens
N. splanchnicus major
Cisterna chyli
Medulla spinalis
Processus spinosus

Linea alba
Peritonaeum parietale
Aorta abdominalis
Intestinum tenue
M. obliquus abdominis externus
M. obliquus abdominis internus
M. transversus abdominis
Colon transversum
Colon descendens
A.V.N. intercostalis
Mm. intercostales
Ren sinister
Costa
M. latissimus dorsi
V. renalis
A. renalis
M. psoas major
M. erector trunci
Corpus vertebrae (L₁₋₂)

Fig. 330. Anatomical chart

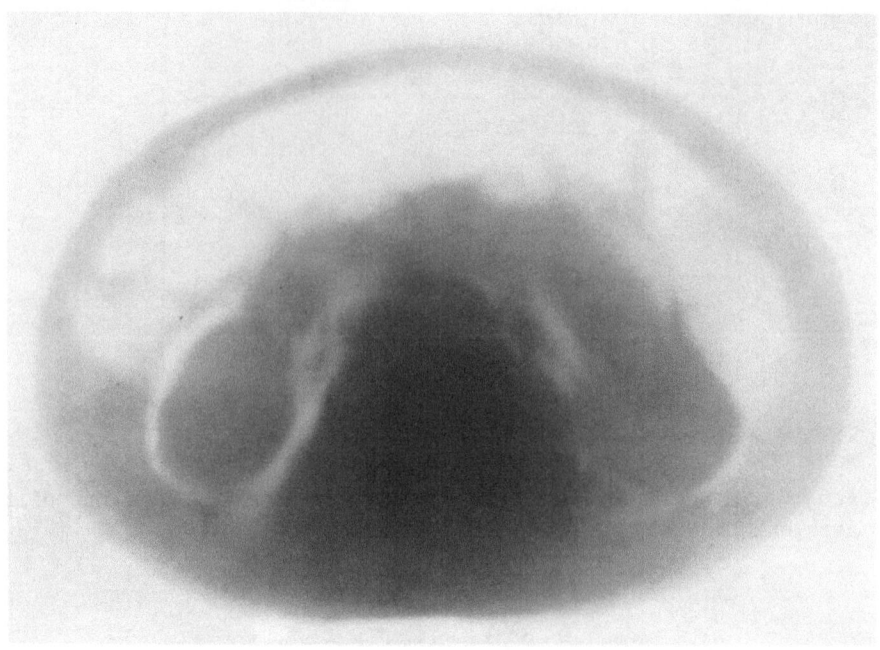

Fig. 331. Axial transverse tomogram

Colon ascendens   Ren dexter   Colon transversum   Duodenum   Intestinum tenue   Colon descendens

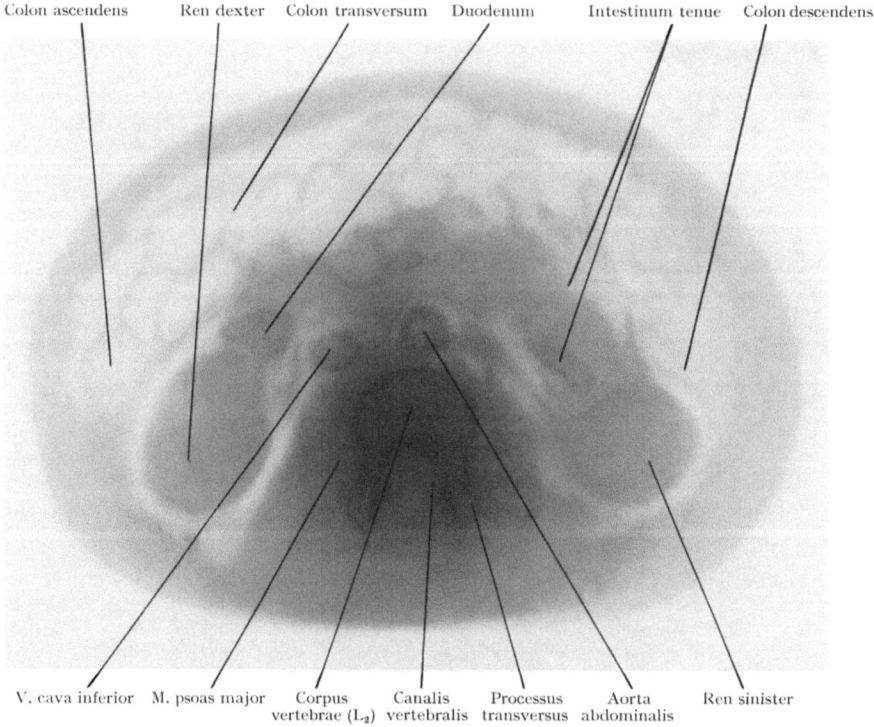

V. cava inferior   M. psoas major   Corpus vertebrae (L₂)   Canalis vertebralis   Processus transversus   Aorta abdominalis   Ren sinister

Fig. 332. Interpretation

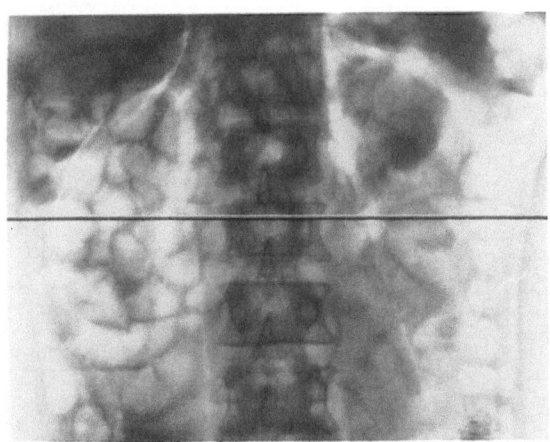

Fig. 333. Normal roentgenogram. Horizontal line showing the level tomographed

Fig. 334. Schematic drawing of the level tomographed

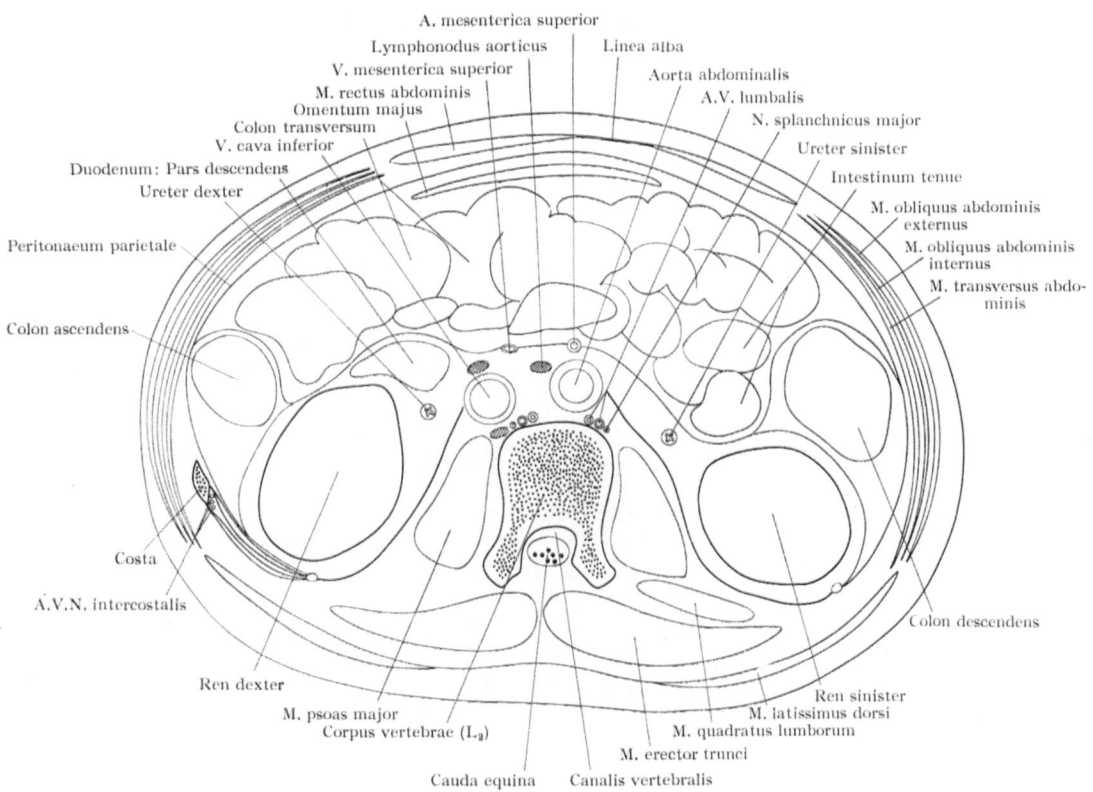

A. mesenterica superior
Lymphonodus aorticus
V. mesenterica superior
M. rectus abdominis
Omentum majus
Colon transversum
V. cava inferior
Duodenum: Pars descendens
Ureter dexter

Linea alba
Aorta abdominalis
A.V. lumbalis
N. splanchnicus major
Ureter sinister
Intestinum tenue
M. obliquus abdominis externus
M. obliquus abdominis internus
M. transversus abdominis

Peritonaeum parietale

Colon ascendens

Costa

A.V.N. intercostalis

Colon descendens

Ren dexter

Ren sinister
M. latissimus dorsi
M. quadratus lumborum
M. erector trunci
Canalis vertebralis

M. psoas major
Corpus vertebrae (L₃)

Cauda equina

Fig. 335. Anatomical chart

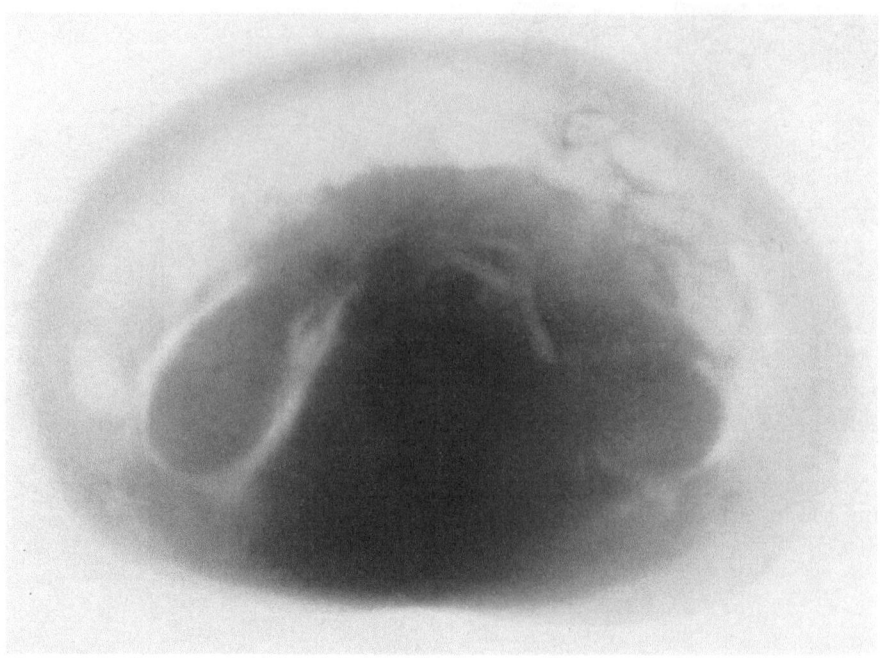

Fig. 336. Axial transverse tomogram

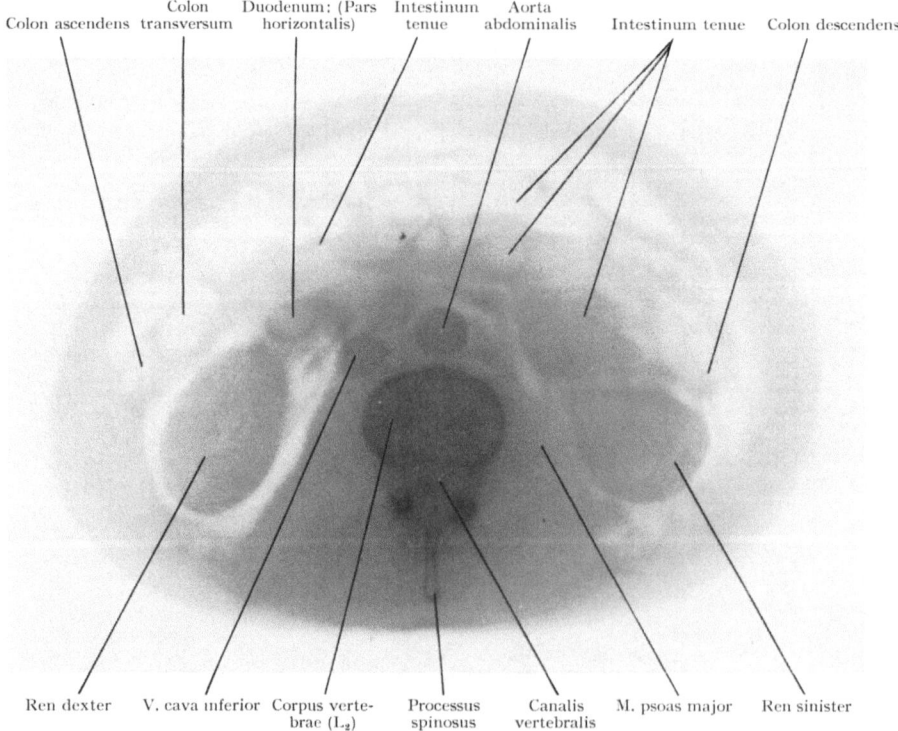

Fig. 337. Interpretation

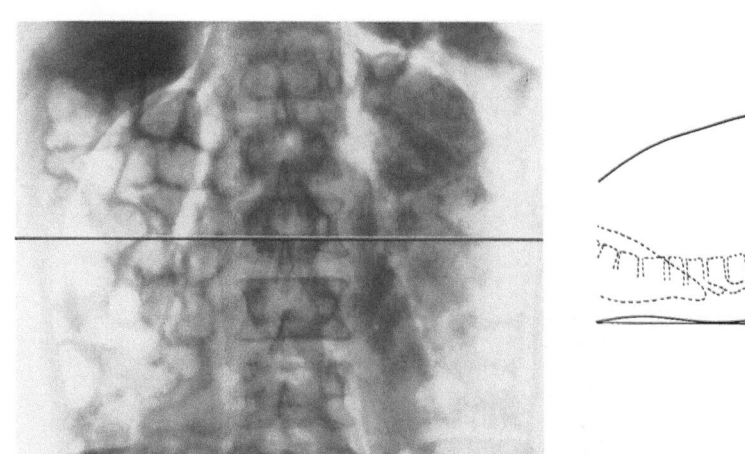

Fig. 338. Normal roentgenogram. Horizontal line showing the level tomographed

Fig. 339. Schematic drawing of the level tomographed

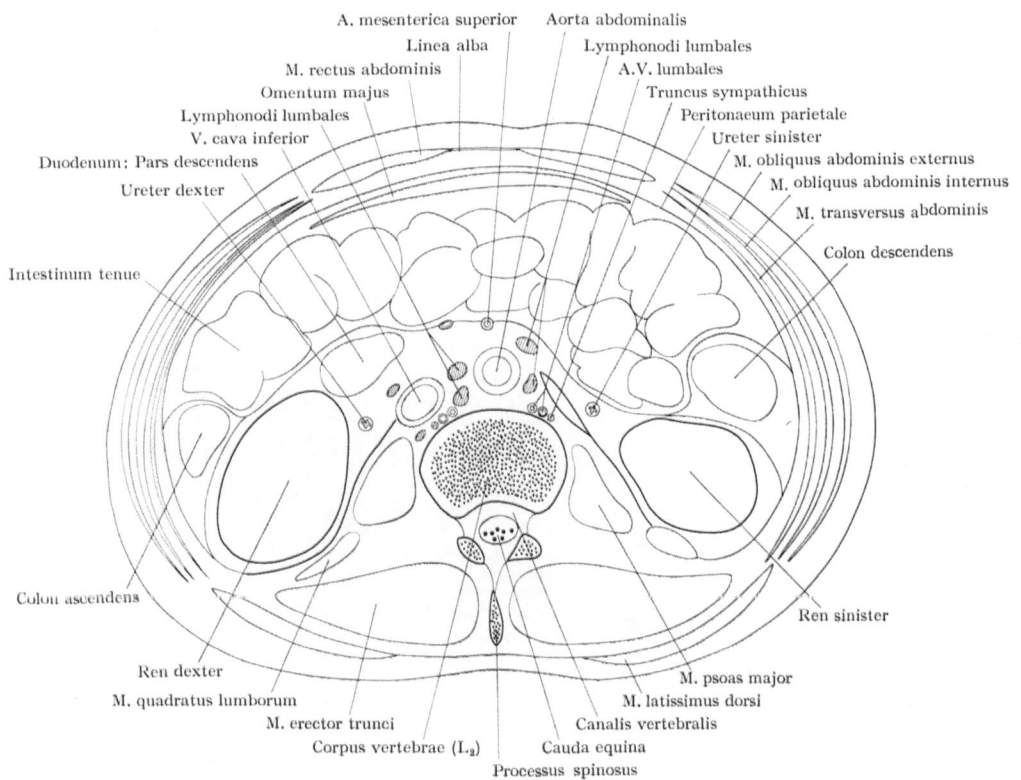

A. mesenterica superior
Linea alba
M. rectus abdominis
Omentum majus
Lymphonodi lumbales
V. cava inferior
Duodenum: Pars descendens
Ureter dexter
Intestinum tenue
Aorta abdominalis
Lymphonodi lumbales
A.V. lumbales
Truncus sympathicus
Peritonaeum parietale
Ureter sinister
M. obliquus abdominis externus
M. obliquus abdominis internus
M. transversus abdominis
Colon descendens
Colon ascendens
Ren sinister
Ren dexter
M. quadratus lumborum
M. erector trunci
Corpus vertebrae (L₃)
Processus spinosus
Cauda equina
Canalis vertebralis
M. latissimus dorsi
M. psoas major

Fig. 340. Anatomical chart

161

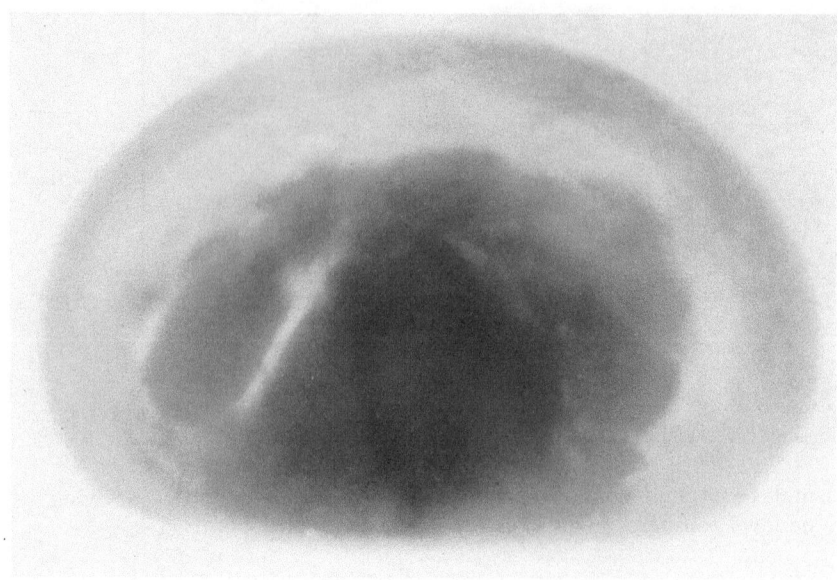

Fig. 341. Axial transverse tomogram

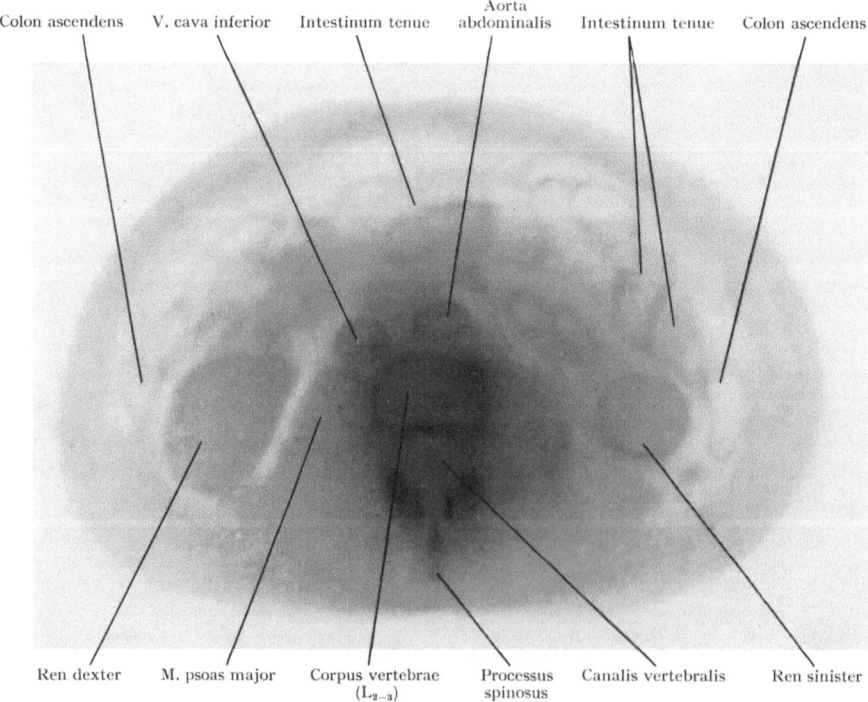

Fig. 342. Interpretation

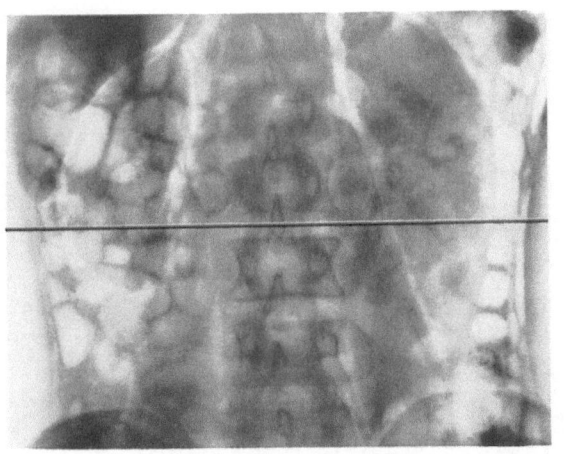

Fig. 343. Normal roentgenogram. Horizontal line showing the level tomographed

Fig. 344. Schematic drawing of the level tomographed

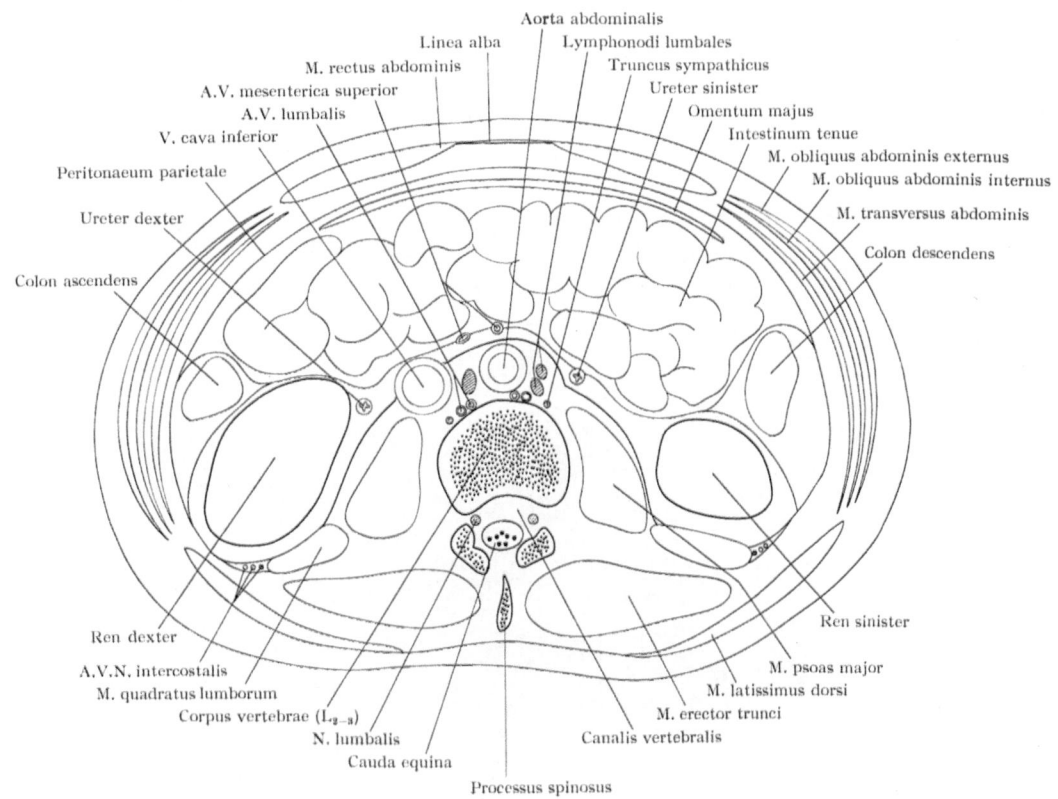

Fig. 345. Anatomical chart

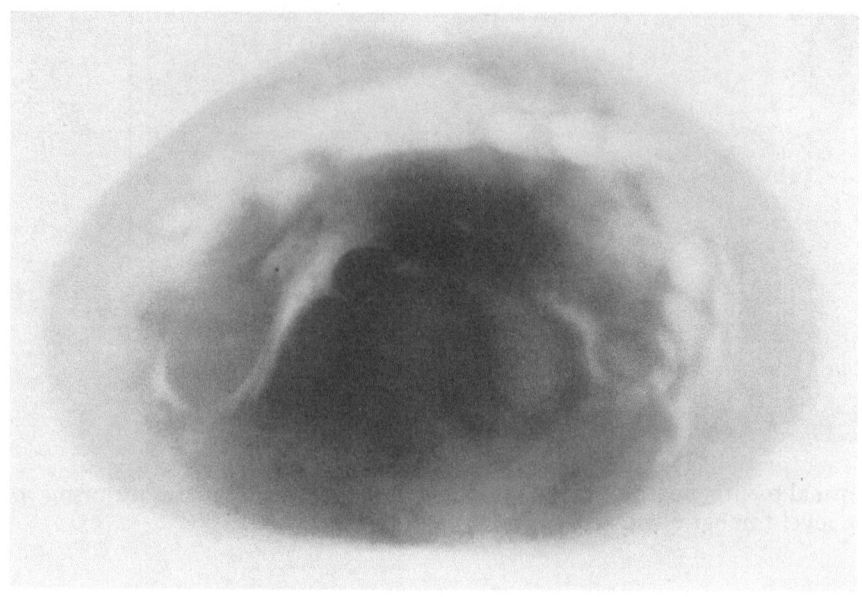

Fig. 346. Axial transverse tomogram

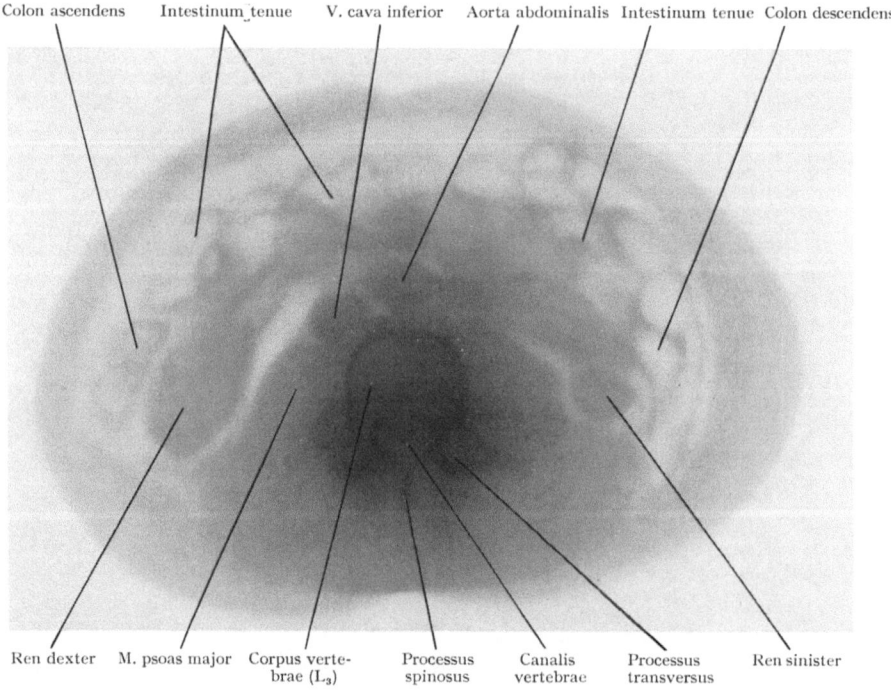

Colon ascendens   Intestinum tenue   V. cava inferior   Aorta abdominalis   Intestinum tenue   Colon descendens

Ren dexter   M. psoas major   Corpus verte-   Processus   Canalis   Processus   Ren sinister
brae (L$_3$)   spinosus   vertebrae   transversus

Fig. 347. Interpretation

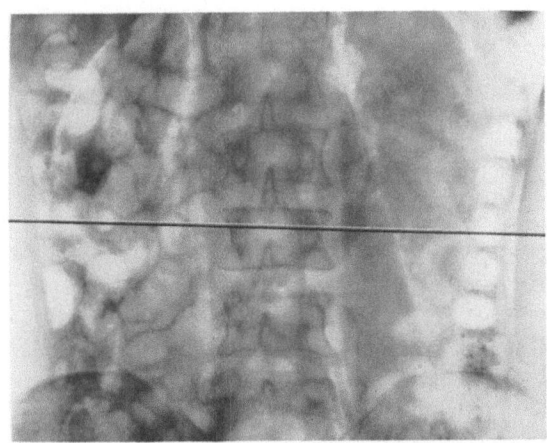
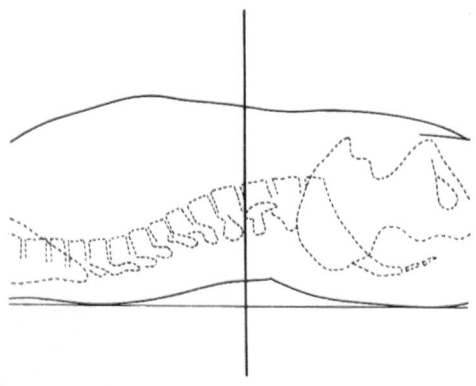

Fig. 348. Normal roentgenogram. Horizontal line showing the level tomographed

Fig. 349. Schematic drawing of the level tomographed

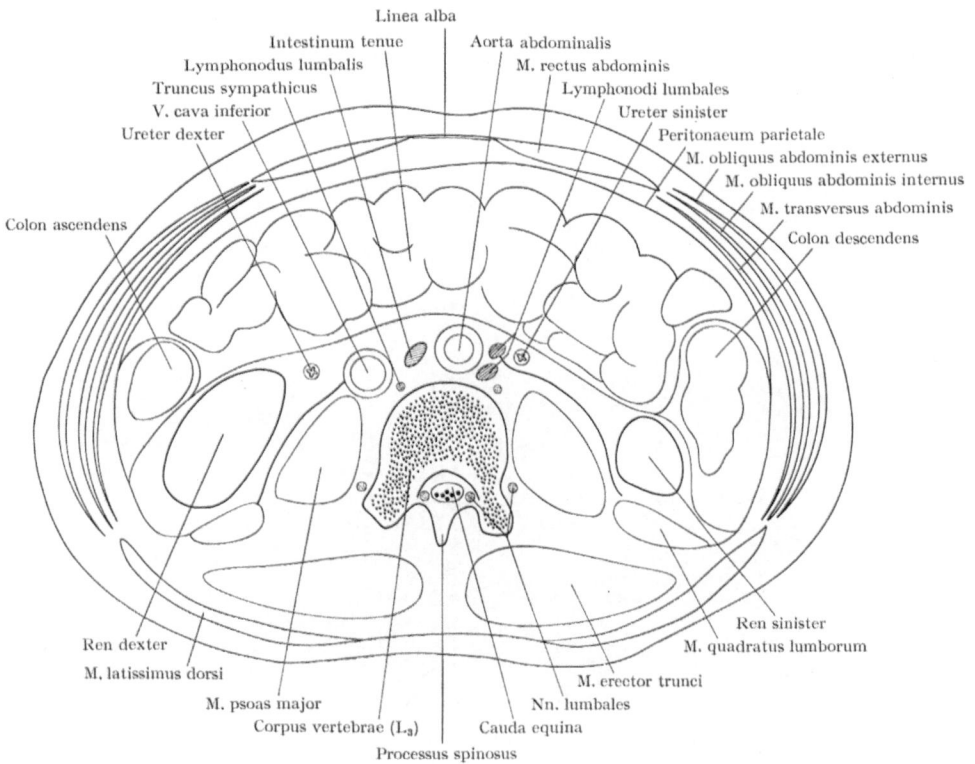

Linea alba

Intestinum tenue

Lymphonodus lumbalis

Truncus sympathicus

V. cava inferior

Ureter dexter

Aorta abdominalis

M. rectus abdominis

Lymphonodi lumbales

Ureter sinister

Peritonaeum parietale

M. obliquus abdominis externus

M. obliquus abdominis internus

M. transversus abdominis

Colon descendens

Colon ascendens

Ren sinister

M. quadratus lumborum

Ren dexter

M. latissimus dorsi

M. psoas major

Corpus vertebrae (L₃)

Processus spinosus

Cauda equina

Nn. lumbales

M. erector trunci

Fig. 350. Anatomical chart

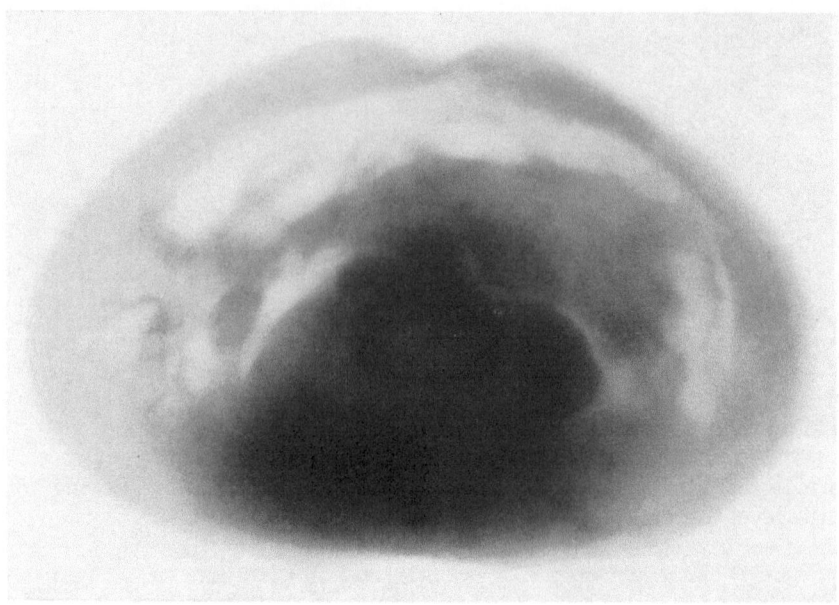

Fig. 351. Axial transverse tomogram

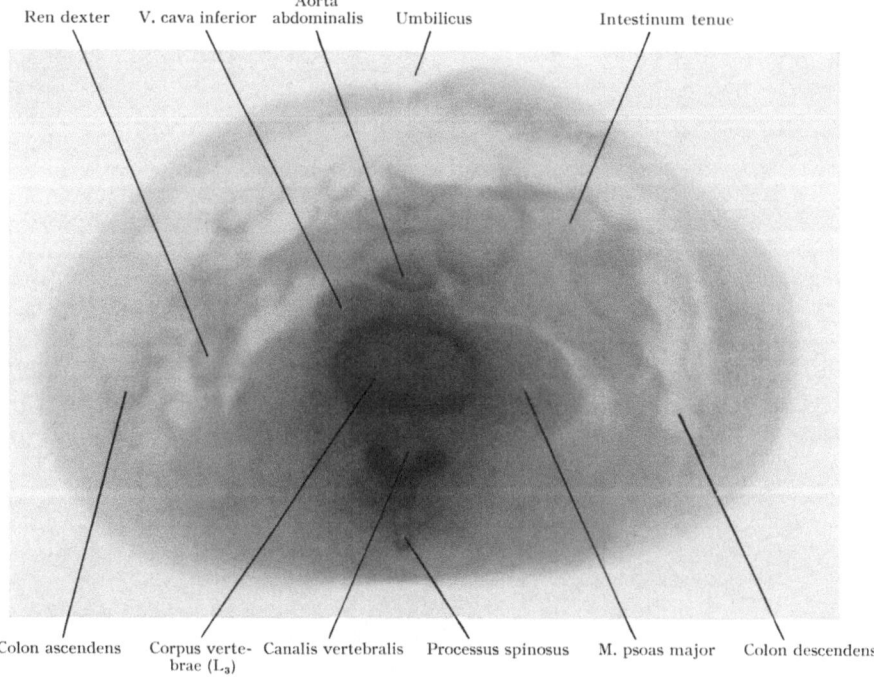

Fig. 352. Interpretation

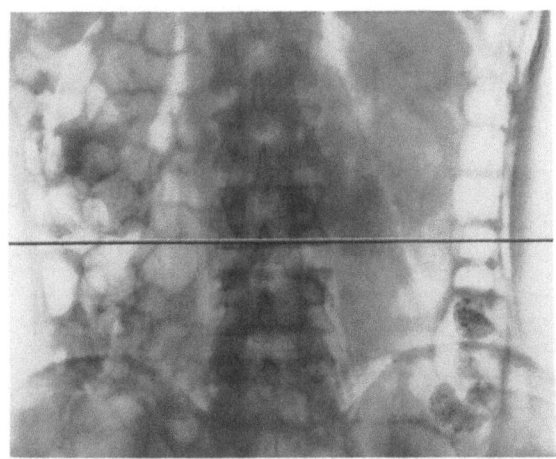

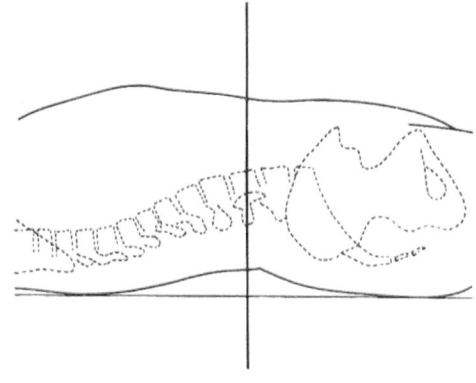

Fig. 353. Normal roentgenogram. Horizontal line showing the level tomographed

Fig. 354. Schematic drawing of the level tomographed

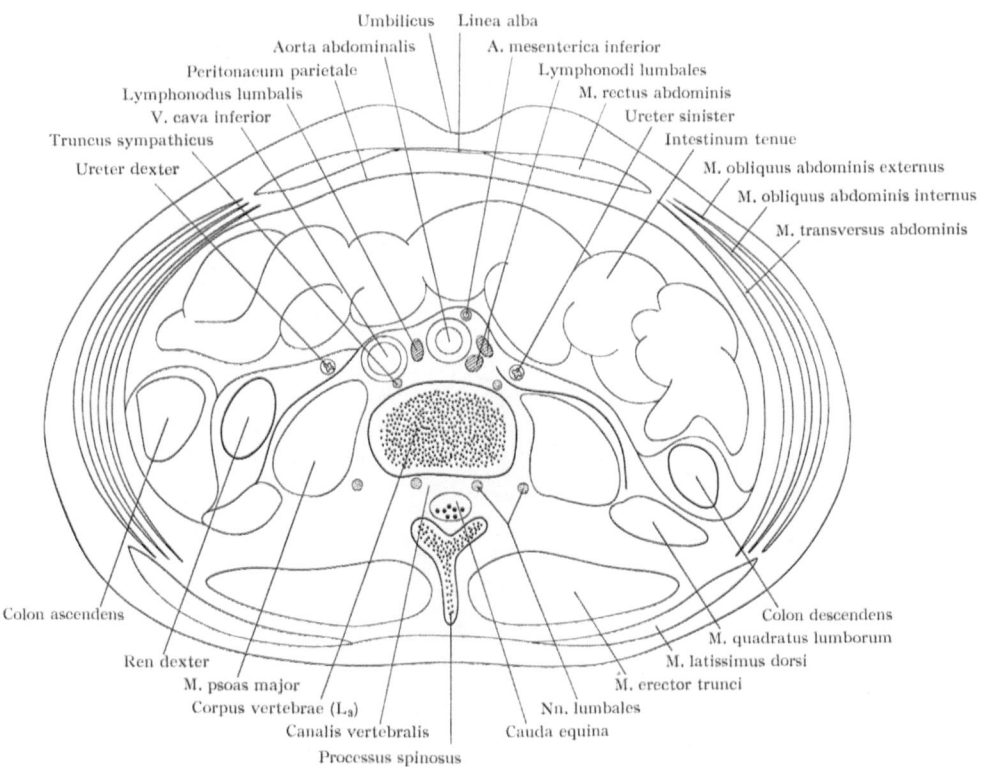

Fig. 355. Anatomical chart

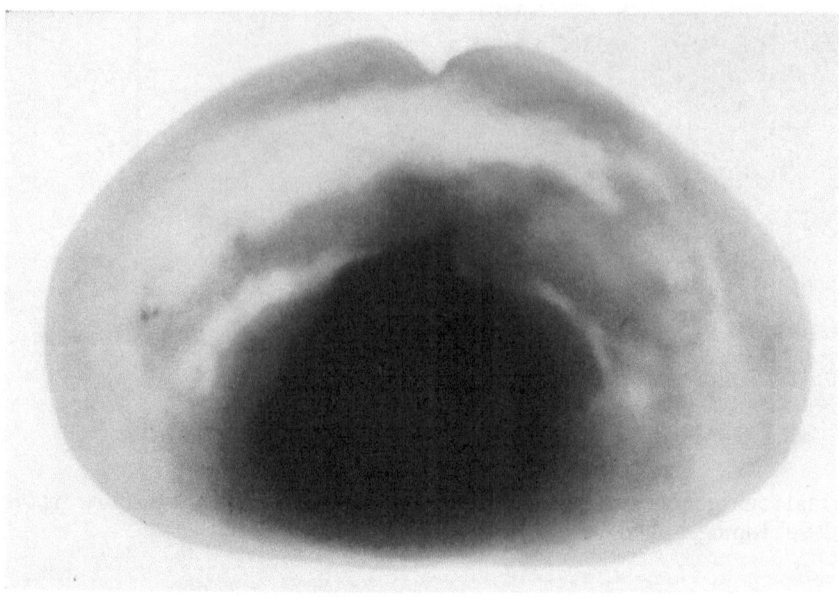

Fig. 356. Axial transverse tomogram

Colon ascendens   Intestinum tenue   V. cava inferior   Umbilicus   Aorta abdominalis   Colon transversum

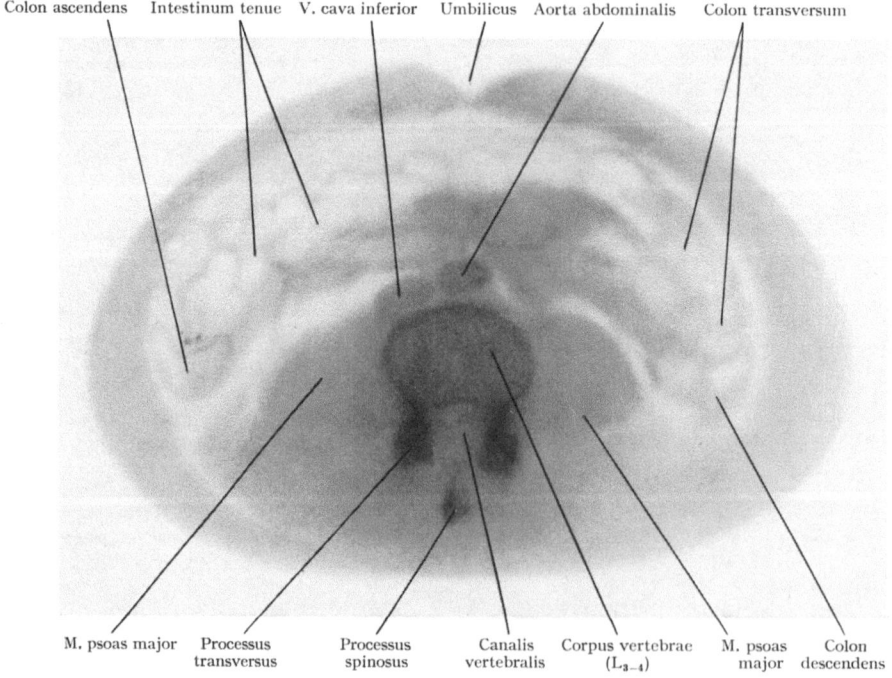

M. psoas major   Processus   Processus   Canalis   Corpus vertebrae   M. psoas   Colon
                 transversus   spinosus   vertebralis   (L$_{3-4}$)   major   descendens

Fig. 357. Interpretation

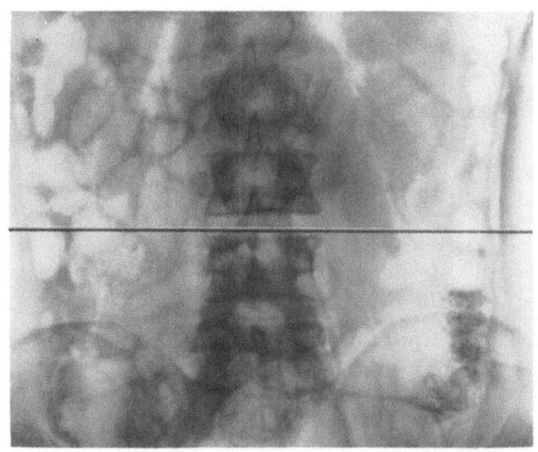

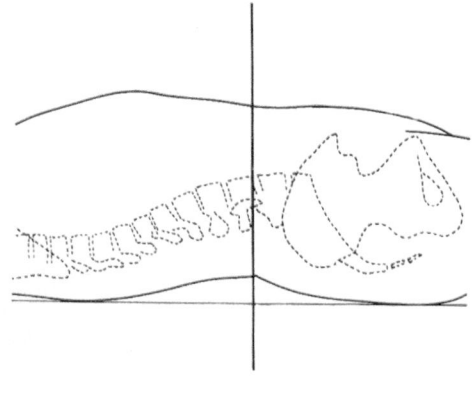

Fig. 358. Normal roentgenogram. Horizontal line showing the level tomographed

Fig. 359. Schematic drawing of the level tomographed

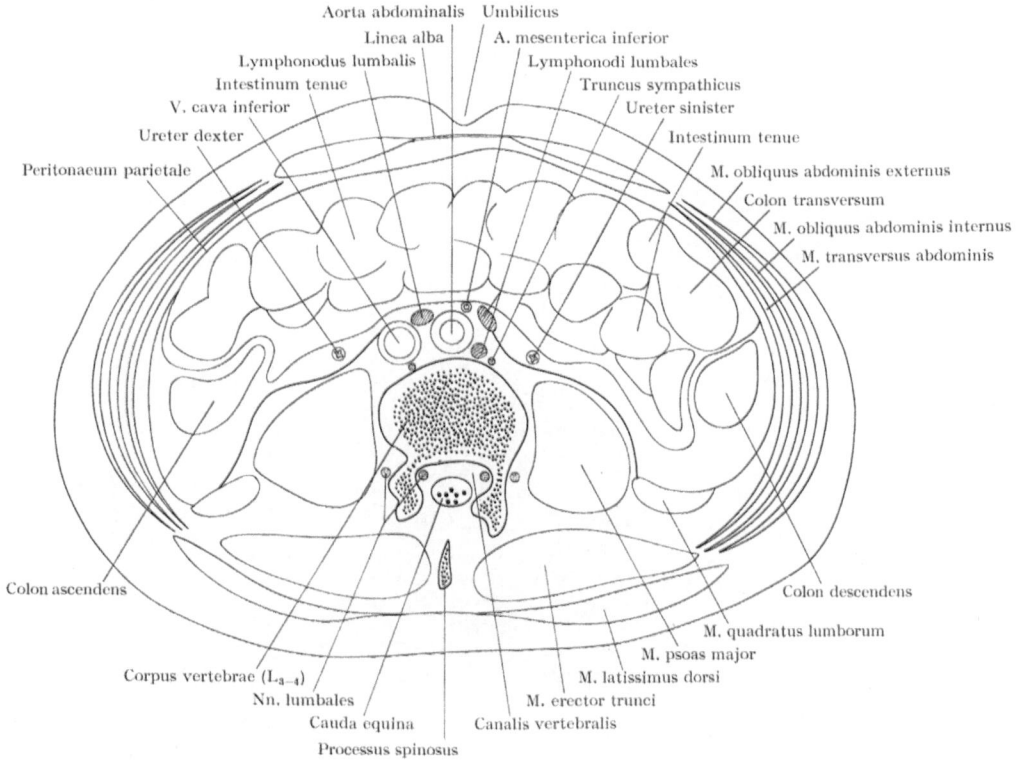

Fig. 360. Anatomical chart

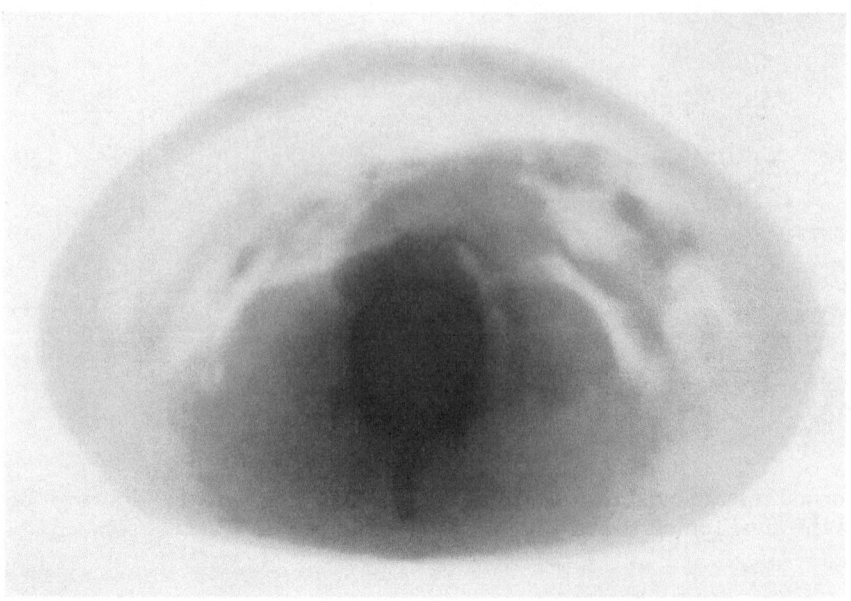

Fig. 361. Axial transverse tomogram

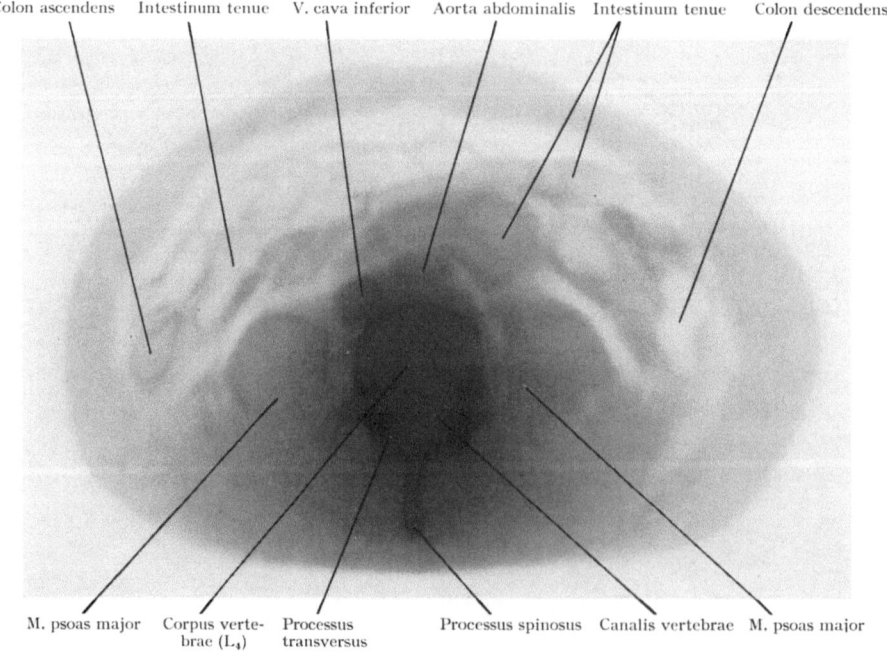

Colon ascendens   Intestinum tenue   V. cava inferior   Aorta abdominalis   Intestinum tenue   Colon descendens

M. psoas major   Corpus verte-   Processus   Processus spinosus   Canalis vertebrae   M. psoas major
                 brae (L$_4$)   transversus

Fig. 362. Interpretation

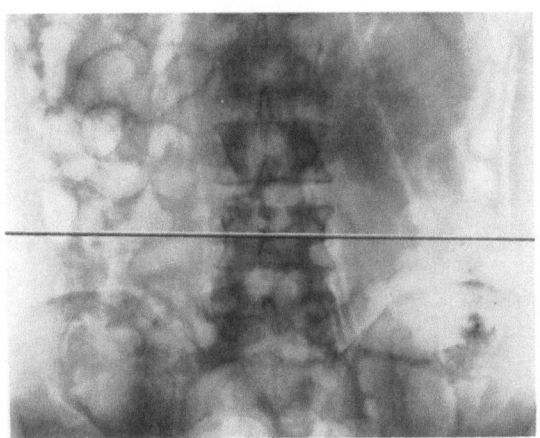

Fig. 363. Normal roentgenogram. Horizontal line showing the level tomographed

Fig. 364. Schematic drawing of the level tomographed

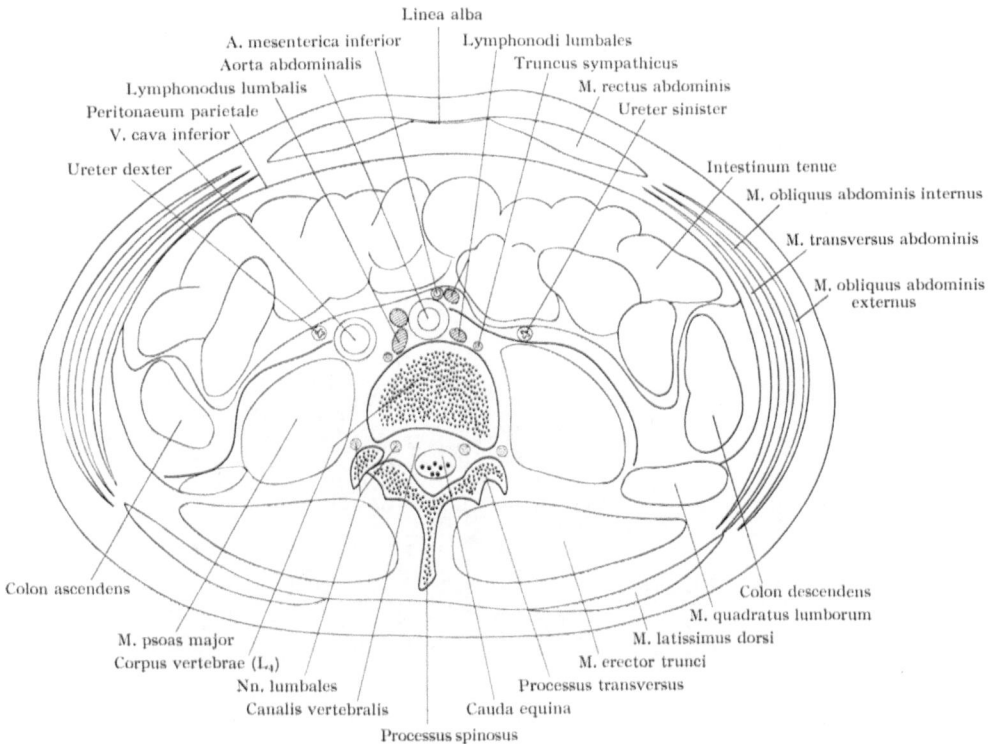

Linea alba
A. mesenterica inferior
Aorta abdominalis
Lymphonodus lumbalis
Peritonaeum parietale
V. cava inferior
Ureter dexter

Lymphonodi lumbales
Truncus sympathicus
M. rectus abdominis
Ureter sinister
Intestinum tenue
M. obliquus abdominis internus
M. transversus abdominis
M. obliquus abdominis externus

Colon ascendens
M. psoas major
Corpus vertebrae (L₄)
Nn. lumbales
Canalis vertebralis
Processus spinosus

Colon descendens
M. quadratus lumborum
M. latissimus dorsi
M. erector trunci
Processus transversus
Cauda equina

Fig. 365. Anatomical chart

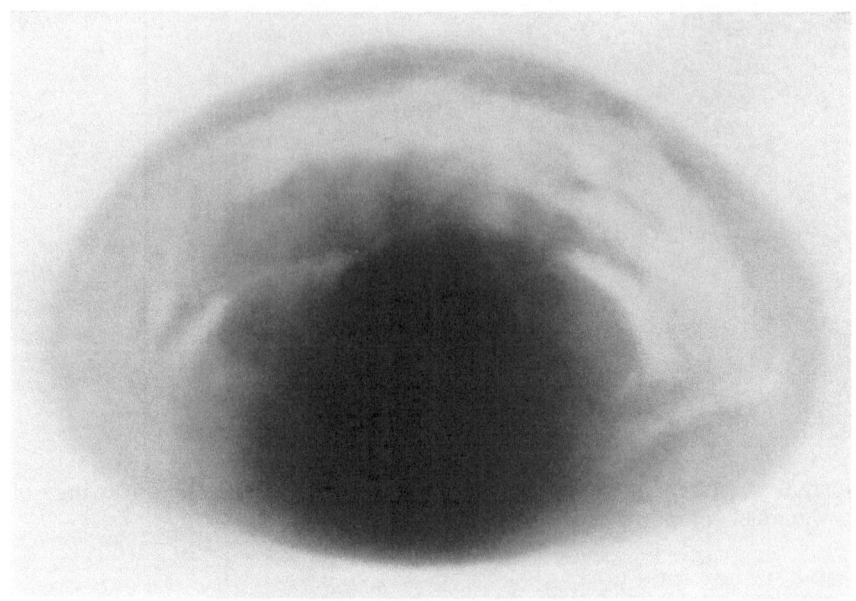

Fig. 366. Axial transverse tomogram

Colon ascendens   M. psoas major   V. cava inferior   Aorta abdominalis   Intestinum tenue

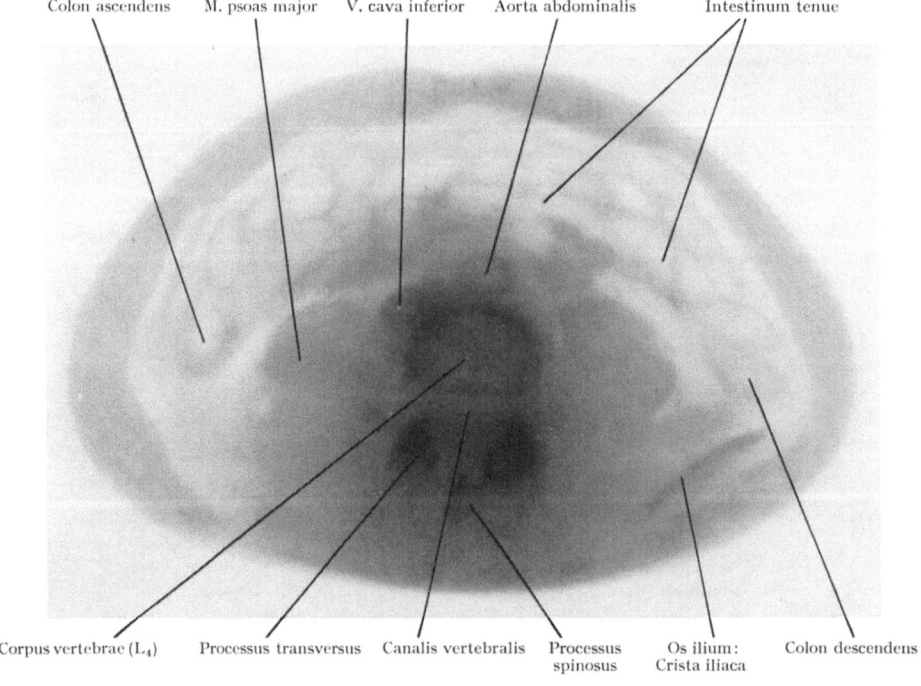

Corpus vertebrae (L$_4$)   Processus transversus   Canalis vertebralis   Processus spinosus   Os ilium: Crista iliaca   Colon descendens

Fig. 367. Interpretation

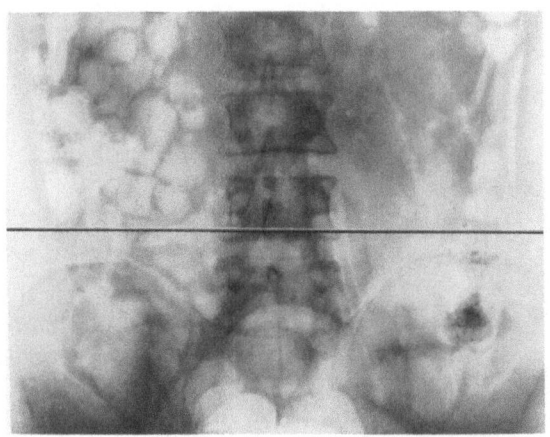

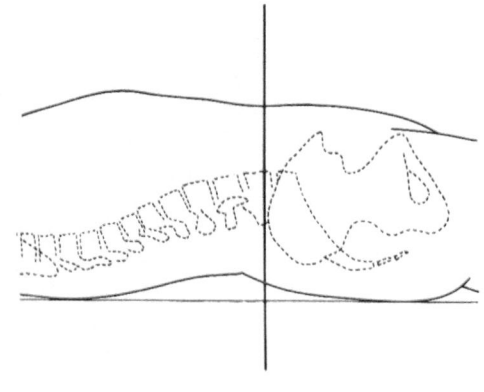

Fig. 368. Normal roentgenogram. Horizontal line showing the level tomographed

Fig. 369. Schematic drawing of the level tomographed

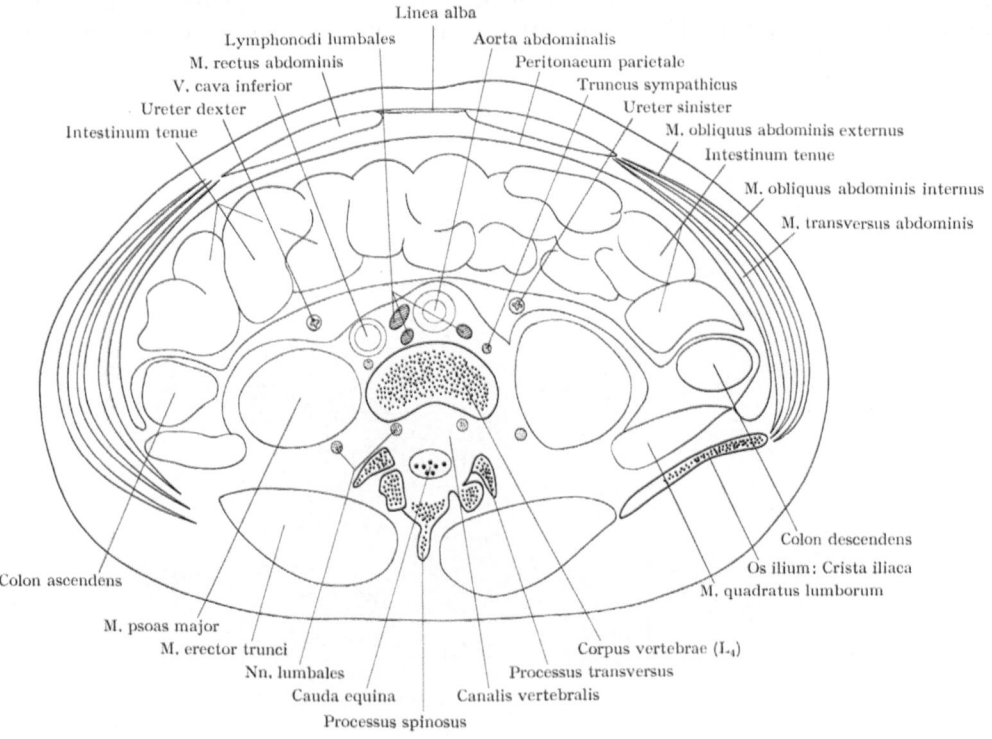

Fig. 370. Anatomical chart

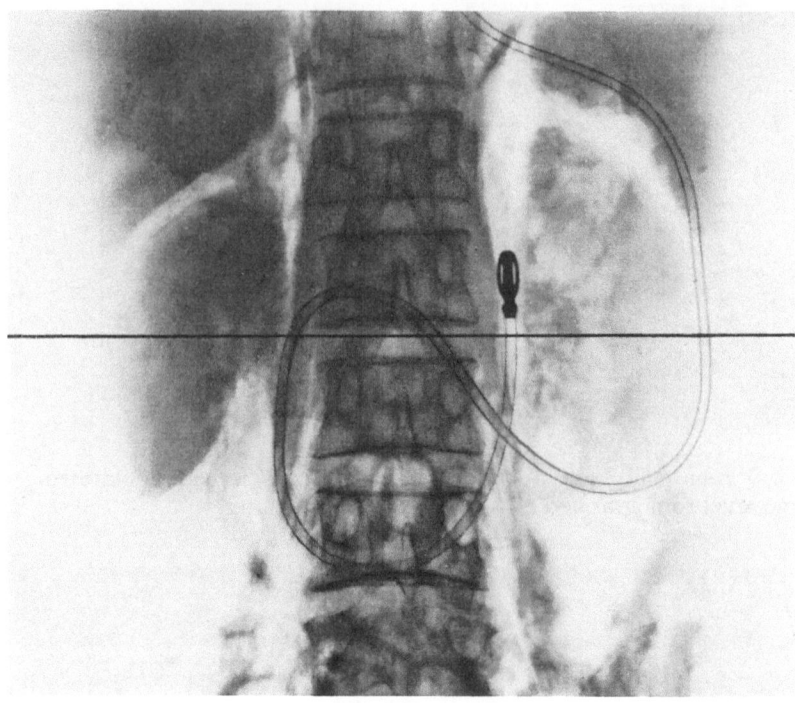

Fig. 371. Normal roentgenogram of the duodenum. The tip of the duodenal tube is located at the flexura duodenojejunalis. The retroperitoneal space is insufflated with air. The horizontal line shows the level tomographed

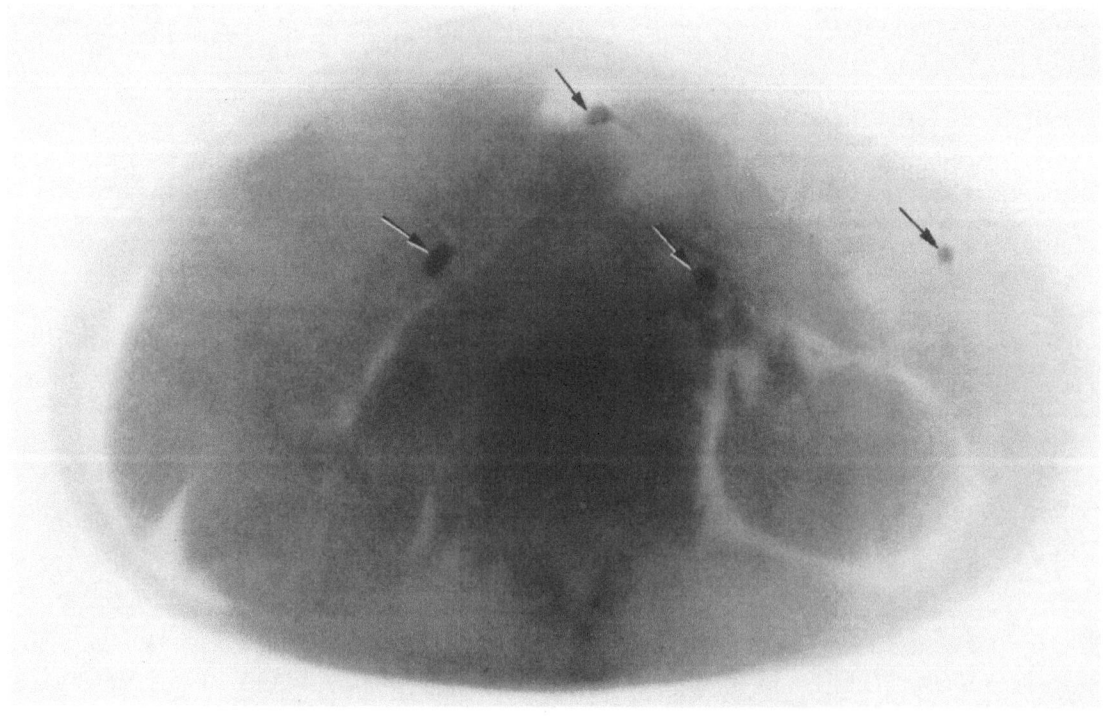

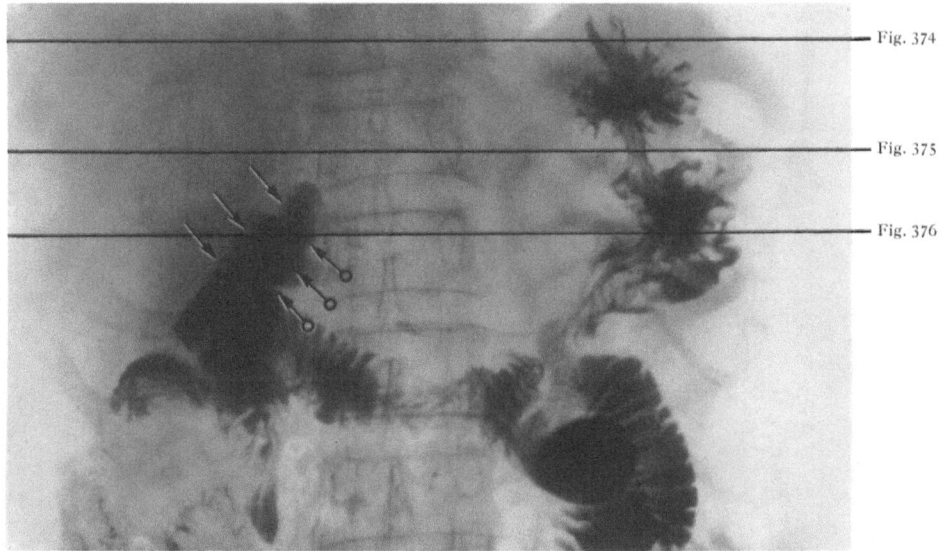

Fig. 374

Fig. 375

Fig. 376

Fig. 373. Normal roentgenogram of the upper abdomen taken following the introduction of contrast media into the stomach, gallbladder and urinary pelvis, without air insufflation of the retroperitoneal space. Horizontal lines showing the levels tomographed

Fig. 372. Axial transverse tomogram shows the cross-section images of the duodenal tube seen (⟋) in the body and pylorus of the stomach and in the descending and ascending duodenum (see Figs. 306—310, 311—315, 316—320, 321—325, 326—330)

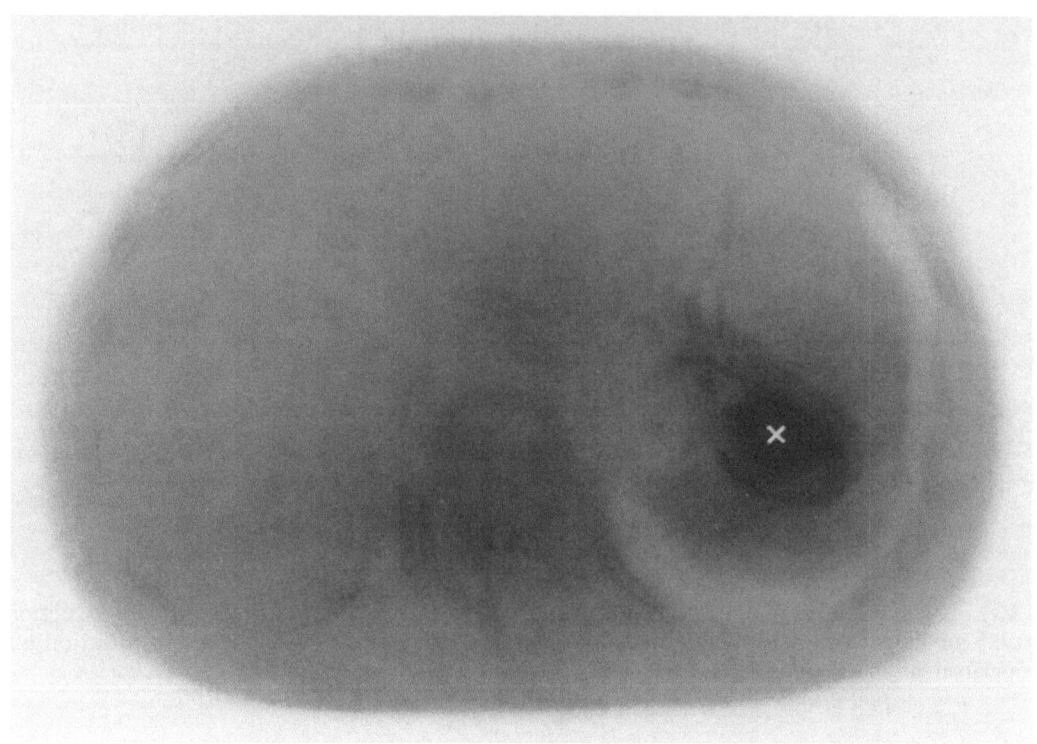

Fig. 374. Axial transverse tomogram shows the cardia (✕) of the stomach (see Figs. 286—290)

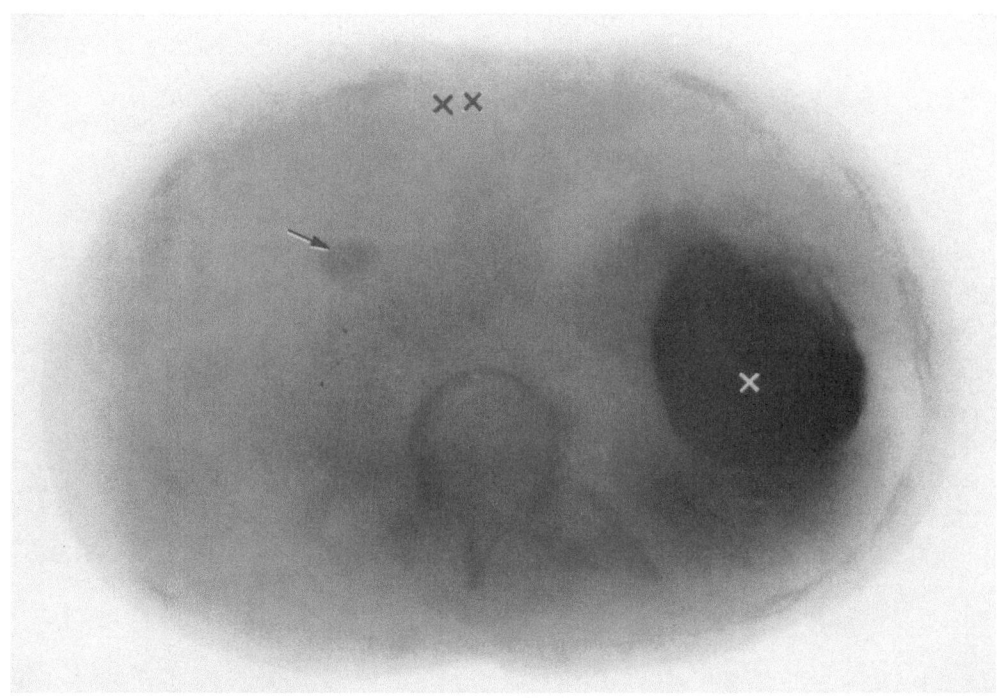

Fig. 375. Axial transverse tomogram shows the body (✕) and pylorus (✕✕) of the stomach and the upper part of the gallbladder (╱) (see Figs. 295, 300, 305, 310)

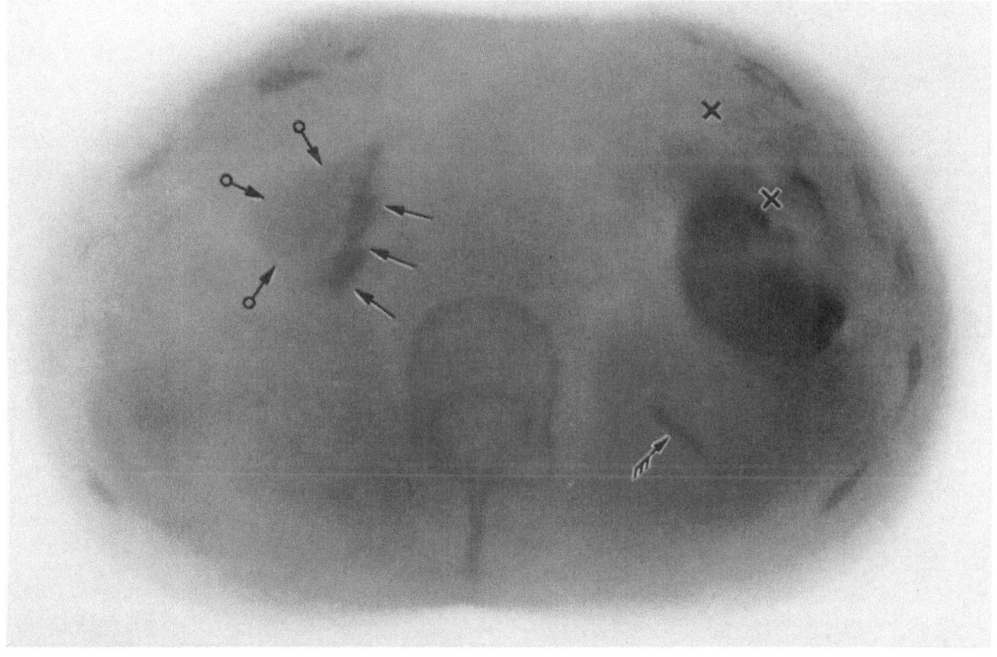

Fig. 376. Axial transverse tomogram shows the antrum (✕) of the stomach, duodenum (╱), gallbladder (✓) and renal pelvis (✓) (see Figs. 310, 315)

Lower Abdomen

Six axial transverse tomograms of female subject with the rectum, the vagina and the bladder contrasted by air

and

Five axial transverse tomograms of male subject.

Appendices:
1. Axial transverse tomogram of urethra with catheter introduced.
2. Axial transverse tomogram of iliac artery with catheter introduced.

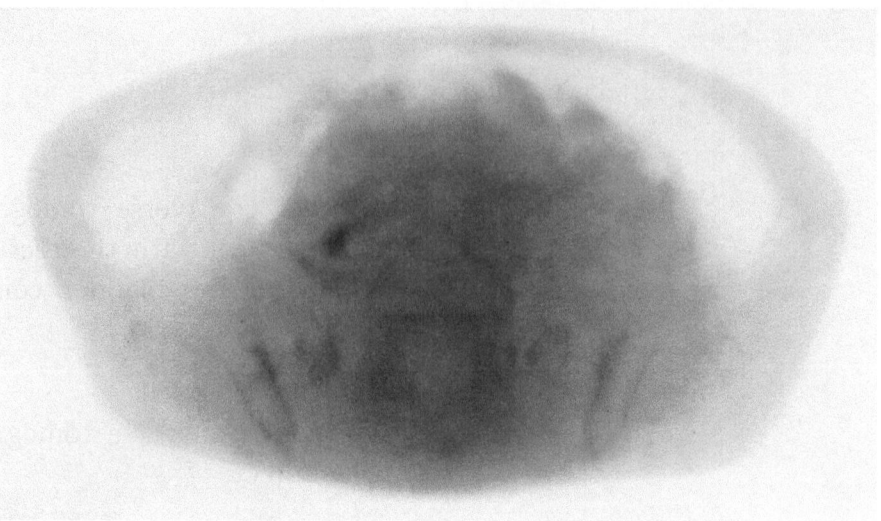

Fig. 377. Axial transverse tomogram

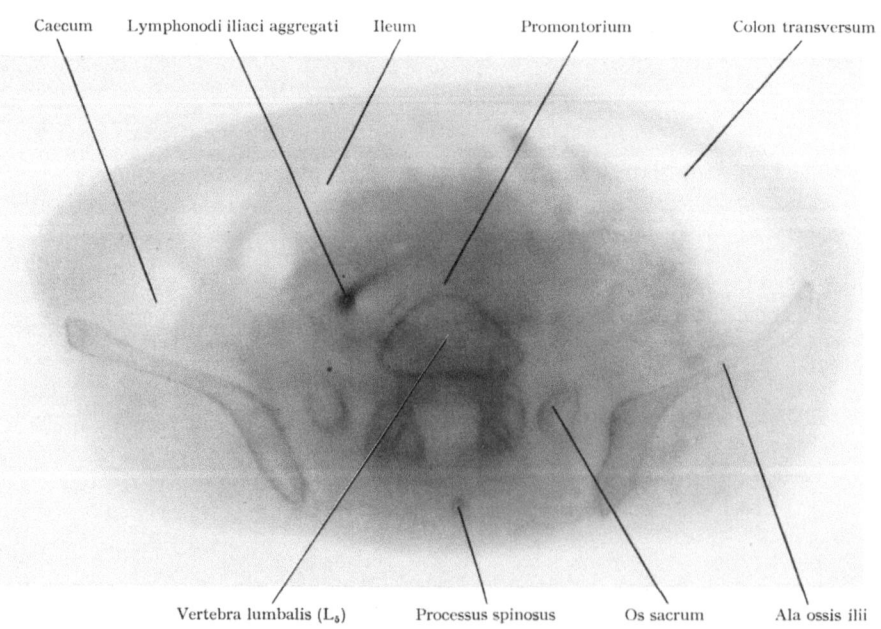

Caecum   Lymphonodi iliaci aggregati   Ileum   Promontorium   Colon transversum

Vertebra lumbalis (L$_5$)   Processus spinosus   Os sacrum   Ala ossis ilii

Fig. 378. Interpretation

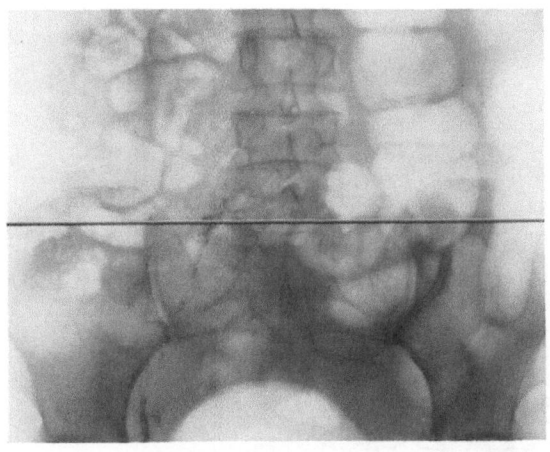

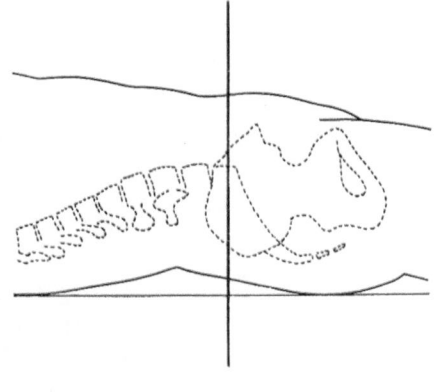

Fig. 379. Normal roentgenogram. Horizontal line showing the level tomographed

Fig. 380. Schematic drawing of the level tomographed

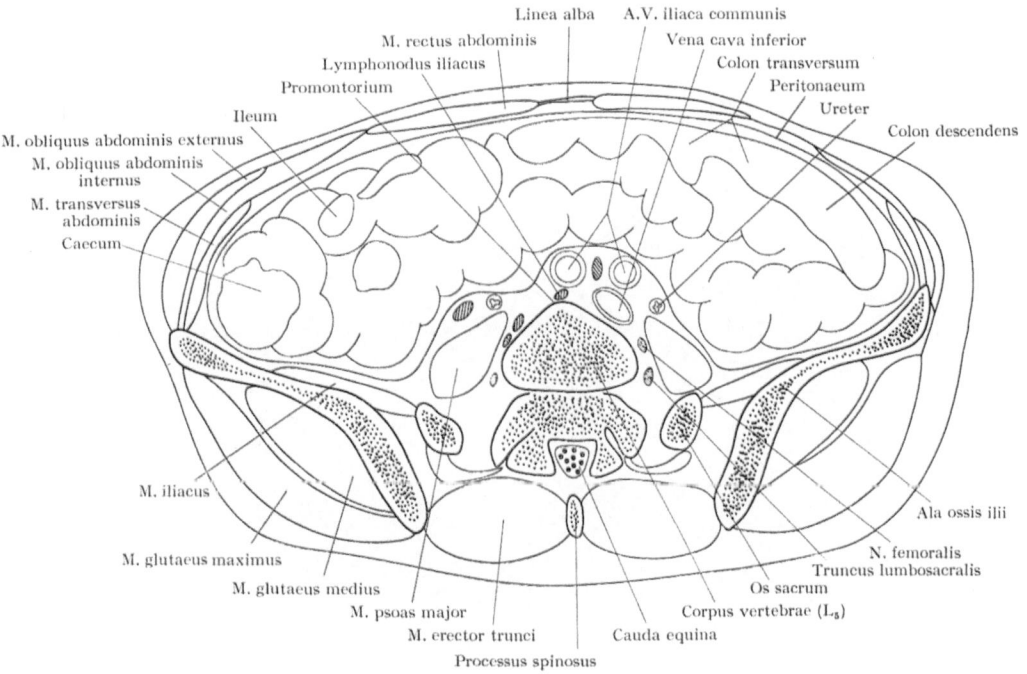

Fig. 381. Anatomical chart

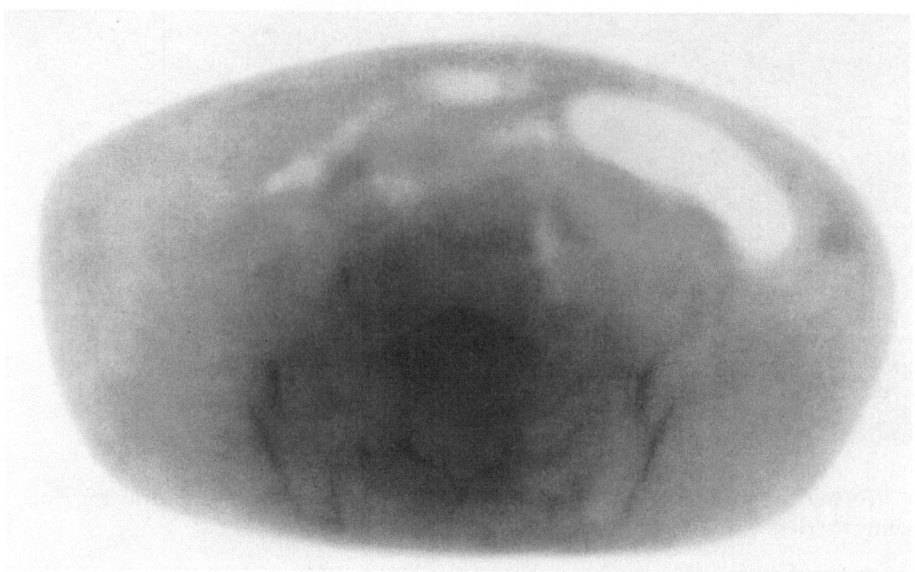

Fig. 382. Axial transverse tomogram

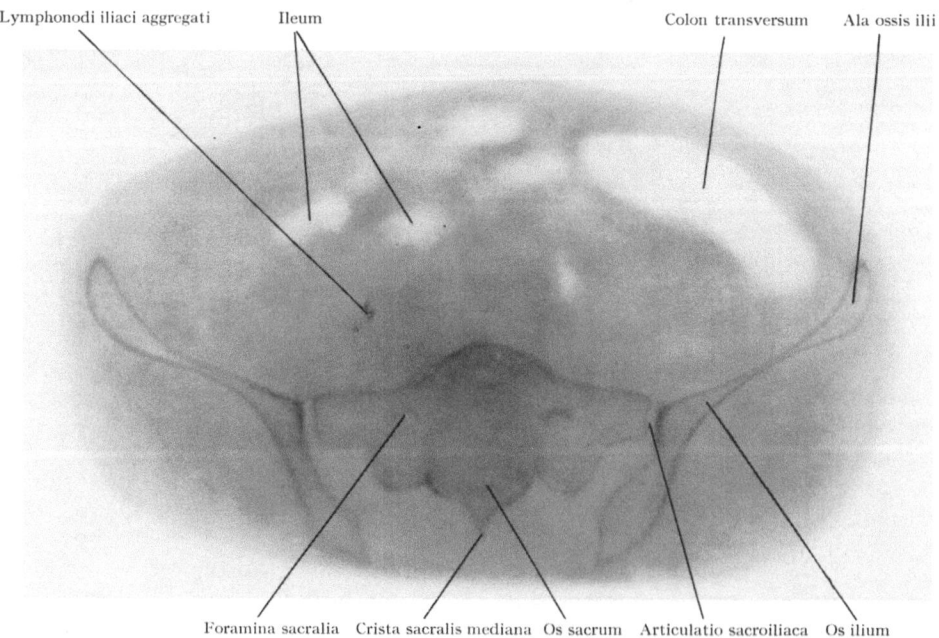

Fig. 383. Interpretation

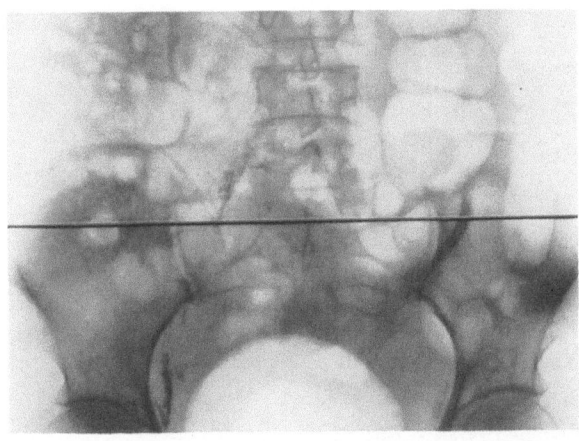
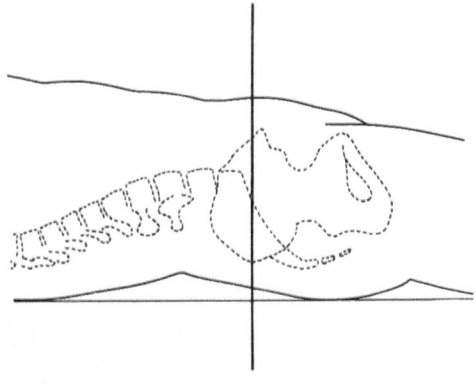

Fig. 384. Normal roentgenogram. Horizontal line showing the level tomographed

Fig. 385. Schematic drawing of the level tomographed

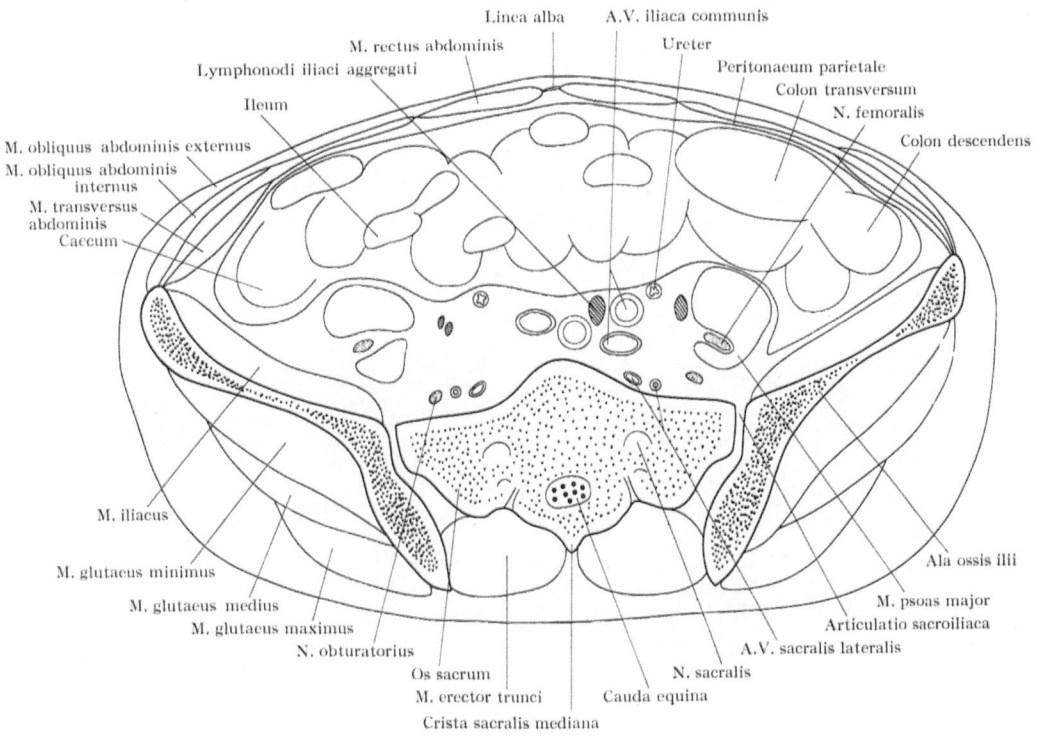

Fig. 386. Anatomical chart

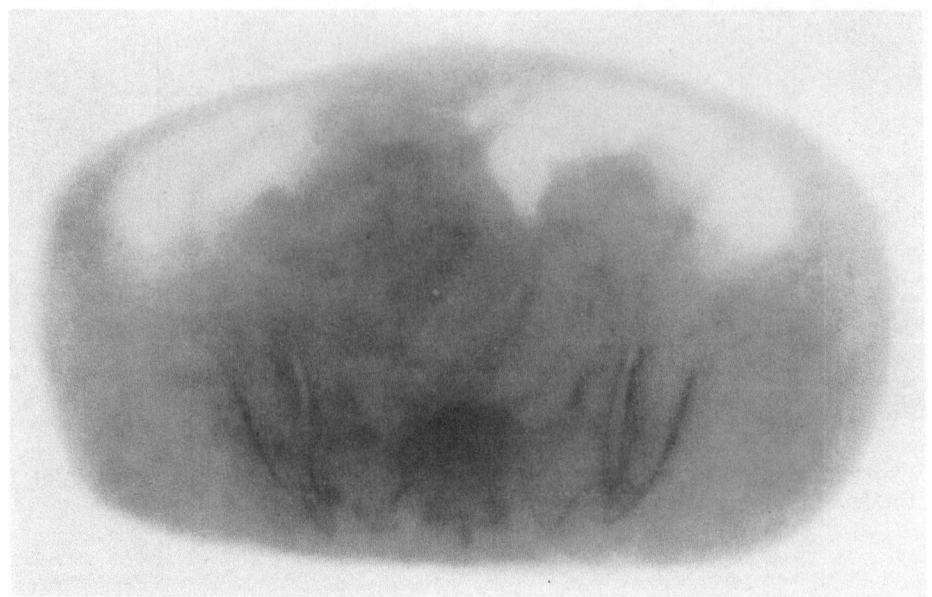

Fig. 387. Axial transverse tomogram

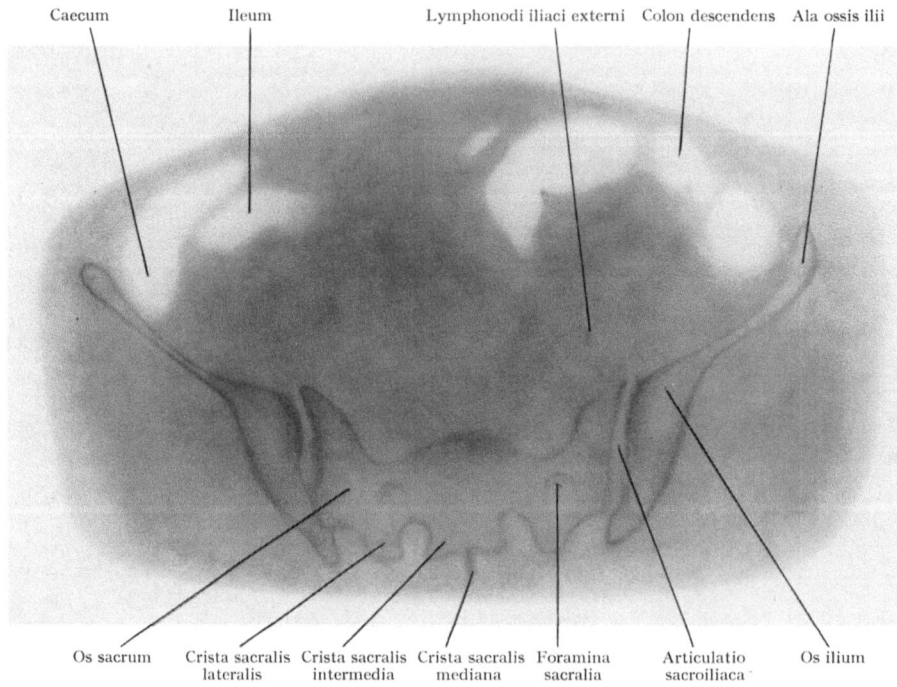

Caecum   Ileum   Lymphonodi iliaci externi Colon descendens Ala ossis ilii

Os sacrum   Crista sacralis   Crista sacralis   Crista sacralis   Foramina   Articulatio   Os ilium
             lateralis   intermedia   mediana   sacralia   sacroiliaca

Fig. 388. Interpretation

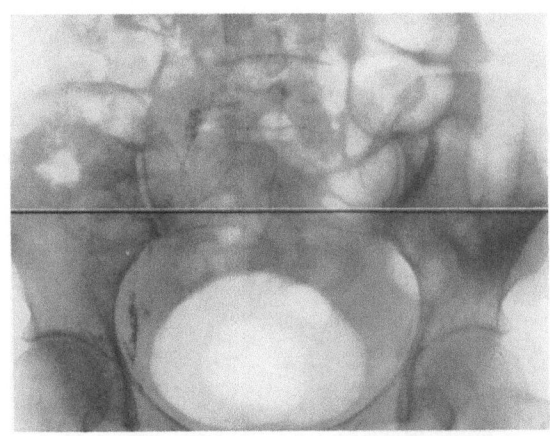

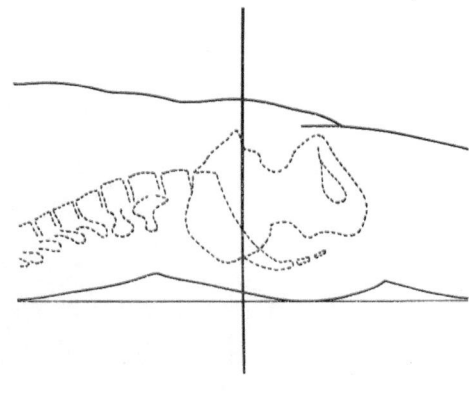

Fig. 389. Normal roentgenogram. Horizontal line showing the level tomographed

Fig. 390. Schematic drawing of the level tomographed

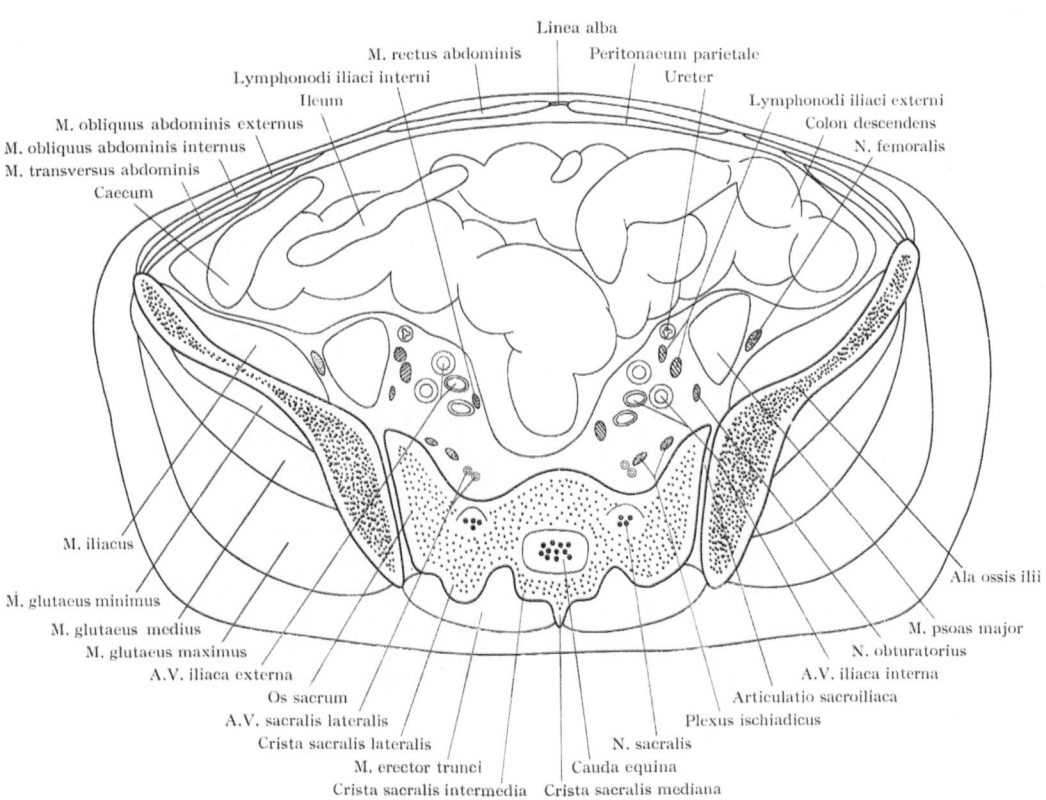

Fig. 391. Anatomical chart

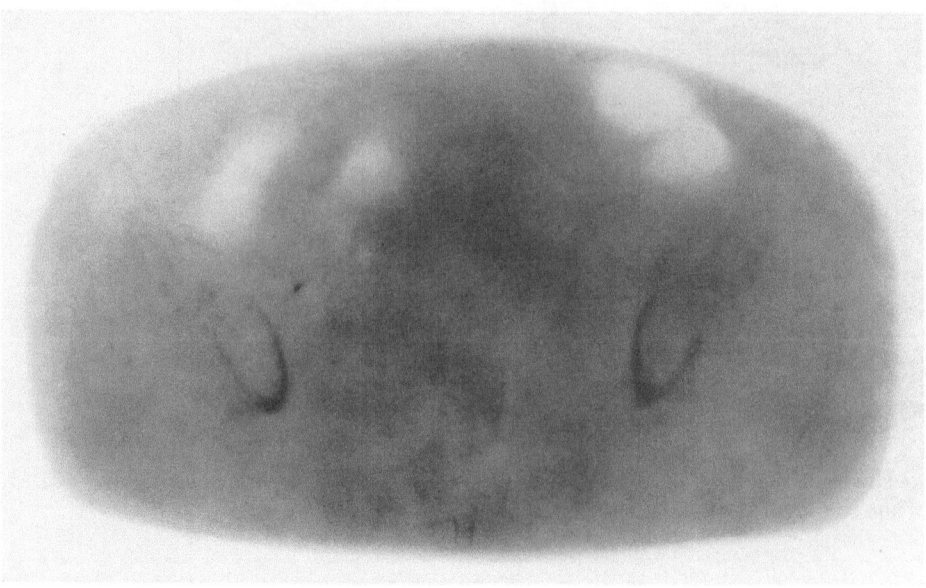

Fig. 392. Axial transverse tomogram

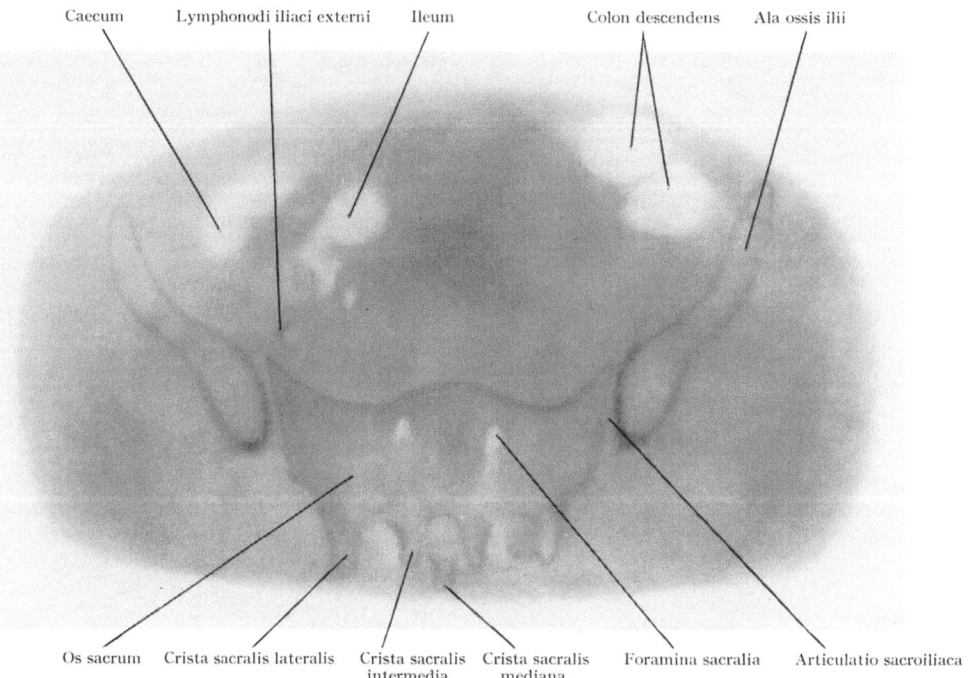

Caecum   Lymphonodi iliaci externi   Ileum   Colon descendens   Ala ossis ilii

Os sacrum   Crista sacralis lateralis   Crista sacralis   Crista sacralis   Foramina sacralia   Articulatio sacroiliaca
                                          intermedia   mediana

Fig. 393. Interpretation

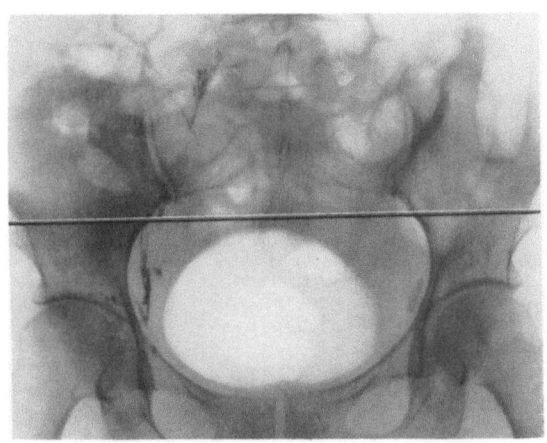

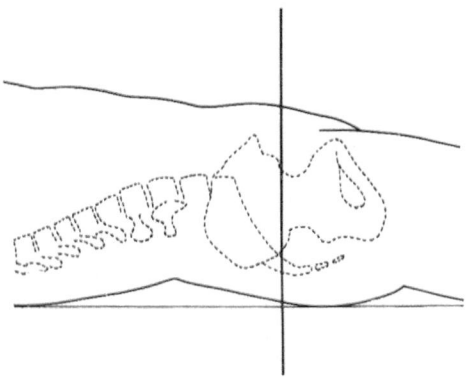

Fig. 394. Normal roentgenogram. Horizontal line showing the level tomographed

Fig. 395. Schematic drawing of the level tomographed

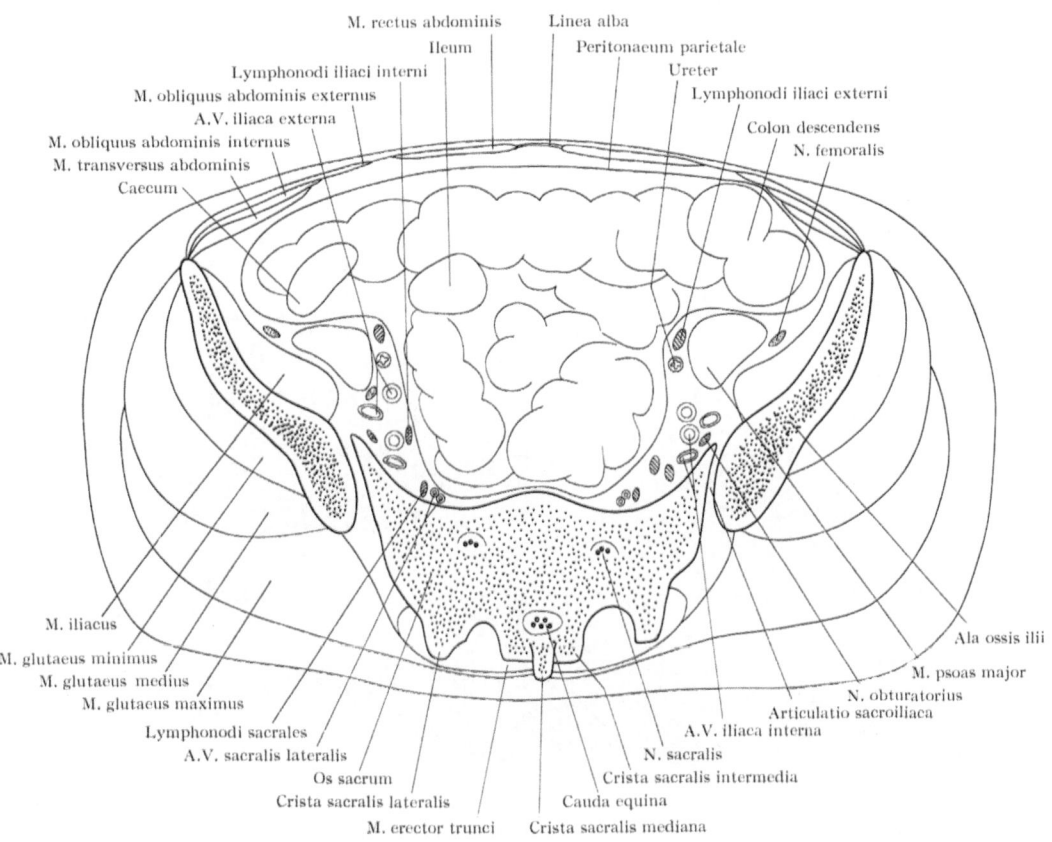

187

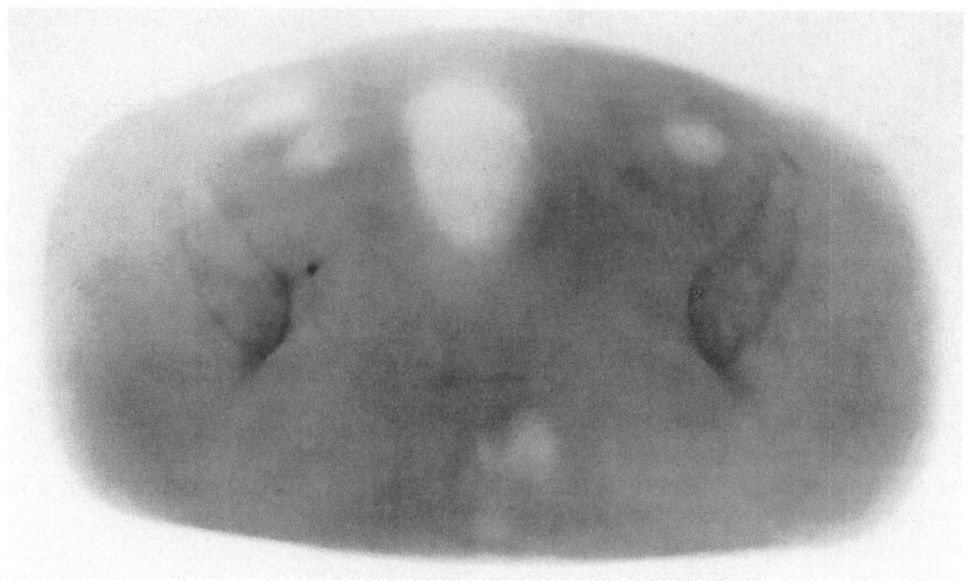

Fig. 397. Axial transverse tomogram

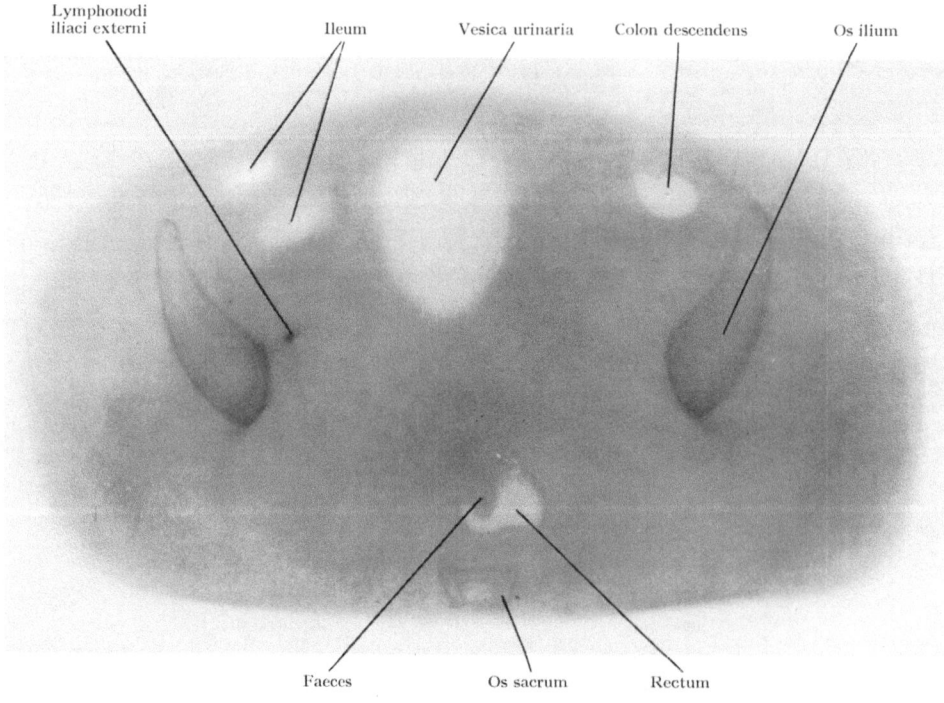

Fig. 398. Interpretation

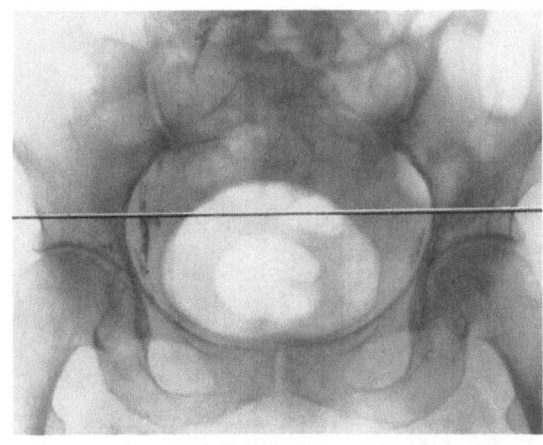

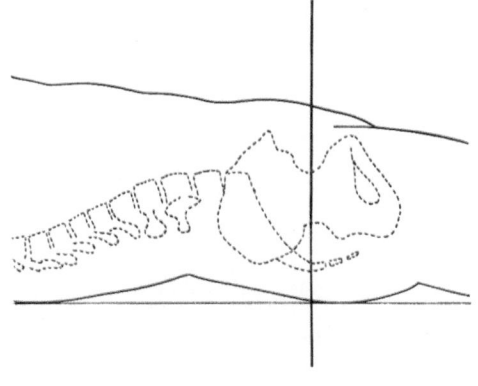

Fig. 399. Normal roentgenogram. Horizontal line showing the level tomographed

Fig. 400. Schematic drawing of the level tomographed

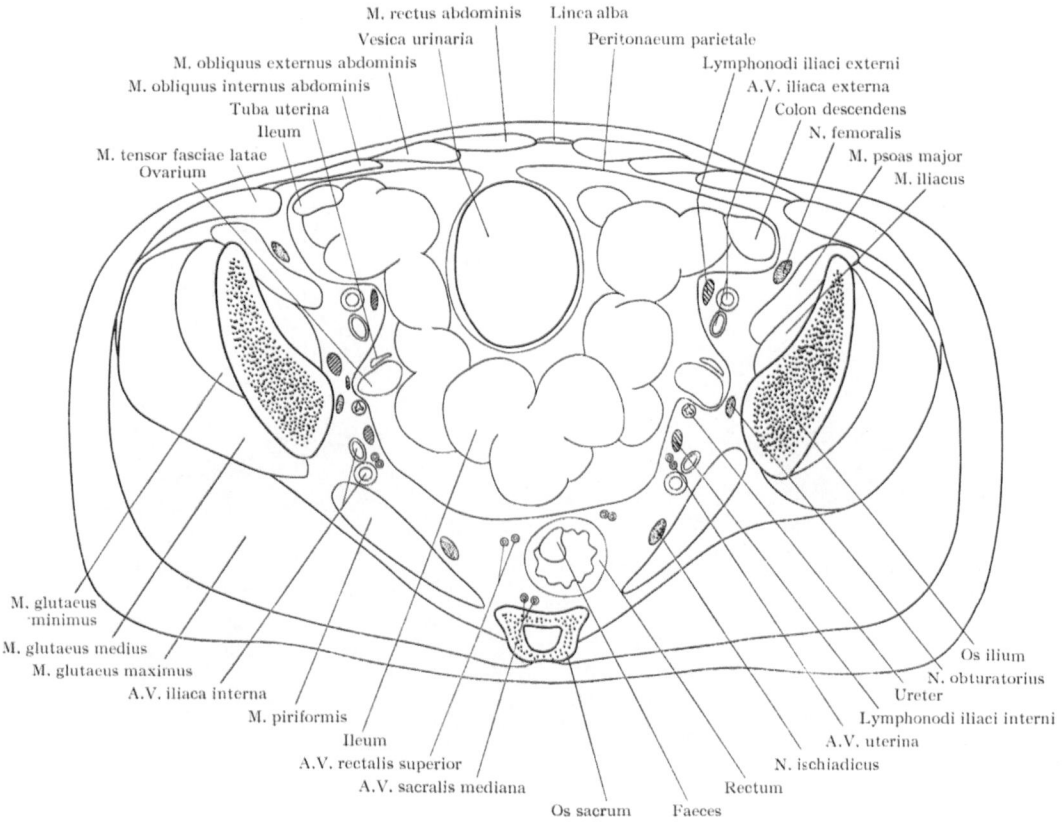

Fig. 401. Anatomical chart

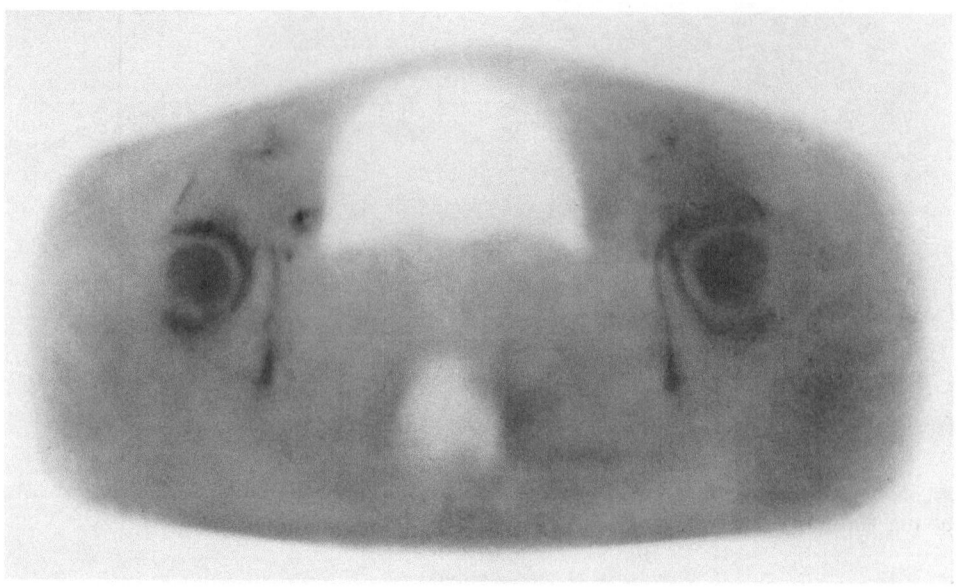

Fig. 402. Axial transverse tomogram

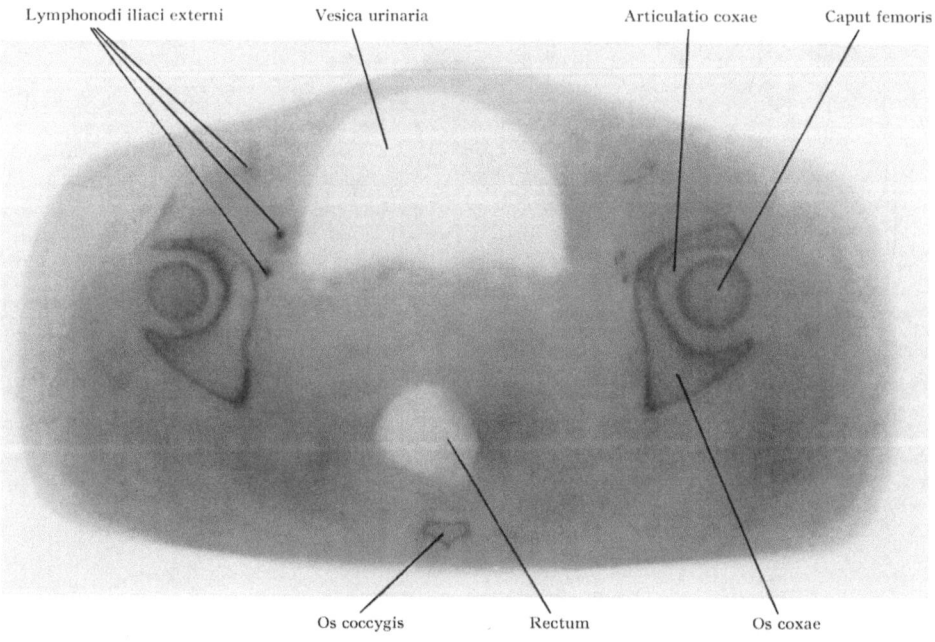

Lymphonodi iliaci externi   Vesica urinaria   Articulatio coxae   Caput femoris

Os coccygis   Rectum   Os coxae

Fig. 403. Interpretation

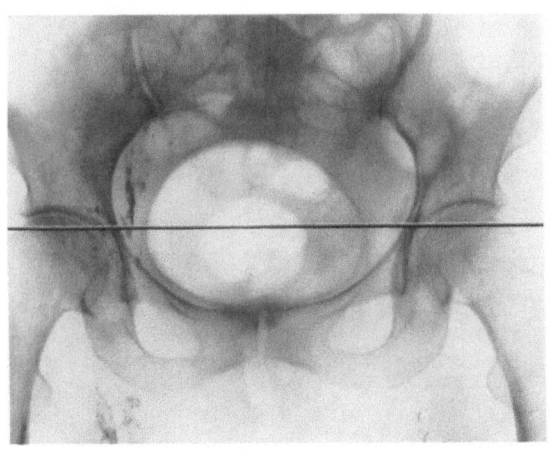

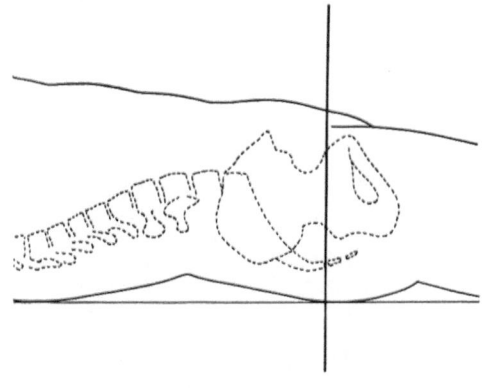

Fig. 404. Normal roentgenogram. Horizontal line showing the level tomographed

Fig. 405. Schematic drawing of the level tomographed

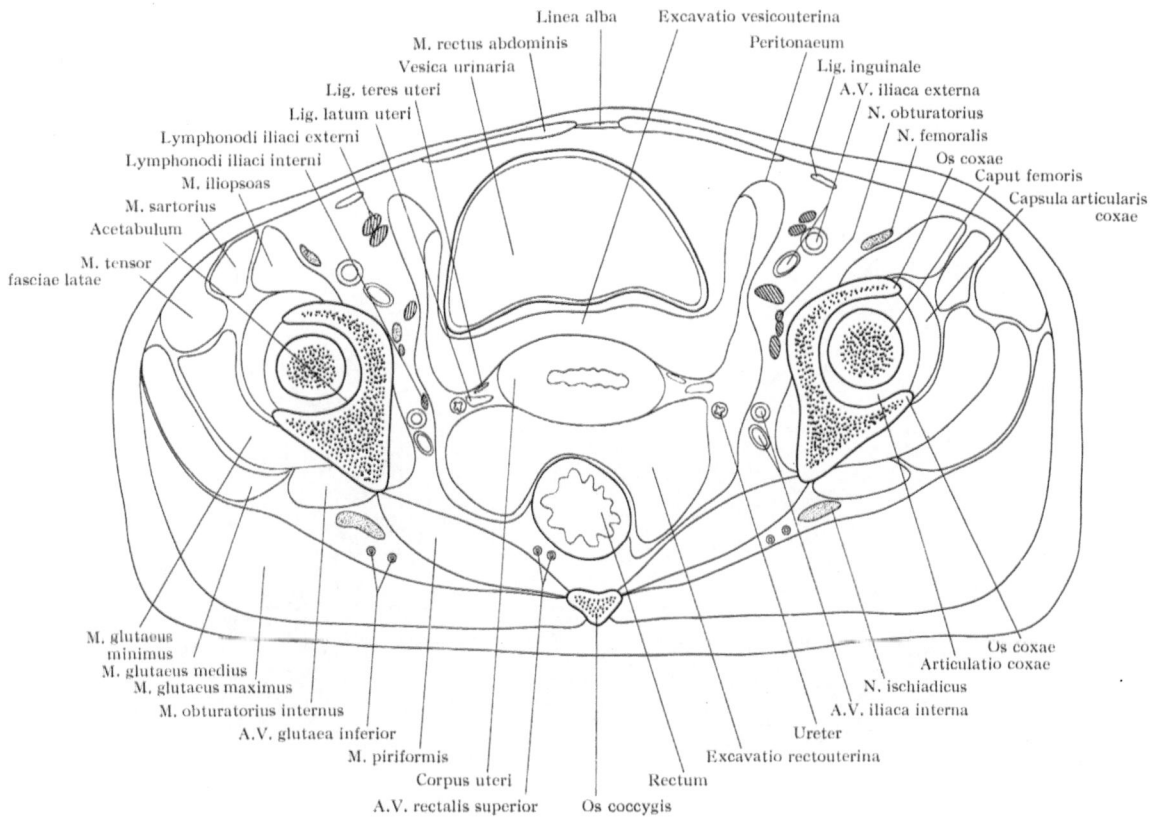

Fig. 406. Anatomical chart

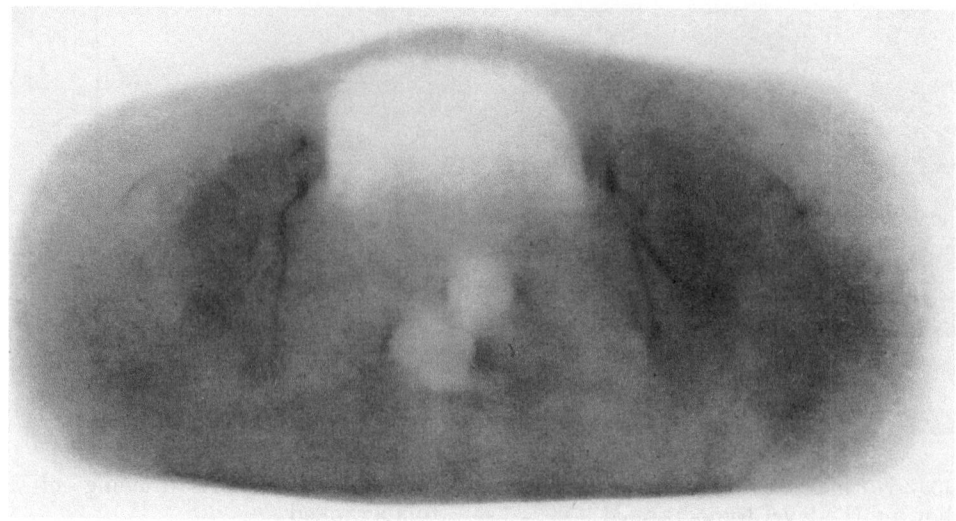

Fig. 407. Axial transverse tomogram

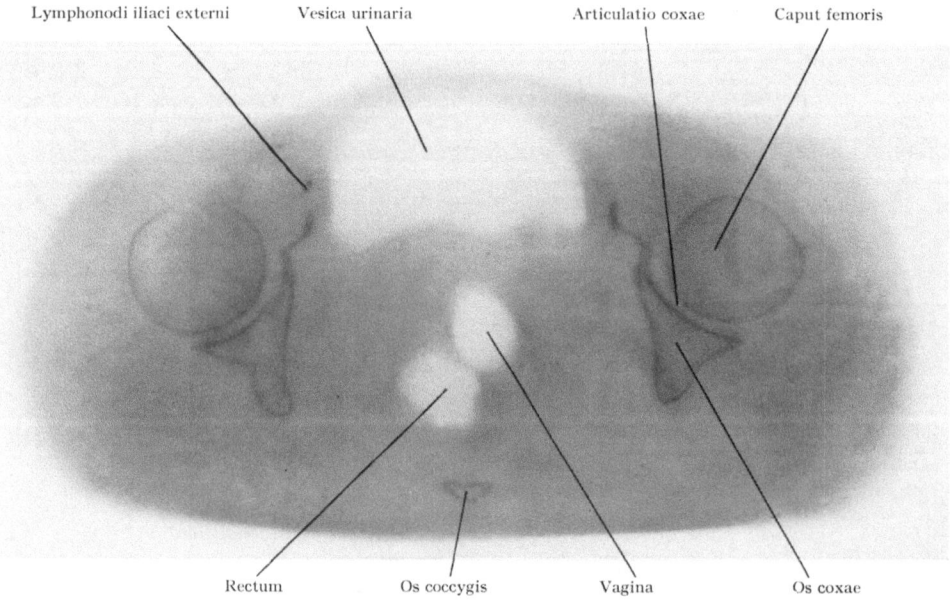

Fig. 408. Interpretation

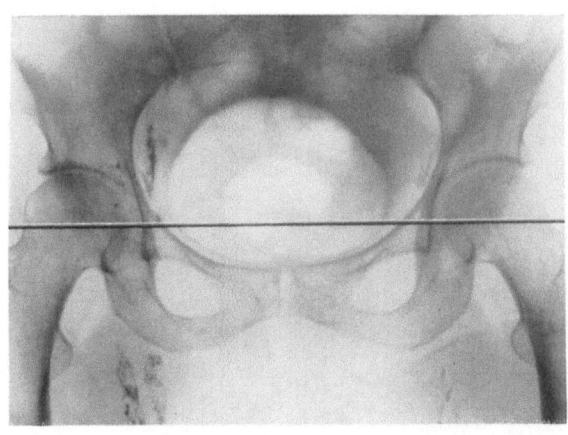

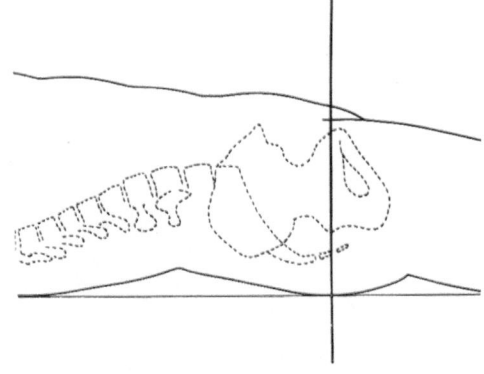

Fig. 409. Normal roentgenogram. Horizontal line showing the level tomographed

Fig. 410. Schematic drawing of the level tomographed

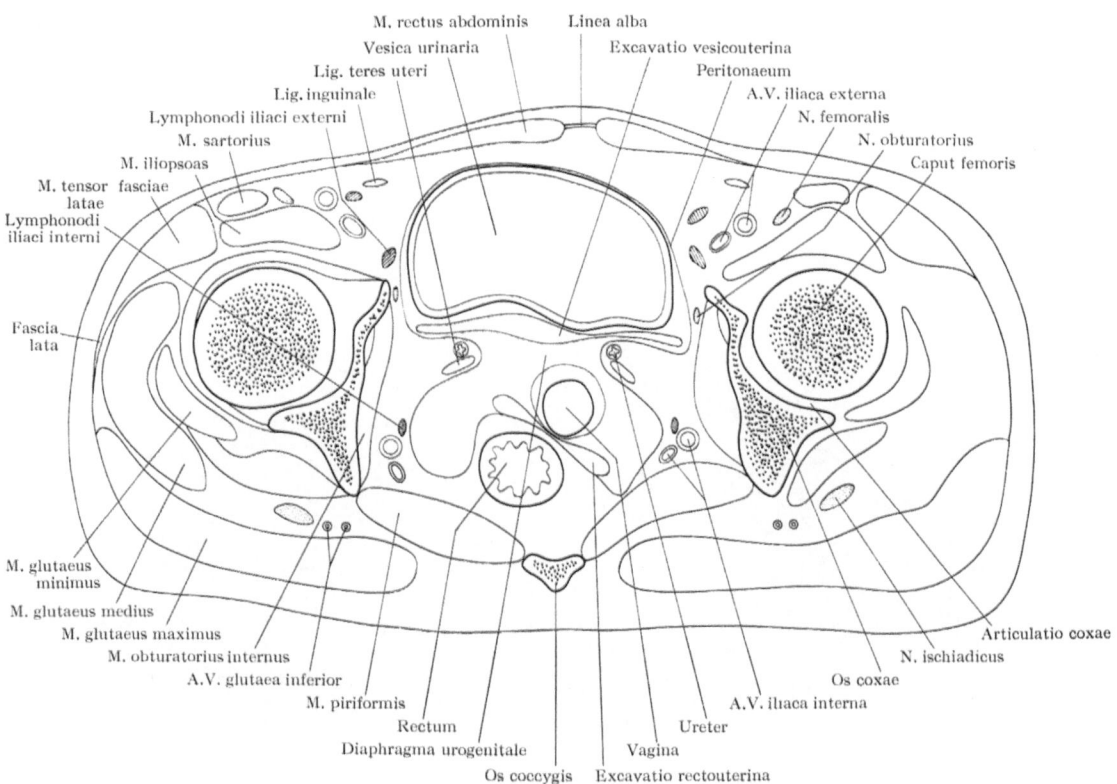

Fig. 411. Anatomical chart

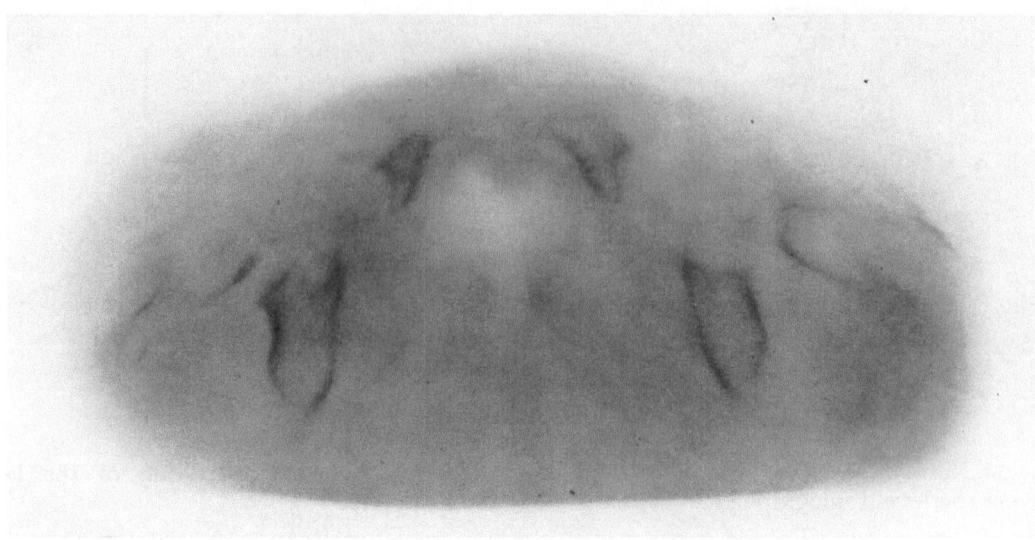

Fig. 412. Axial transverse tomogram

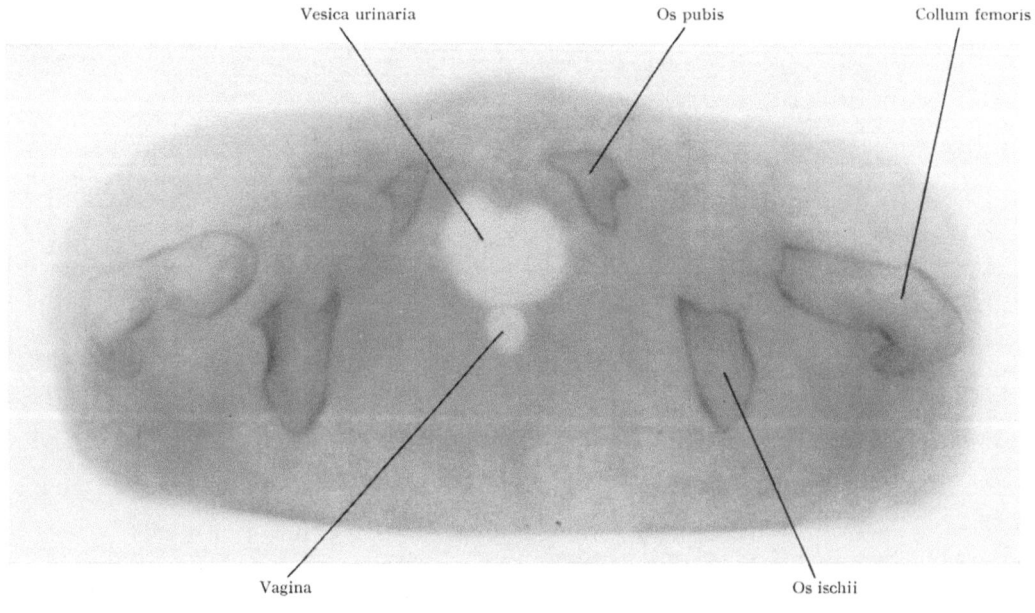

Fig. 413. Interpretation

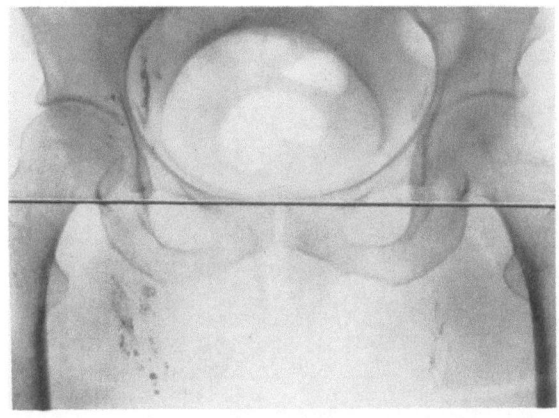

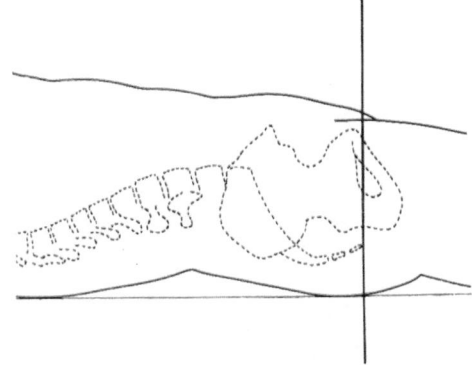

Fig. 414. Normal roentgenogram. Horizontal line showing the level tomographed

Fig. 415. Schematic drawing of the level tomographed

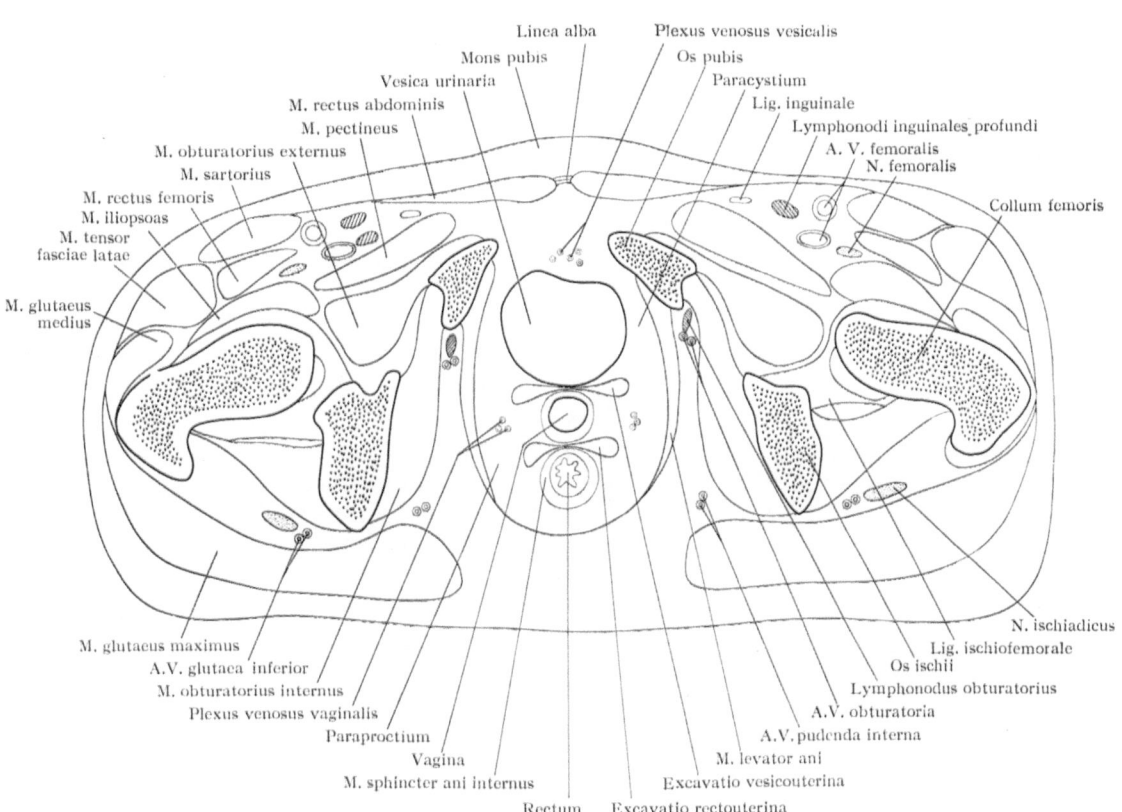

Fig. 416. Anatomical chart

195

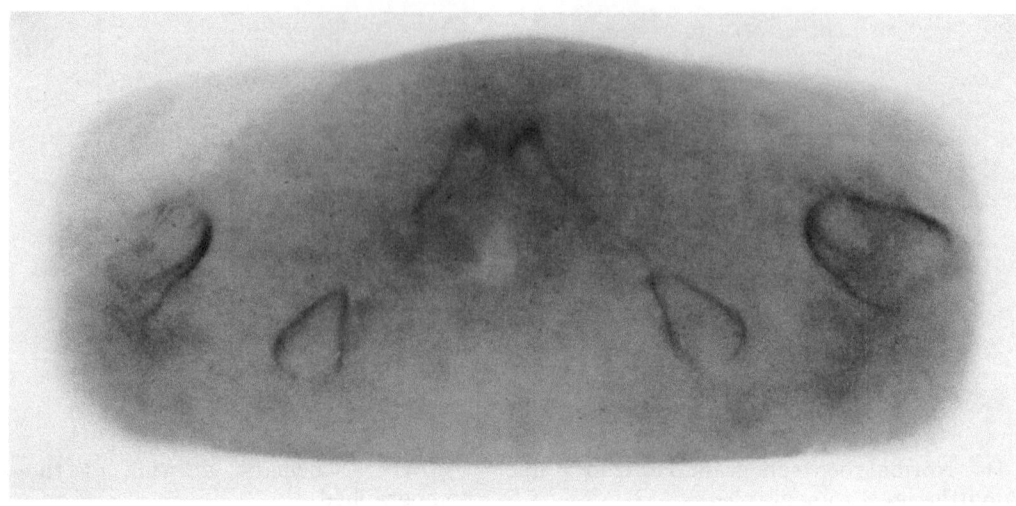

Fig. 417. Axial transverse tomogram

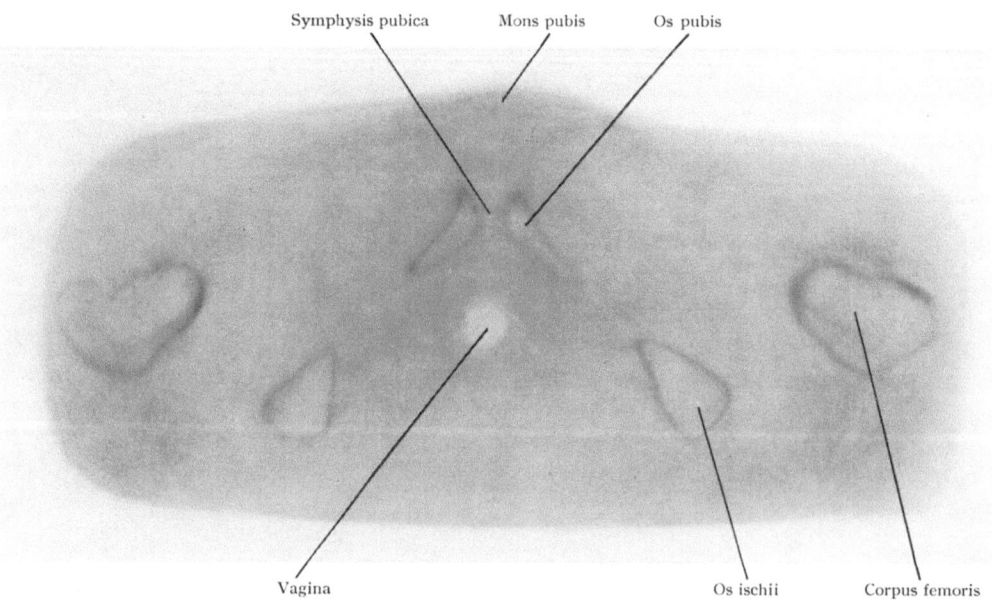

Fig. 418. Interpretation

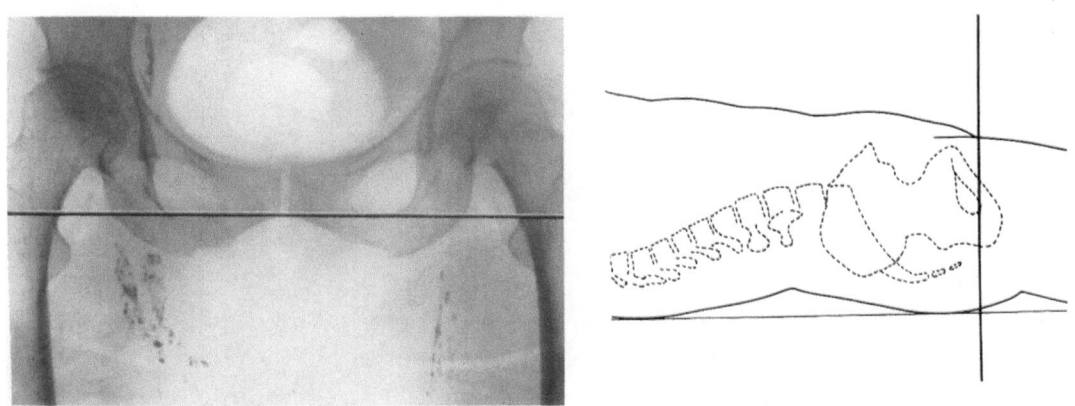

Fig. 419. Normal roentgenogram. Horizontal line showing the level tomographed

Fig. 420. Schematic drawing of the level tomographed

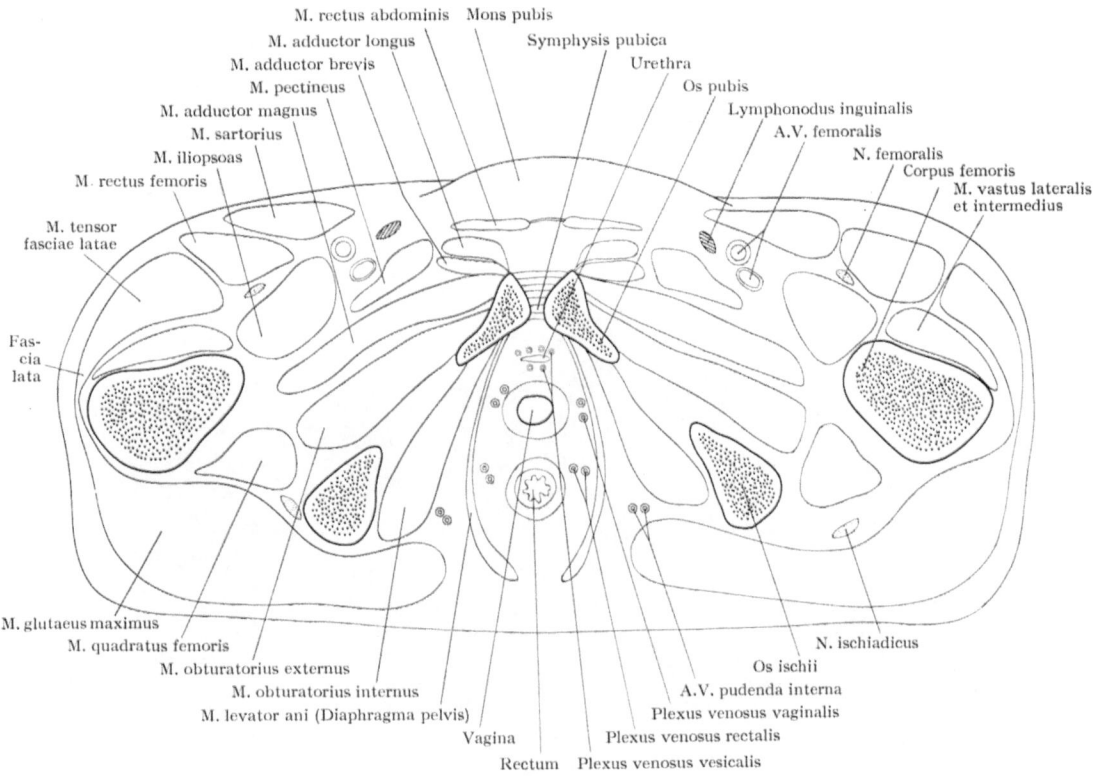

M. rectus abdominis   Mons pubis
M. adductor longus   Symphysis pubica
M. adductor brevis   Urethra
M. pectineus   Os pubis
M. adductor magnus   Lymphonodus inguinalis
M. sartorius   A.V. femoralis
M. iliopsoas   N. femoralis
M. rectus femoris   Corpus femoris
    M. vastus lateralis
M. tensor   et intermedius
fasciae latae

Fas-
cia
lata

M. glutaeus maximus   N. ischiadicus
M. quadratus femoris   Os ischii
M. obturatorius externus   A.V. pudenda interna
M. obturatorius internus   Plexus venosus vaginalis
M. levator ani (Diaphragma pelvis)   Plexus venosus rectalis
Vagina   Plexus venosus vesicalis
Rectum

Fig. 421. Anatomical chart

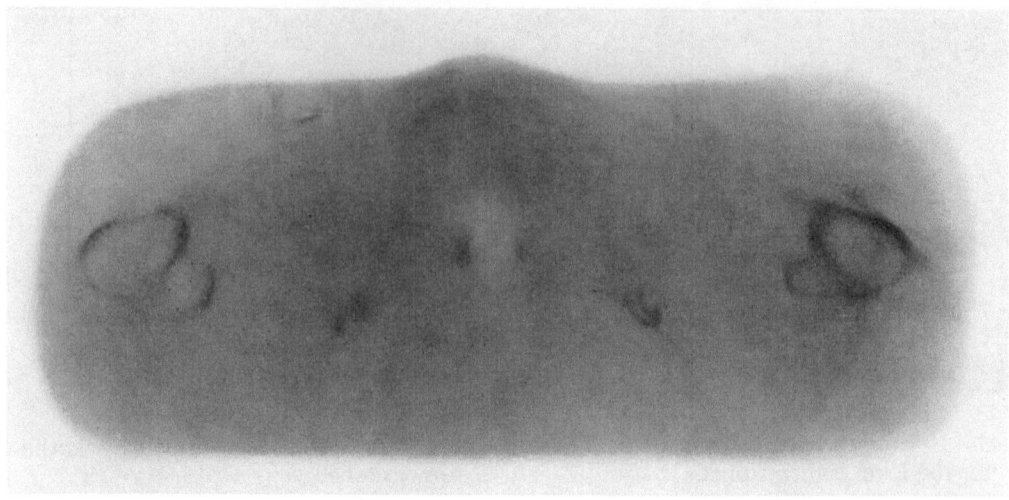

Fig. 422. Axial transverse tomogram

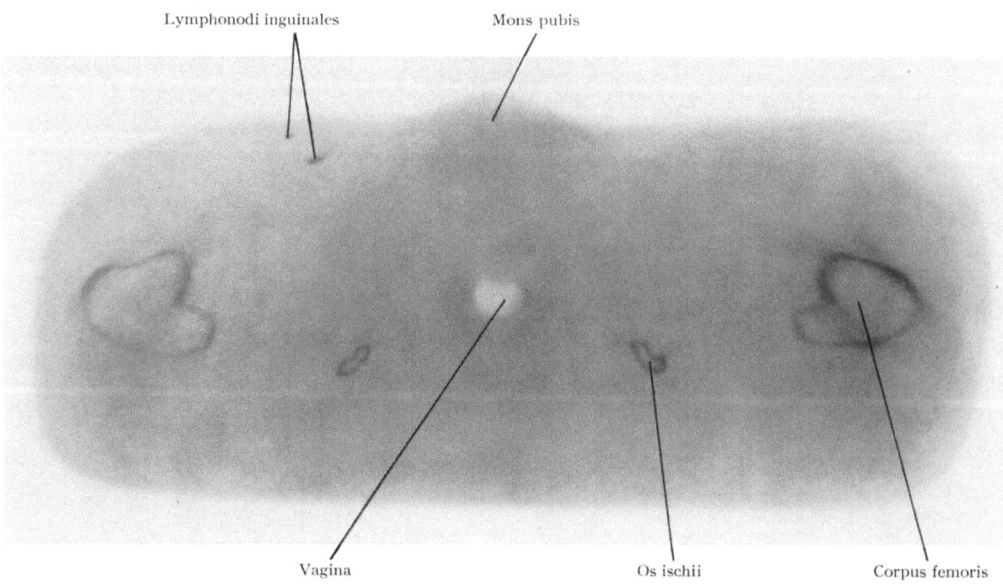

Lymphonodi inguinales   Mons pubis

Vagina   Os ischii   Corpus femoris

Fig. 423. Interpretation

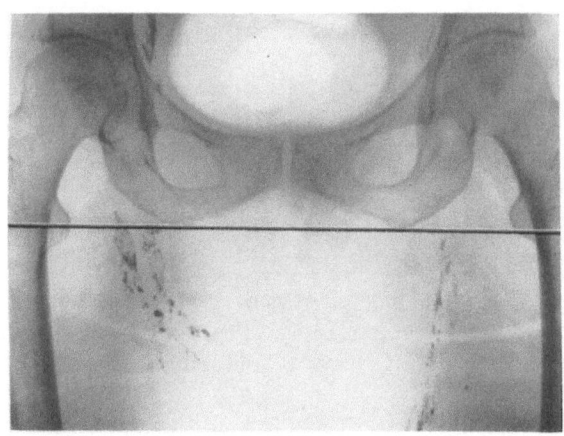

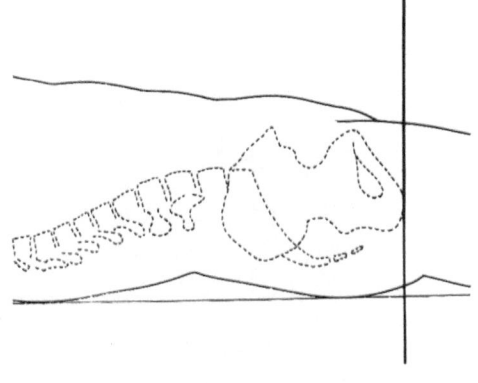

Fig. 424. Normal roentgenogram. Horizontal line showing the level tomographed

Fig. 425. Schematic drawing of the level tomographed

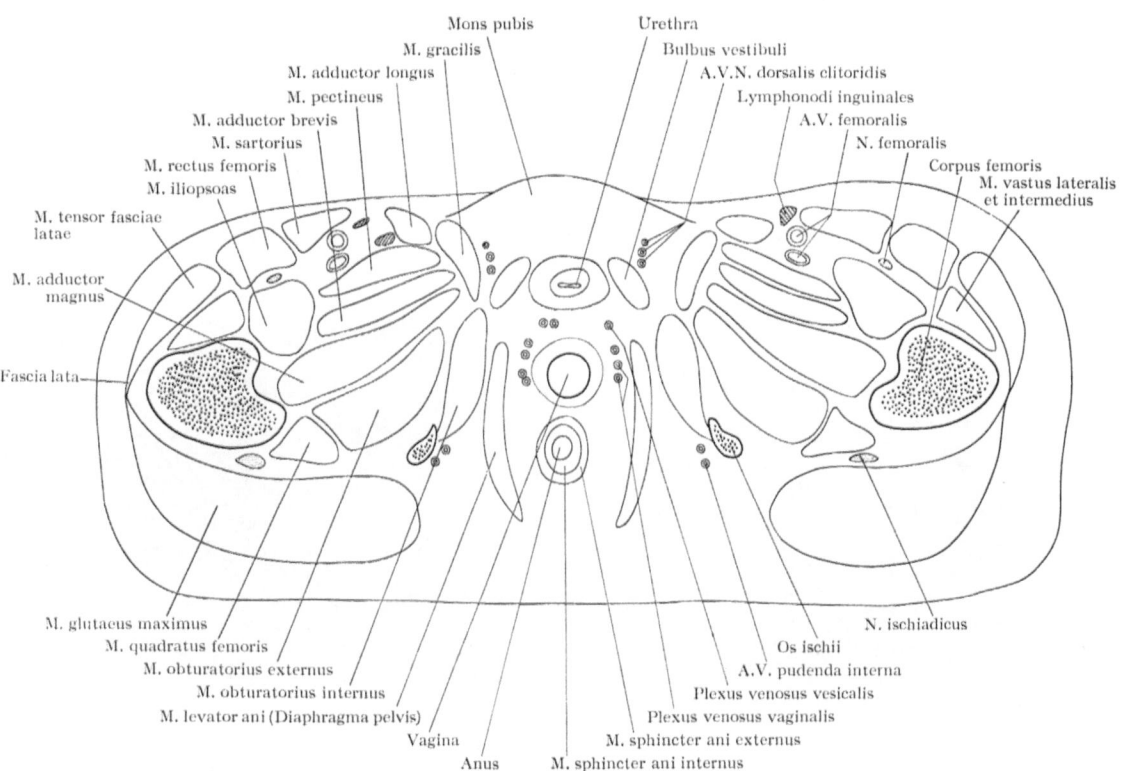

Fig. 426. Anatomical chart

199

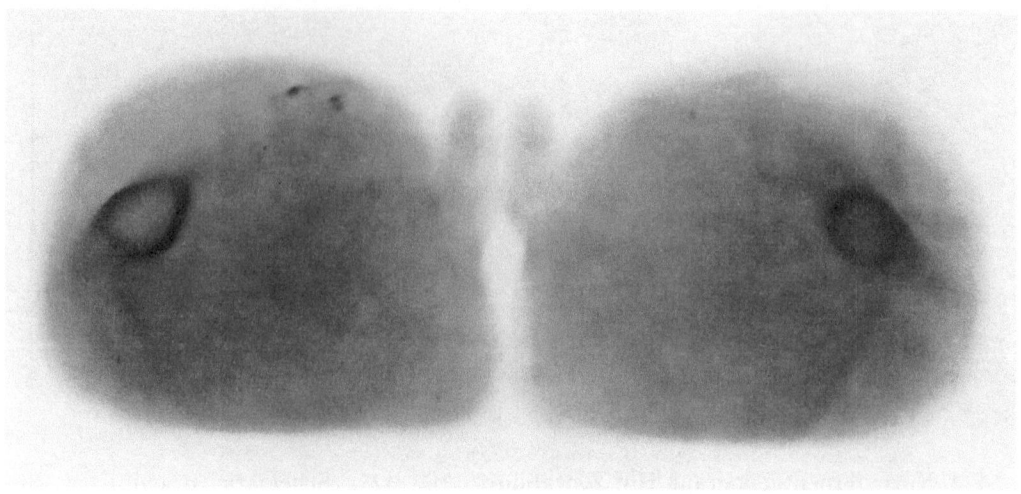

Fig. 427. Axial transverse tomogram

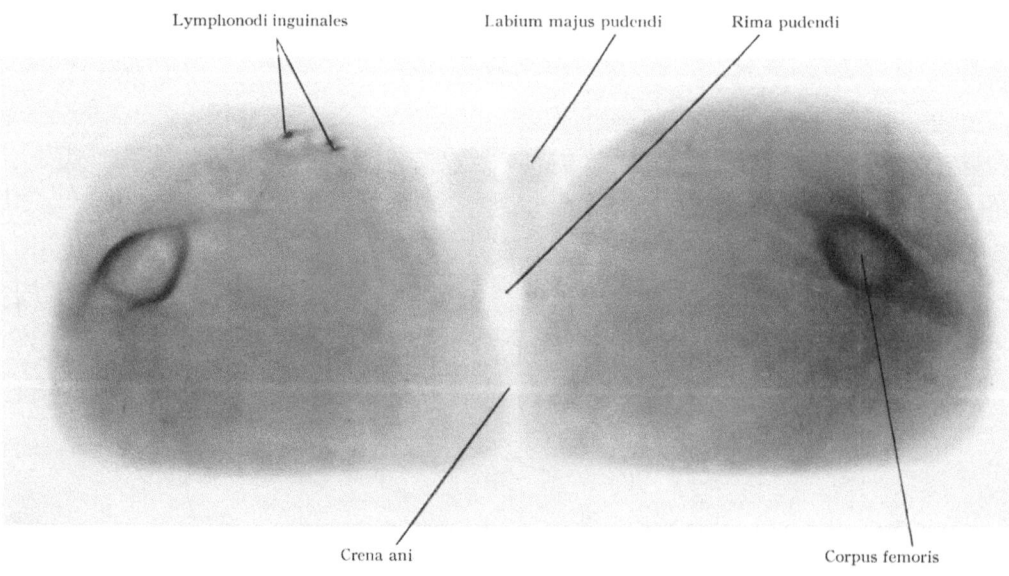

Fig. 428. Interpretation

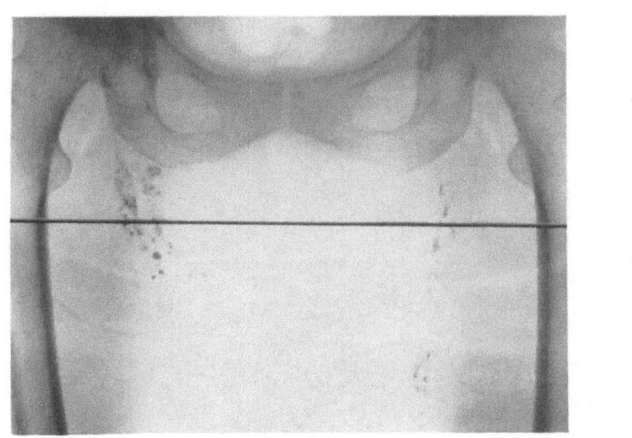

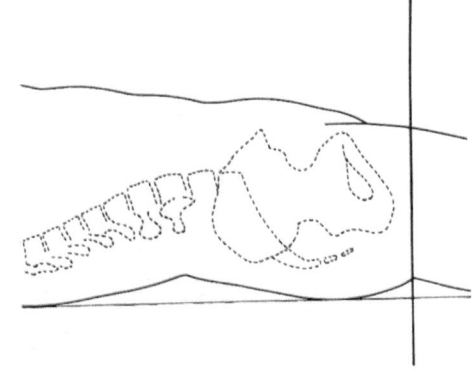

Fig. 429. Normal roentgenogram. Horizontal line showing the level tomographed

Fig. 430. Schematic drawing of the level tomographed

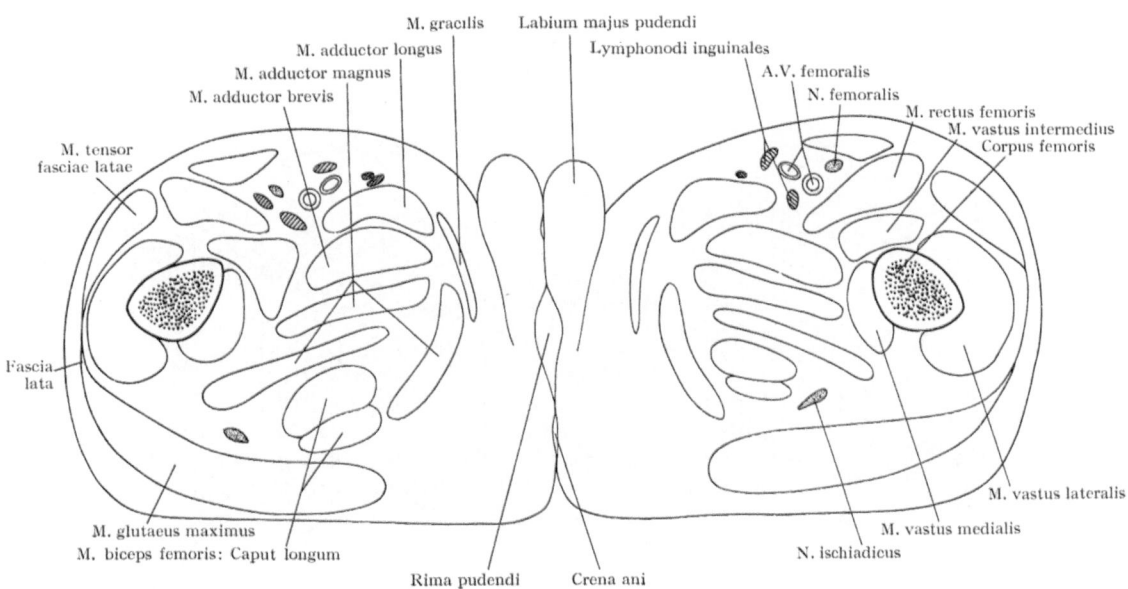

Fig. 431. Anatomical chart

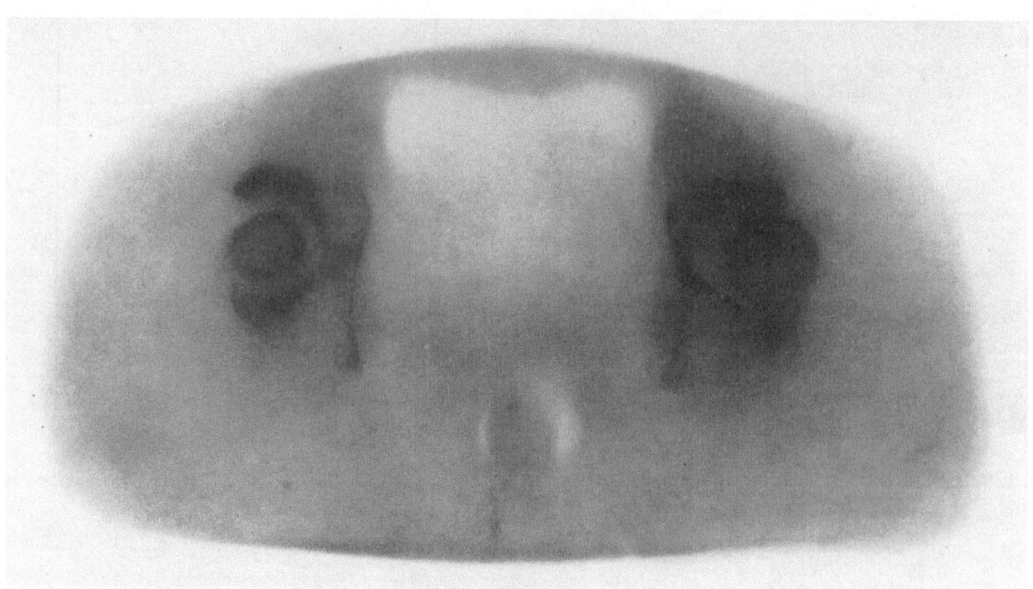

Fig. 432. Axial transverse tomogram

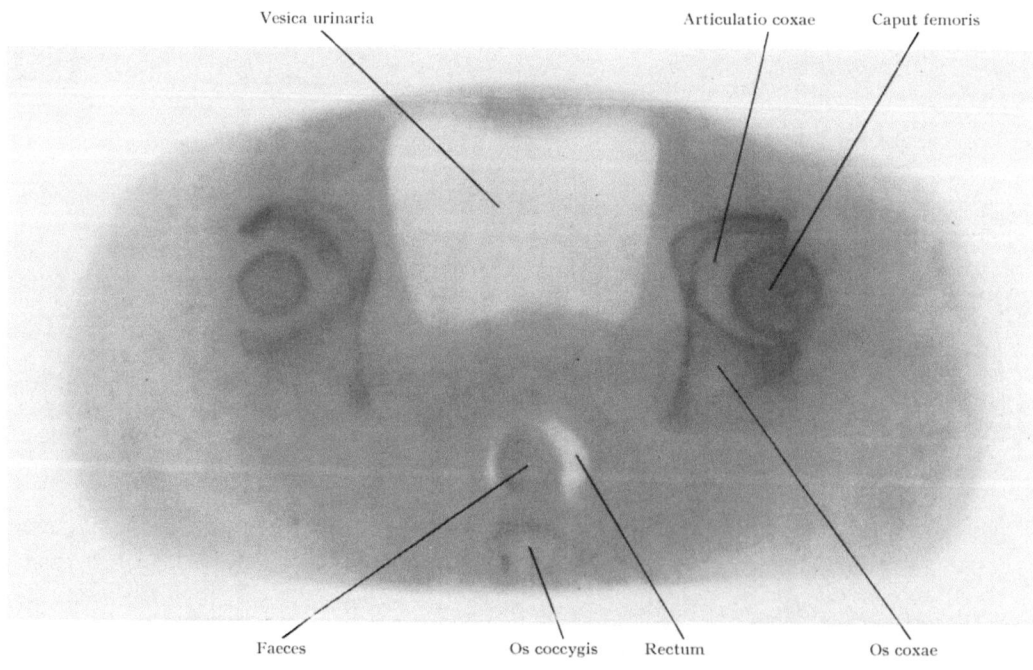

Fig. 433. Interpretation

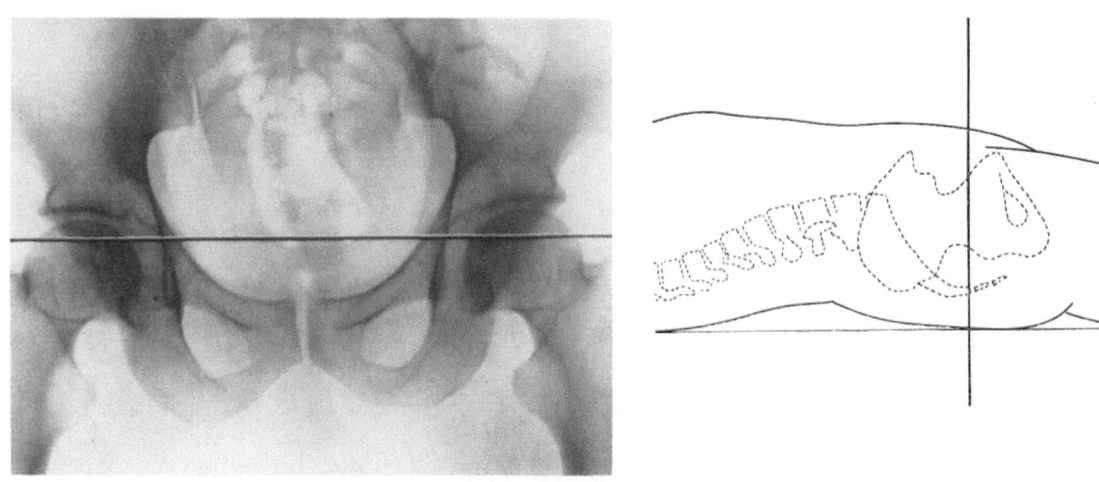

Fig. 434. Normal roentgenogram. Horizontal line showing the level tomographed

Fig. 435. Schematic drawing of the level tomographed

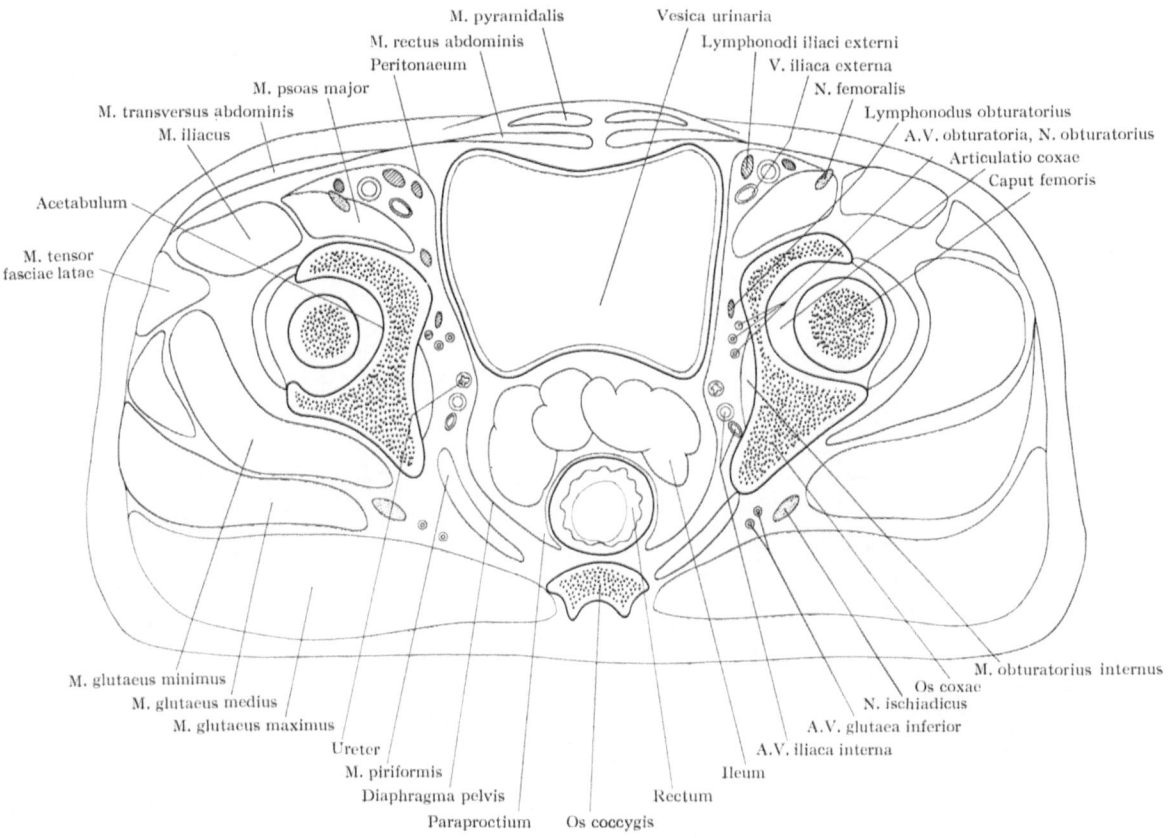

M. pyramidalis
M. rectus abdominis
Peritonaeum
M. psoas major
M. transversus abdominis
M. iliacus
Acetabulum
M. tensor fasciae latae
Vesica urinaria
Lymphonodi iliaci externi
V. iliaca externa
N. femoralis
Lymphonodus obturatorius
A.V. obturatoria, N. obturatorius
Articulatio coxae
Caput femoris
M. glutaeus minimus
M. glutaeus medius
M. glutaeus maximus
Ureter
M. piriformis
Diaphragma pelvis
Paraproctium
Os coccygis
Rectum
Ileum
A.V. iliaca interna
A.V. glutaea inferior
N. ischiadicus
Os coxae
M. obturatorius internus

Fig. 436. Anatomical chart

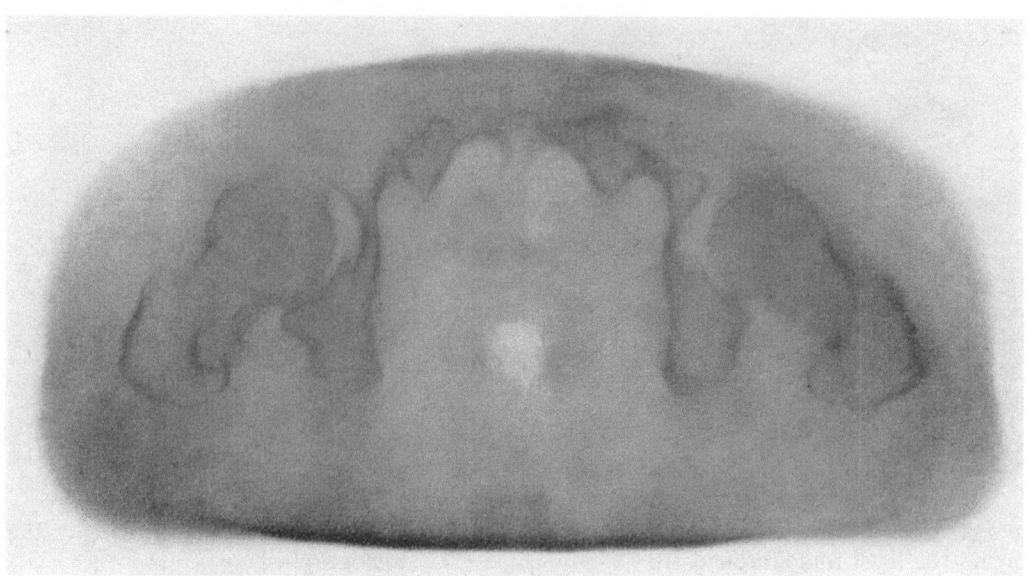

Fig. 437. Axial transverse tomogram

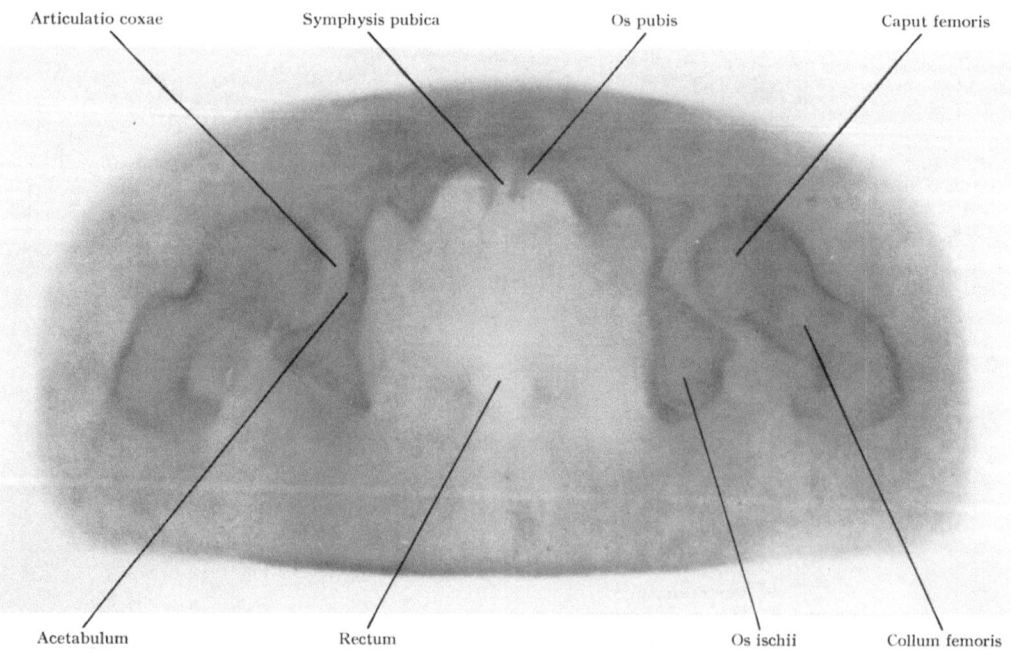

Fig. 438. Interpretation

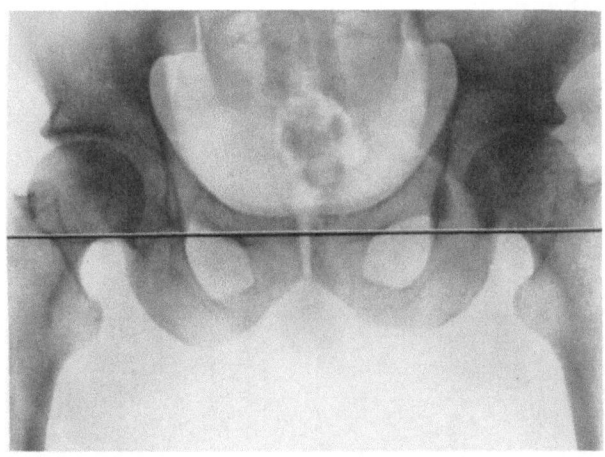

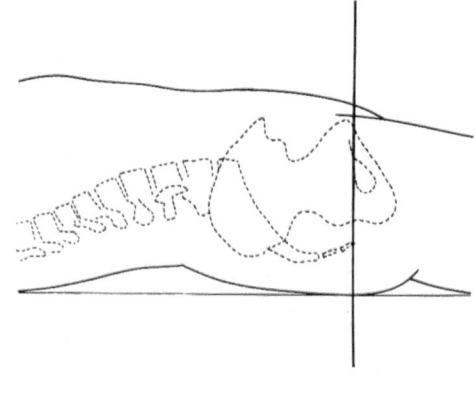

Fig. 439. Normal roentgenogram. Horizontal line showing the level tomographed

Fig. 440. Schematic drawing of the level tomographed

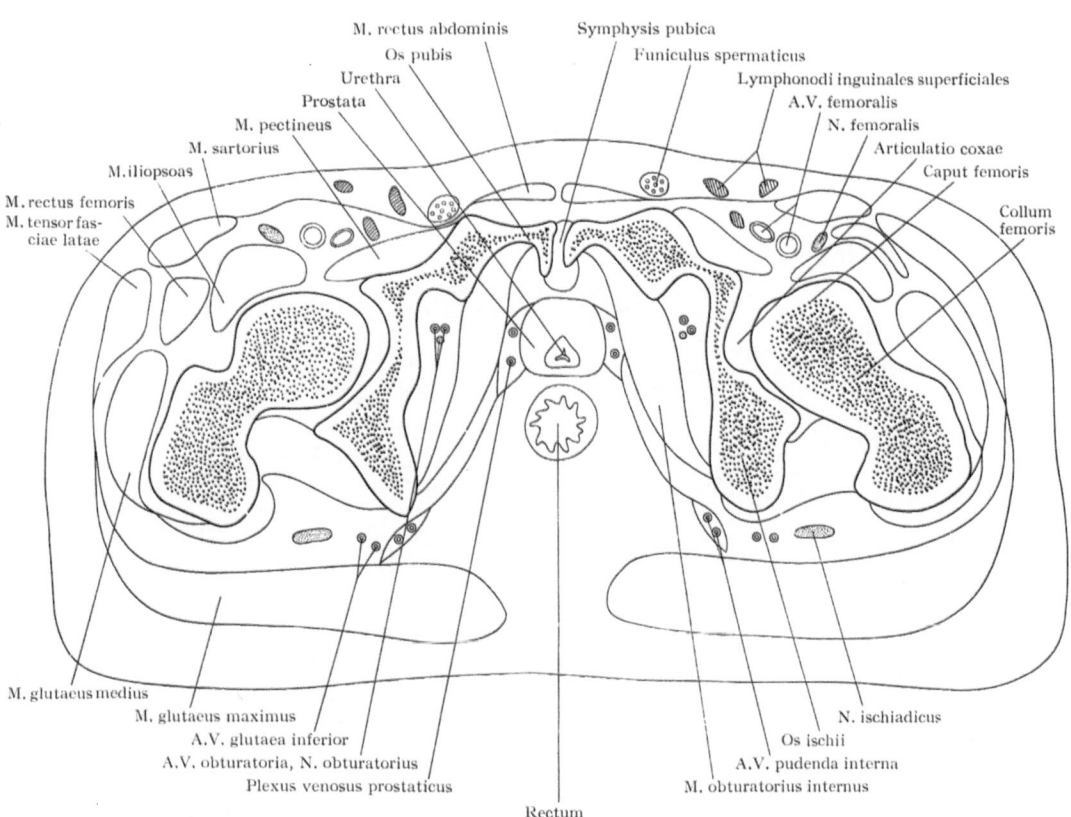

Fig. 441. Anatomical chart

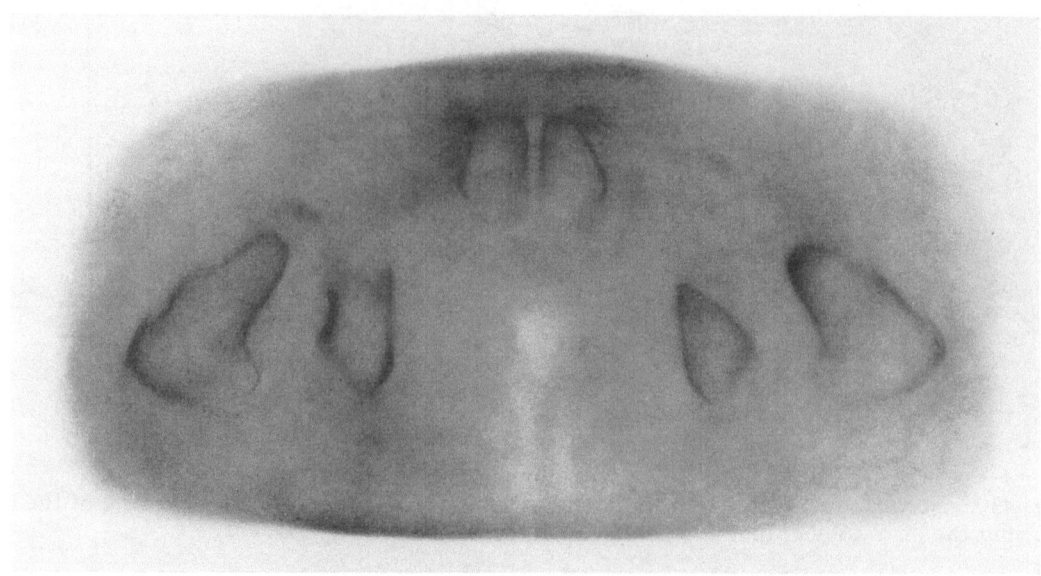

Fig. 442. Axial transverse tomogram

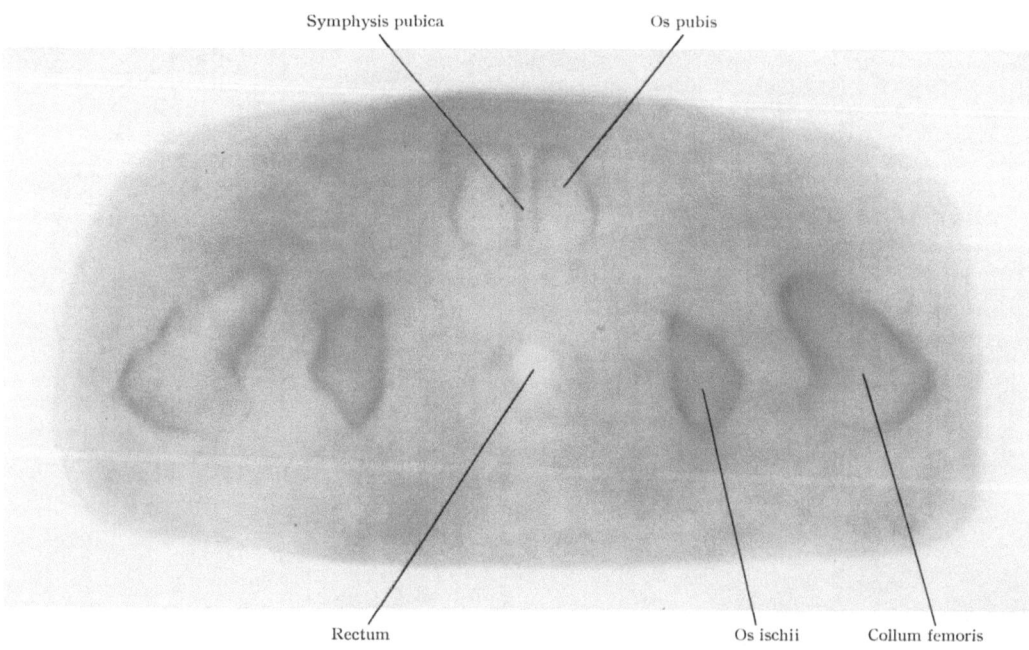

Fig. 443. Interpretation

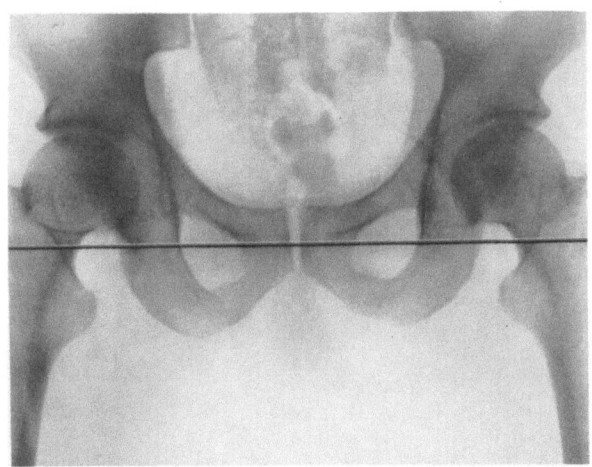

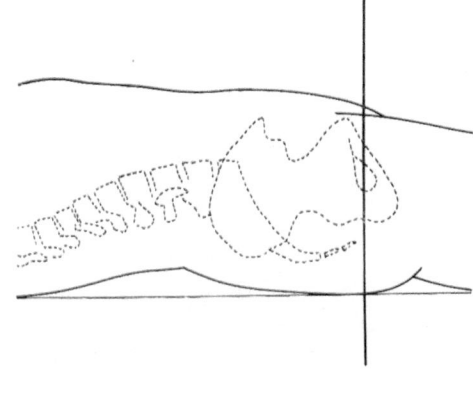

Fig. 444. Normal roentgenogram. Horizontal line showing the level tomographed

Fig. 445. Schematic illustration of the level tomographed

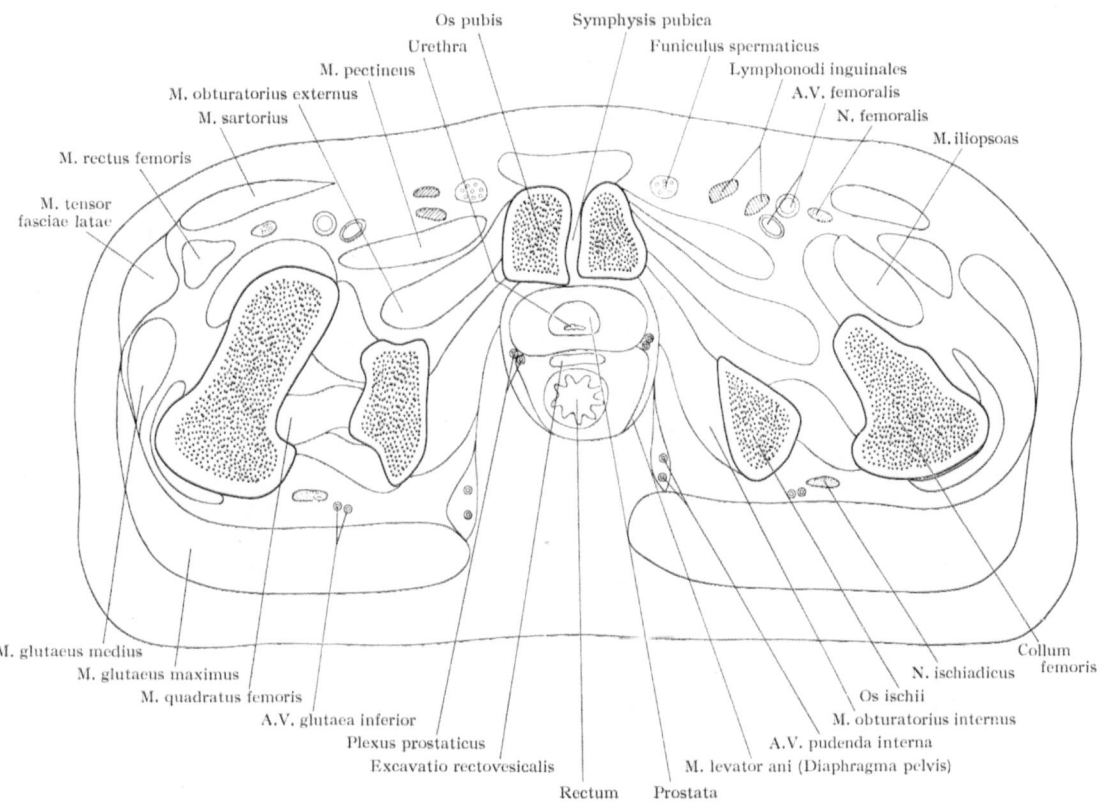

Os pubis
Symphysis pubica
Urethra
Funiculus spermaticus
M. pectineus
Lymphonodi inguinales
M. obturatorius externus
A.V. femoralis
M. sartorius
N. femoralis
M. rectus femoris
M. iliopsoas
M. tensor
fasciae latae

M. glutaeus medius
Collum
femoris
M. glutaeus maximus
N. ischiadicus
M. quadratus femoris
Os ischii
A.V. glutaea inferior
M. obturatorius internus
Plexus prostaticus
A.V. pudenda interna
Excavatio rectovesicalis
M. levator ani (Diaphragma pelvis)
Rectum   Prostata

Fig. 446. Anatomical chart

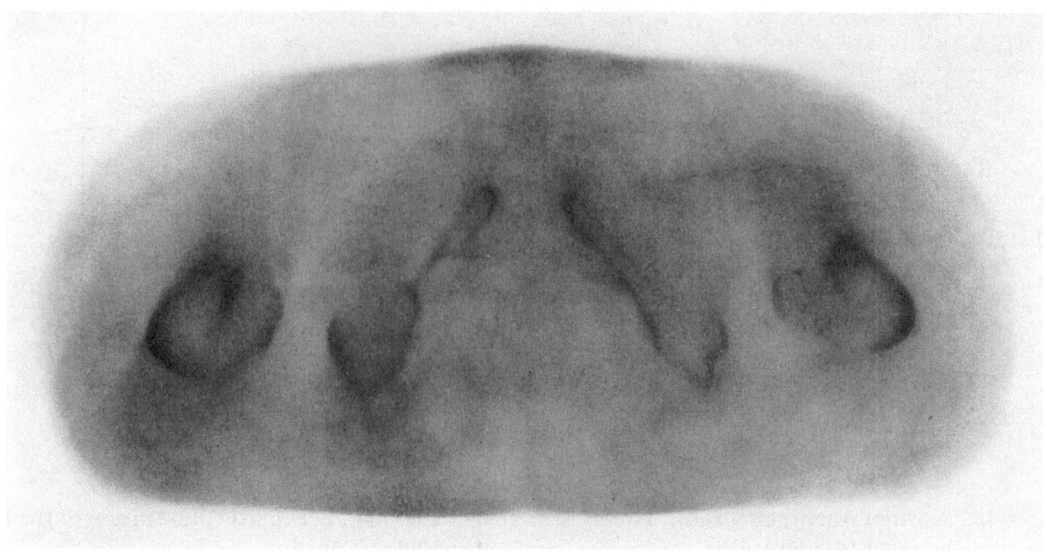

Fig. 447. Axial transverse tomogram

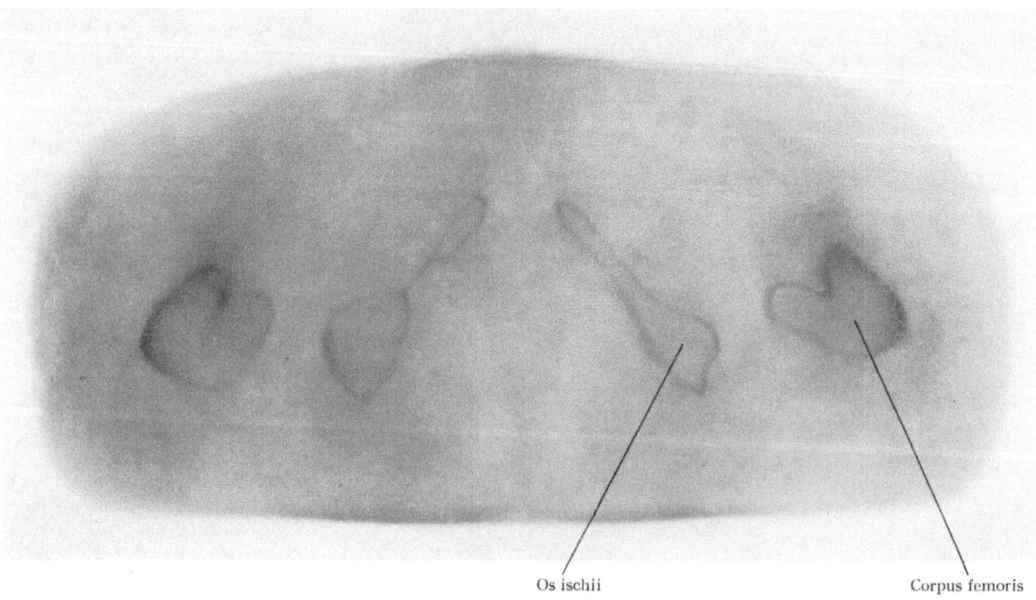

Os ischii   Corpus femoris

Fig. 448. Interpretation

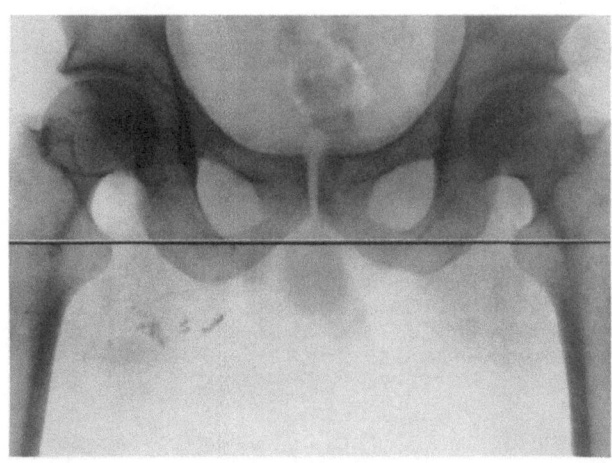

Fig. 449. Normal roentgenogram. Horizontal line showing the level tomographed

Fig. 450. Schematic drawing of the level tomographed

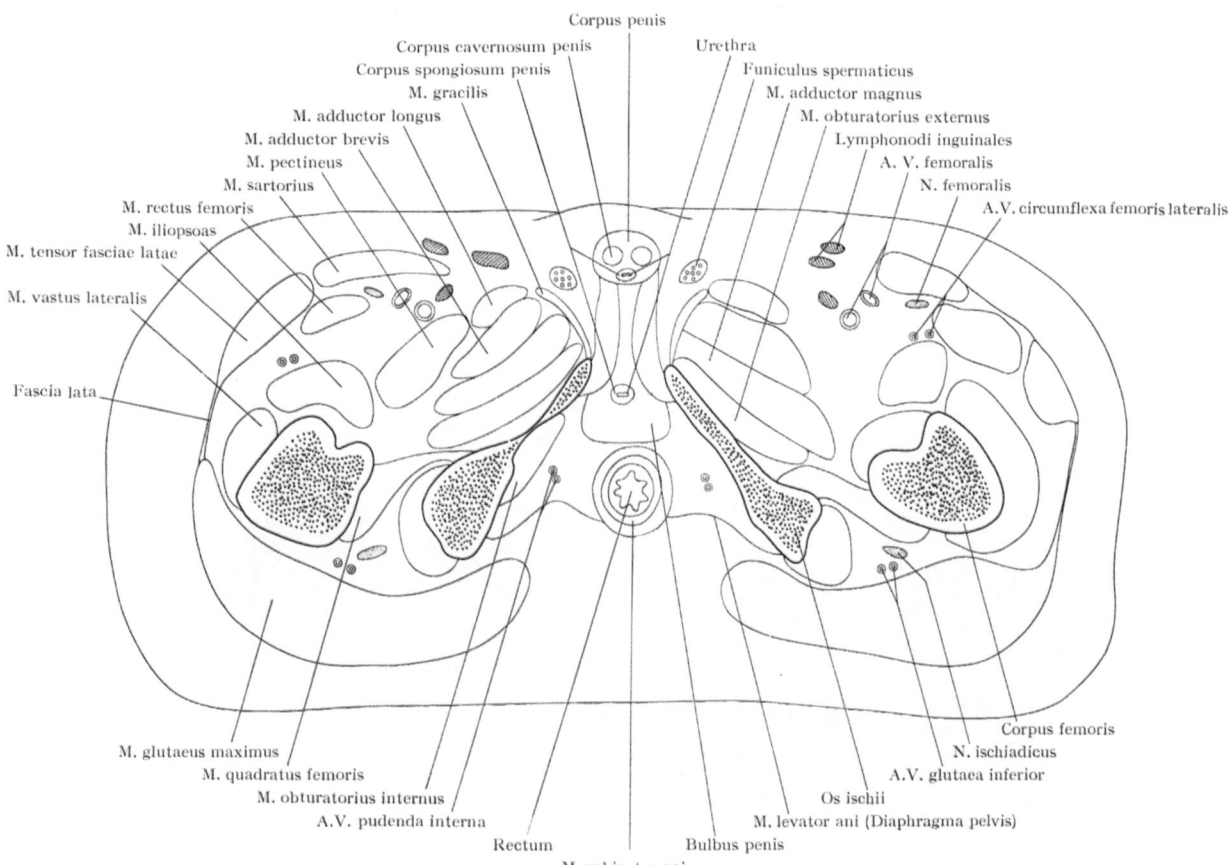

Fig. 451. Anatomical chart

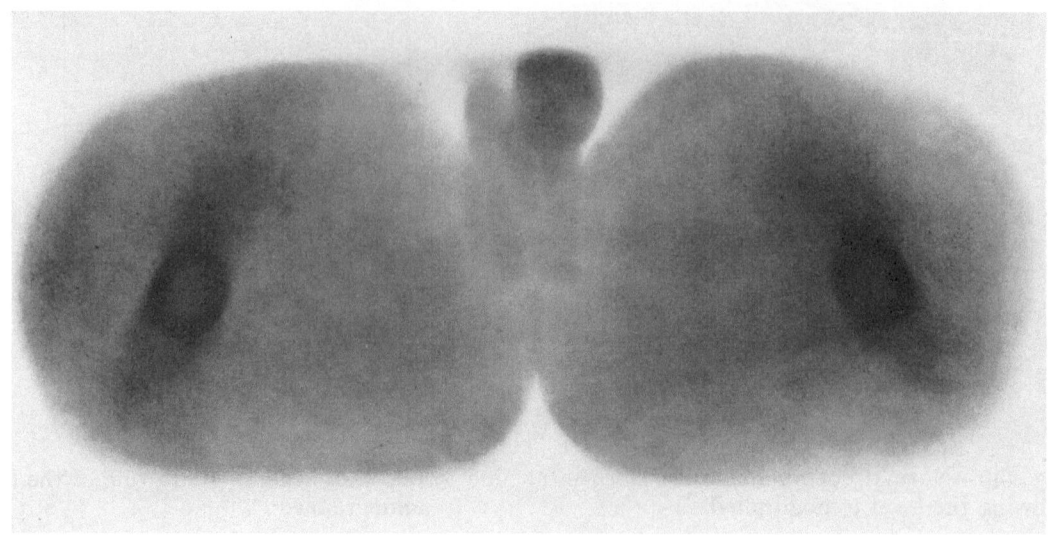

Fig. 452. Axial transverse tomogram

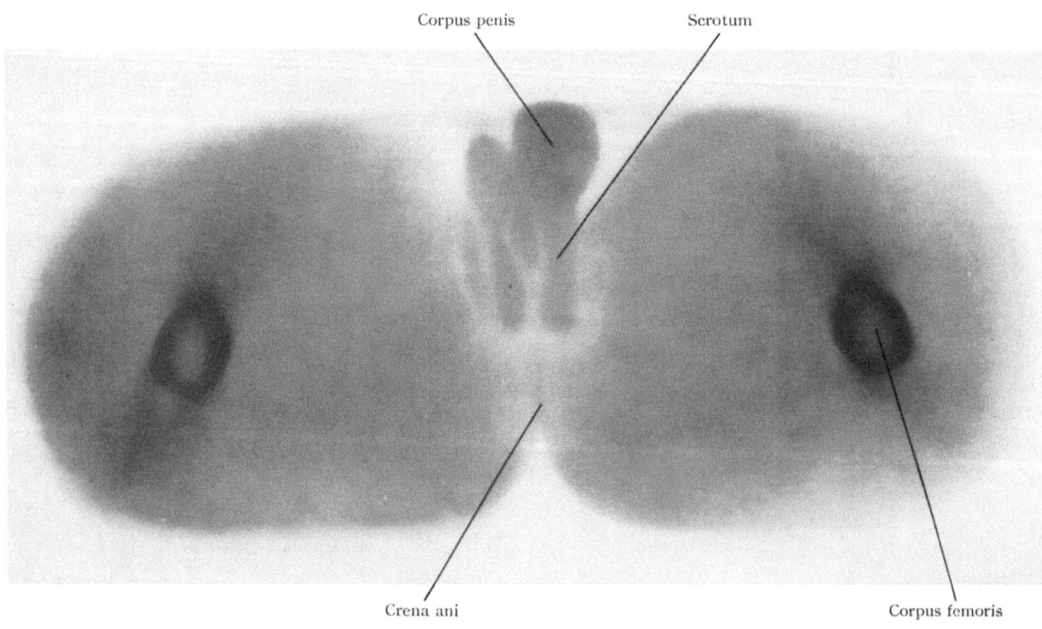

Fig. 453. Interpretation

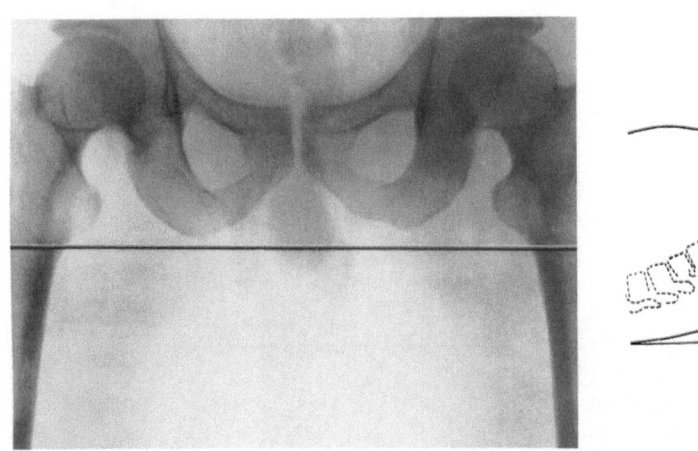

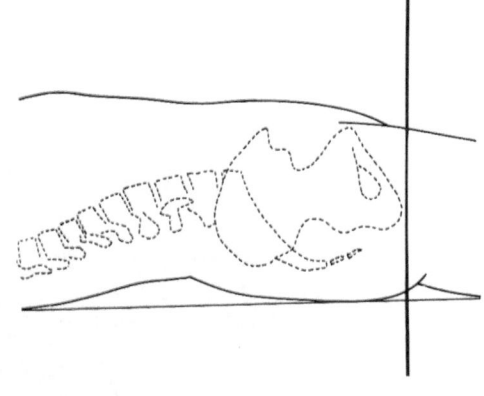

Fig. 454. Normal roentgenogram. Horizontal line showing the level tomographed

Fig. 455. Schematic drawing of the level tomographed

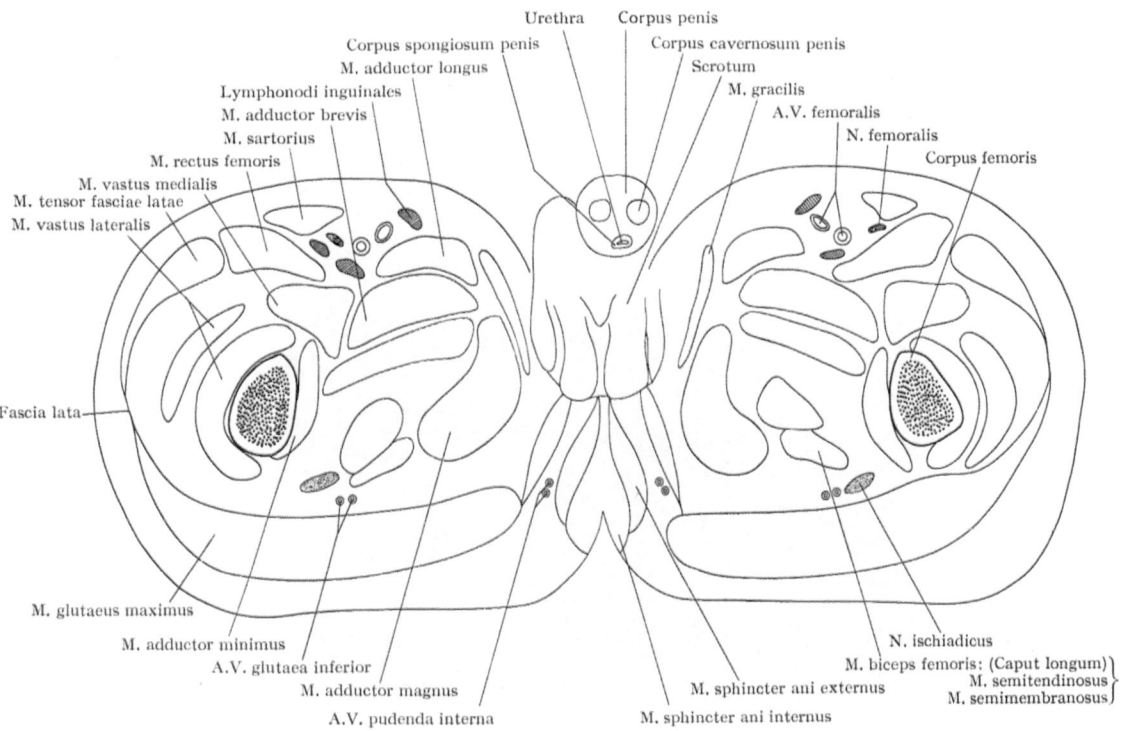

Fig. 456. Anatomical chart

211

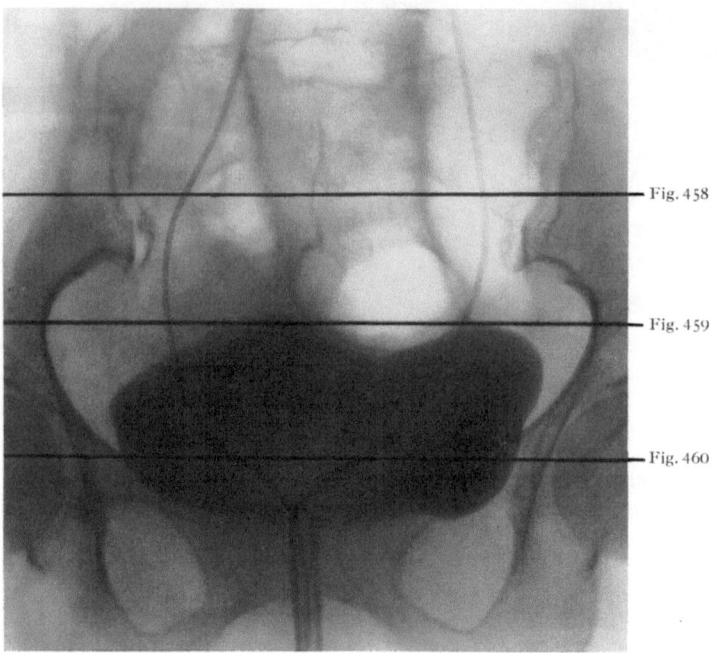

Fig. 457. Normal roentgenogram of the ureter with catheters introduced

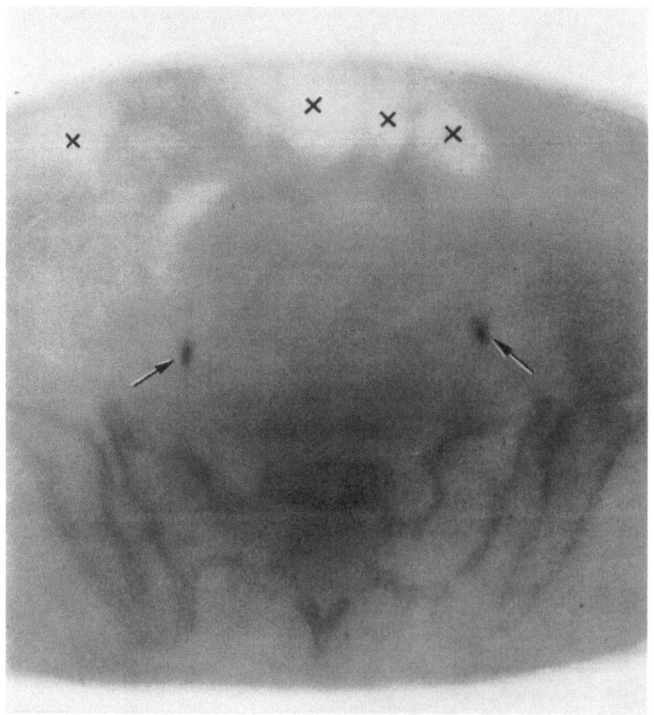

Fig. 458. Axial transverse tomogram of the ureter (↗) (see Figs. 387—391). Colon transversum (✕)

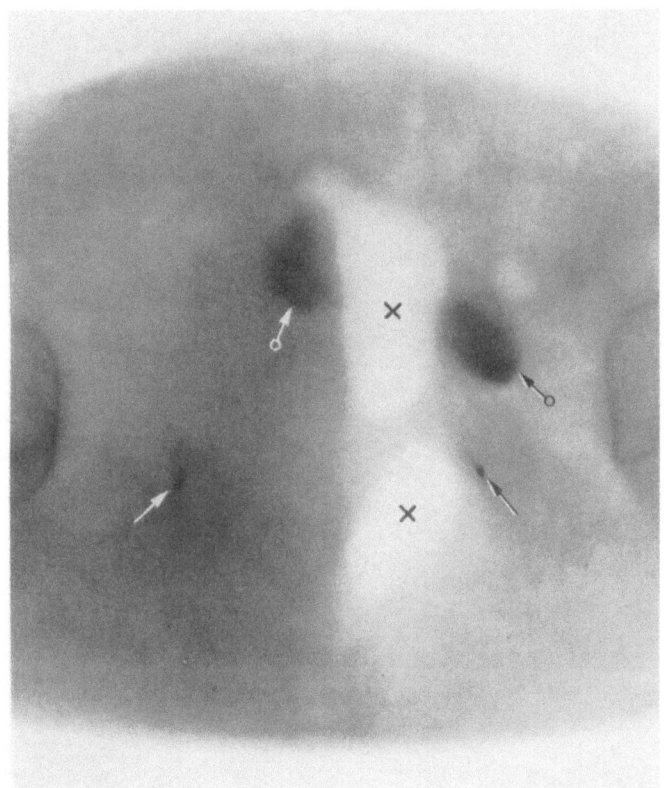

Fig. 459. Axial transverse tomogram of the ureter (↗), colon sigmoideum (✗) and Vesica urinaria (↗). Colon sigmoideum imaged at the middle of the urinary bladder (see Figs. 397—401)

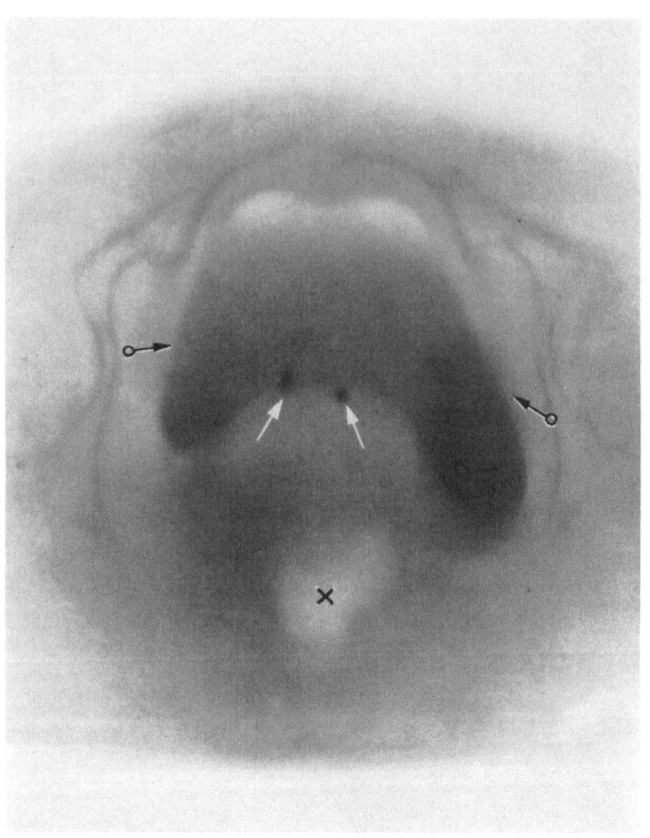

Fig. 460. Axial transverse tomogram. The ureter (⟋) is seen in front of the orifice of the urinary bladder. This image can only be produced by axial transverse tomography (see Figs. 407—411, 437—441). Vesica urinaria (⟋); Rectum (×)

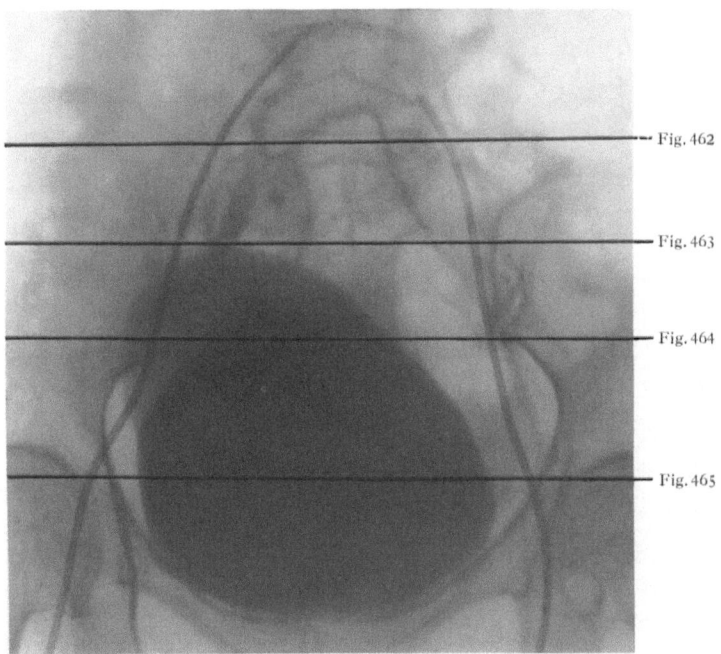

Fig. 461. Normal roentgenogram of the external iliac artery with Oedman-Ledin catheters

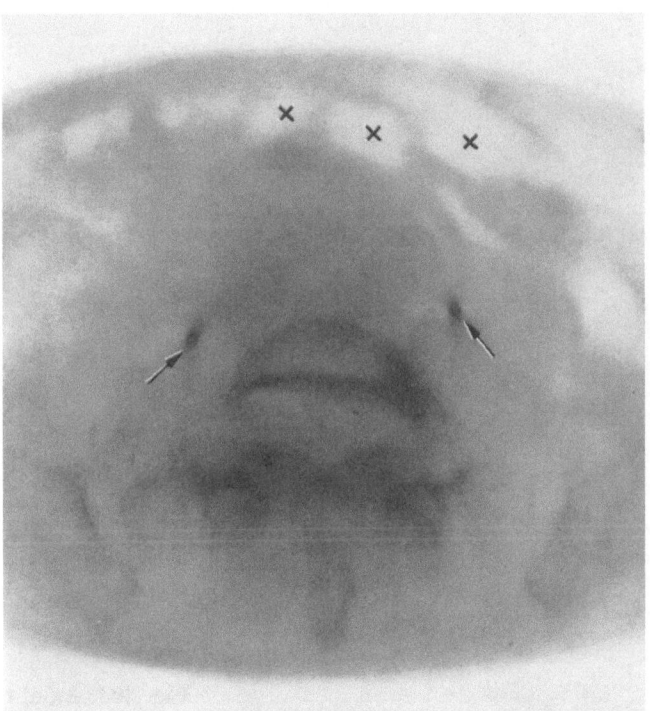

Fig. 462. Axial transverse tomogram of the external iliac artery (╱) (see Figs. 377—381). Colon transversum (✕)

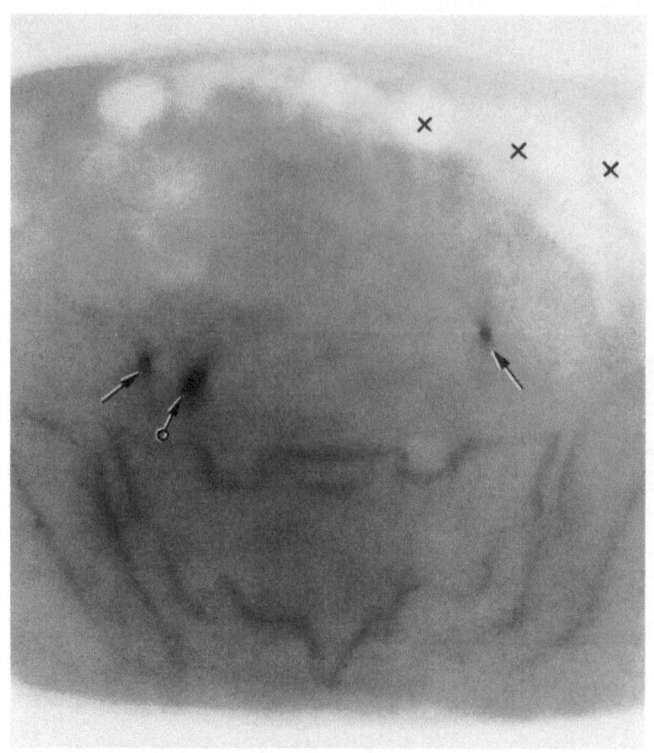

Fig. 463. Axial transverse tomogram of the external iliac artery (↗) (see Figs. 387—391). Colon transversum (×); Ureter dext (↗)

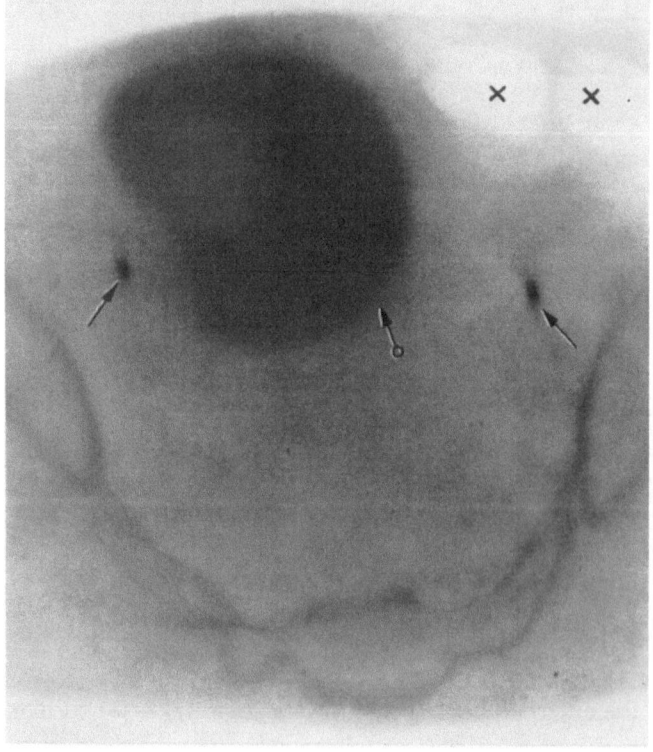

Fig. 464. Axial transverse tomogram of the external iliac artery (↗) (see Figs. 392—401). Colon transversum (×); Vesica urinaria (↗)

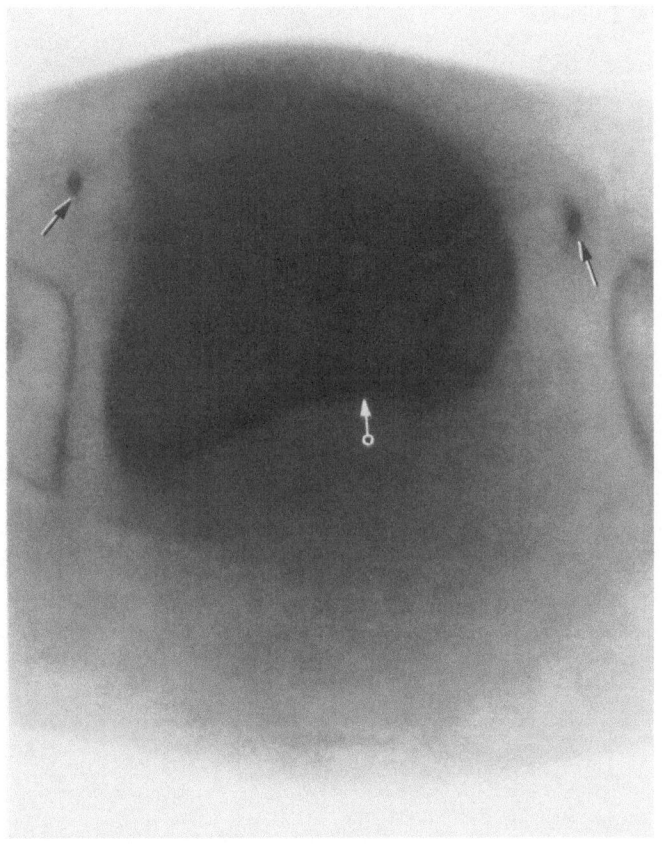

Fig. 465. Axial transverse tomogram of the external iliac artery (↗) (see Figs. 402—406, 432—436). Vesica urinaria (↗)

Arm

Eight axial transverse lympho-tomograms.

Findings visible on the axial transverse tomogram are printed in *italics* in the anatomical chart.

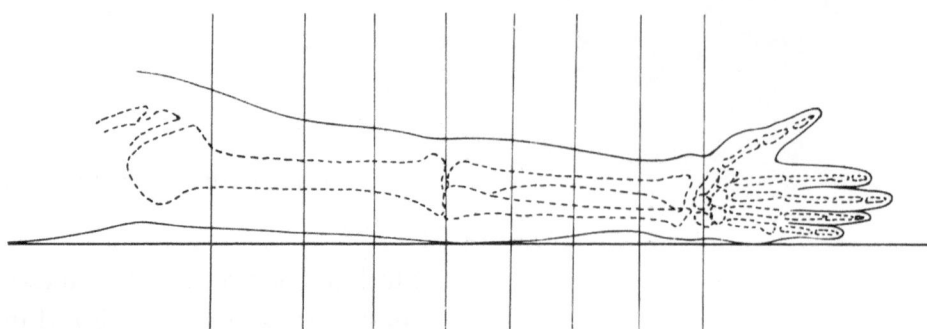

Fig. 466. Schema of tomographed levels

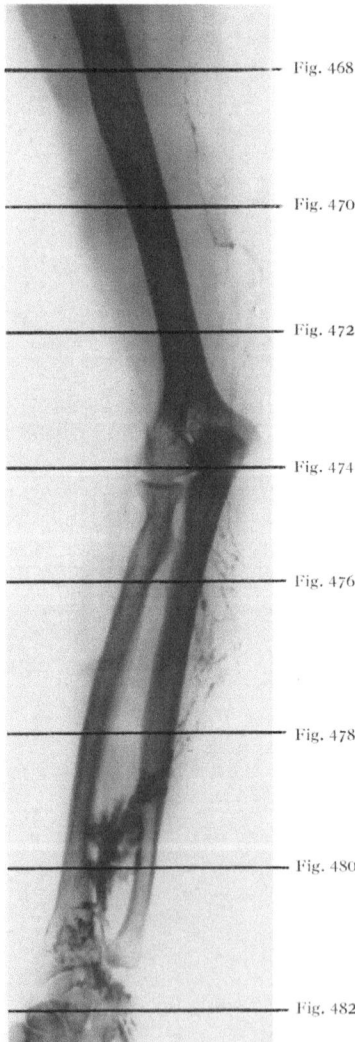

Fig. 467. Normal roentgenogram. Vertical lines showing the levels tomographed

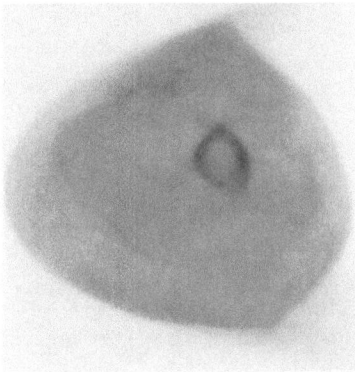

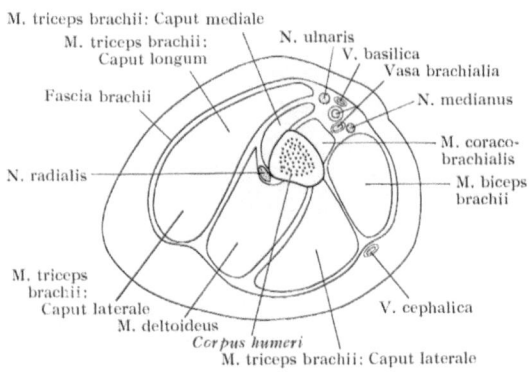

Fig. 468. Axial transverse tomogram

Fig. 469. Anatomical chart

M. triceps brachii: Caput mediale
M. triceps brachii: Caput longum
Fascia brachii
N. radialis
M. triceps brachii: Caput laterale
M. deltoideus
Corpus humeri
M. triceps brachii: Caput laterale
N. ulnaris
V. basilica
Vasa brachialia
N. medianus
M. coraco-brachialis
M. biceps brachii
V. cephalica

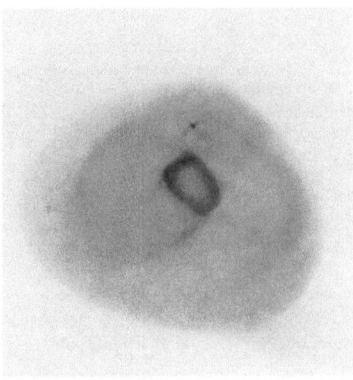

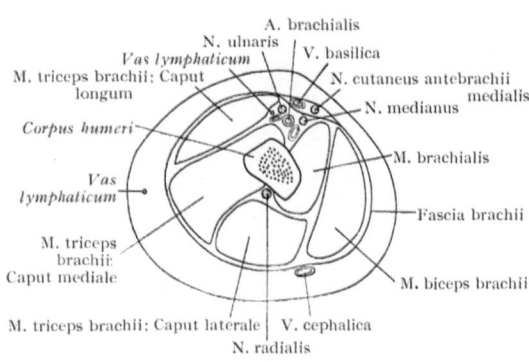

Fig. 470. Axial transverse tomogram

Fig. 471. Anatomical chart

A. brachialis
N. ulnaris
Vas lymphaticum
M. triceps brachii: Caput longum
Corpus humeri
Vas lymphaticum
M. triceps brachii: Caput mediale
M. triceps brachii: Caput laterale
N. radialis
V. basilica
N. cutaneus antebrachii medialis
N. medianus
M. brachialis
Fascia brachii
M. biceps brachii
V. cephalica

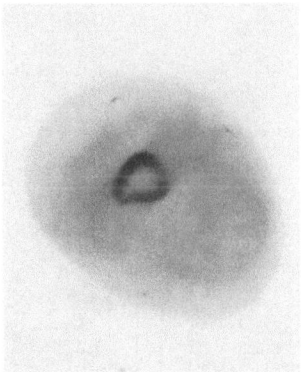

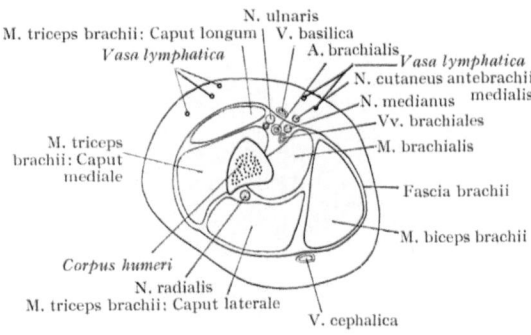

Fig. 472. Axial transverse tomogram

Fig. 473. Anatomical chart

N. ulnaris
M. triceps brachii: Caput longum
V. basilica
Vasa lymphatica
A. brachialis
Vasa lymphatica
N. cutaneus antebrachii medialis
N. medianus
Vv. brachiales
M. triceps brachii: Caput mediale
M. brachialis
Fascia brachii
M. biceps brachii
Corpus humeri
N. radialis
M. triceps brachii: Caput laterale
V. cephalica

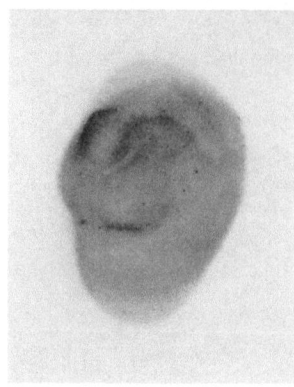

Fig. 474. Axial transverse tomogram

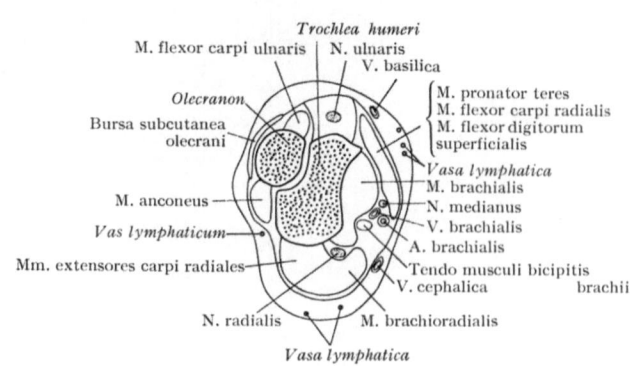

Fig. 475. Anatomical chart

Trochlea humeri
M. flexor carpi ulnaris | N. ulnaris
V. basilica
Olecranon
M. pronator teres
M. flexor carpi radialis
Bursa subcutanea
olecrani
M. flexor digitorum
superficialis
Vasa lymphatica
M. brachialis
M. anconeus
N. medianus
Vas lymphaticum
V. brachialis
A. brachialis
Mm. extensores carpi radiales
Tendo musculi bicipitis
V. cephalica
brachii
N. radialis
M. brachioradialis
Vasa lymphatica

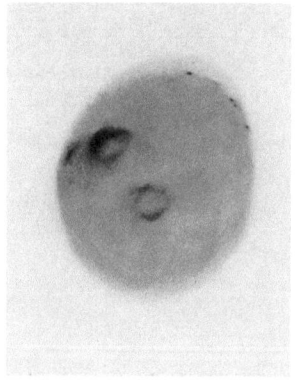

Fig. 476. Axial transverse tomogram

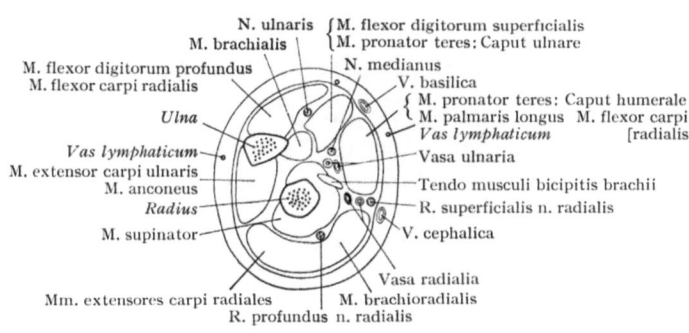

Fig. 477. Anatomical chart

N. ulnaris
M. flexor digitorum superficialis
M. brachialis
M. pronator teres: Caput ulnare
M. flexor digitorum profundus
N. medianus
M. flexor carpi radialis
V. basilica
Ulna
M. pronator teres: Caput humerale
M. palmaris longus   M. flexor carpi
Vas lymphaticum
[radialis
Vas lymphaticum
Vasa ulnaria
M. extensor carpi ulnaris
M. anconeus
Tendo musculi bicipitis brachii
Radius
R. superficialis n. radialis
M. supinator
V. cephalica
Vasa radialia
Mm. extensores carpi radiales
M. brachioradialis
R. profundus n. radialis

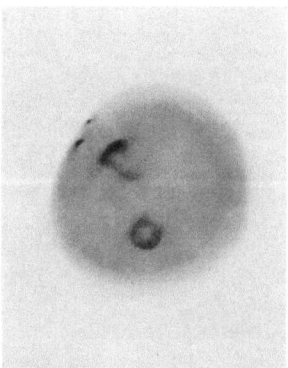

Fig. 478. Axial transverse tomogram

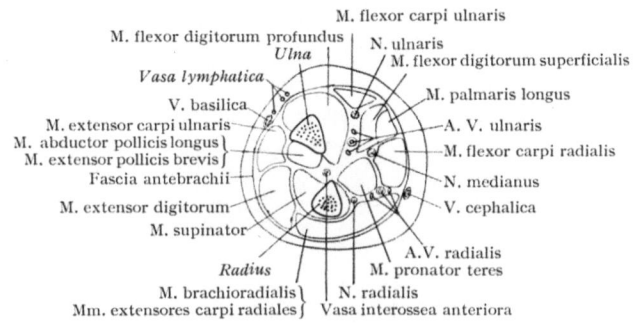

Fig. 479. Anatomical chart

M. flexor carpi ulnaris
M. flexor digitorum profundus
Ulna
N. ulnaris
Vasa lymphatica
M. flexor digitorum superficialis
V. basilica
M. palmaris longus
M. extensor carpi ulnaris
M. abductor pollicis longus
A. V. ulnaris
M. extensor pollicis brevis
M. flexor carpi radialis
Fascia antebrachii
N. medianus
M. extensor digitorum
V. cephalica
M. supinator
A.V. radialis
Radius
M. pronator teres
M. brachioradialis
N. radialis
Mm. extensores carpi radiales
Vasa interossea anteriora

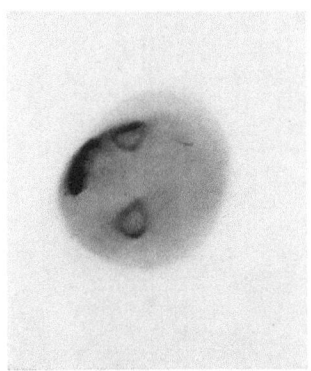

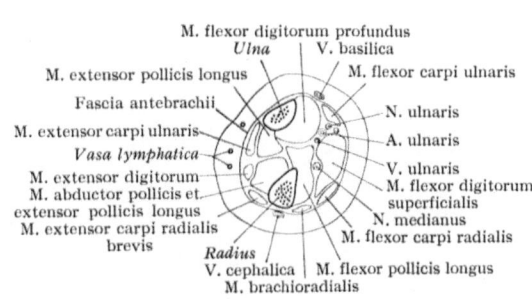

M. flexor digitorum profundus
Ulna V. basilica
M. extensor pollicis longus — M. flexor carpi ulnaris
Fascia antebrachii — N. ulnaris
M. extensor carpi ulnaris — A. ulnaris
Vasa lymphatica — V. ulnaris
M. extensor digitorum — M. flexor digitorum superficialis
M. abductor pollicis et extensor pollicis longus — N. medianus
M. extensor carpi radialis brevis — M. flexor carpi radialis
Radius — M. flexor pollicis longus
V. cephalica — M. brachioradialis

Fig. 480. Axial transverse tomogram   Fig. 481. Anatomical chart

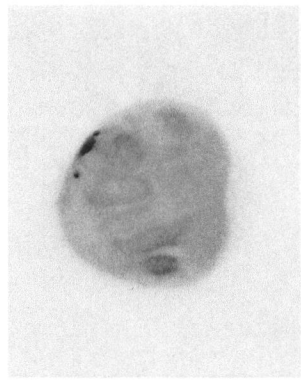

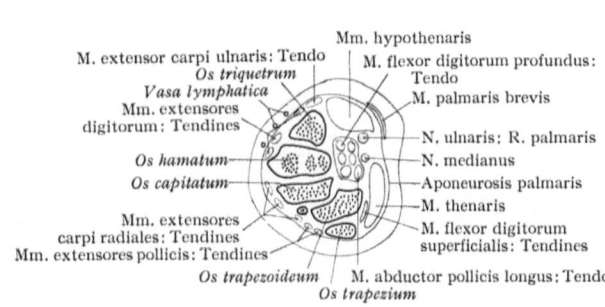

Mm. hypothenaris
M. extensor carpi ulnaris: Tendo — M. flexor digitorum profundus: Tendo
Os triquetrum — M. palmaris brevis
Vasa lymphatica
Mm. extensores digitorum: Tendines — N. ulnaris: R. palmaris
Os hamatum — N. medianus
Os capitatum — Aponeurosis palmaris
Mm. extensores carpi radiales: Tendines — M. thenaris
Mm. extensores pollicis: Tendines — M. flexor digitorum superficialis: Tendines
Os trapezoideum — M. abductor pollicis longus: Tendo
Os trapezium

Fig. 482. Axial transverse tomogram   Fig. 483. Anatomical chart

Leg

Seven axial transverse phlebo- and lympho-tomograms.

Findings visible on the axial transverse tomogram are printed in *italics* in the anatomical chart.

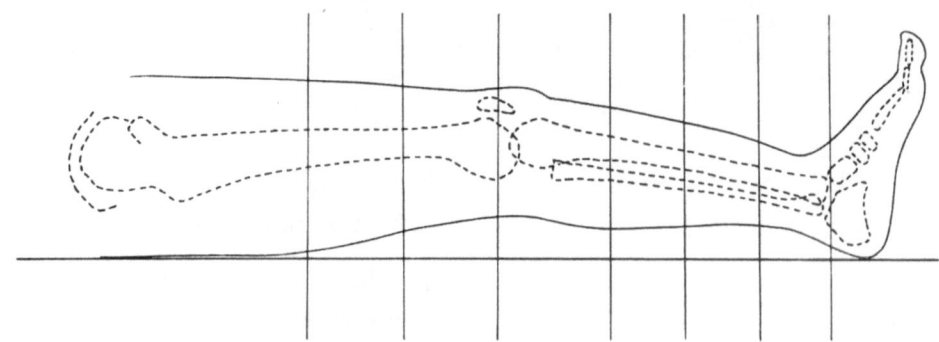

Fig. 484. Schema of tomographed levels

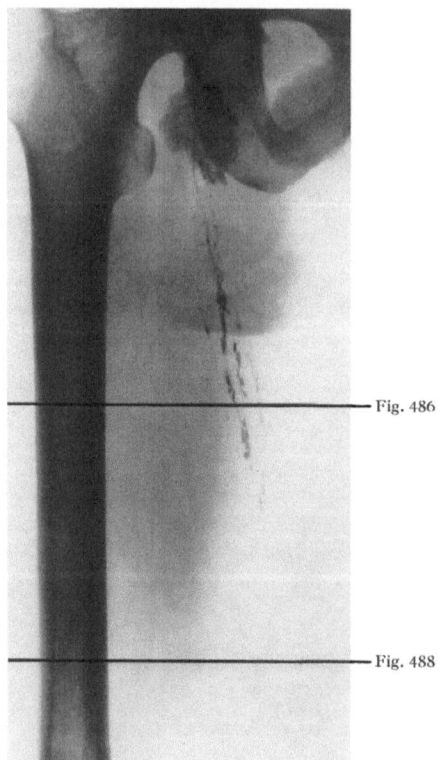

Fig. 486

Fig. 488

Fig. 485. Normal roentgenogram. Horizontal lines showing the levels tomographed

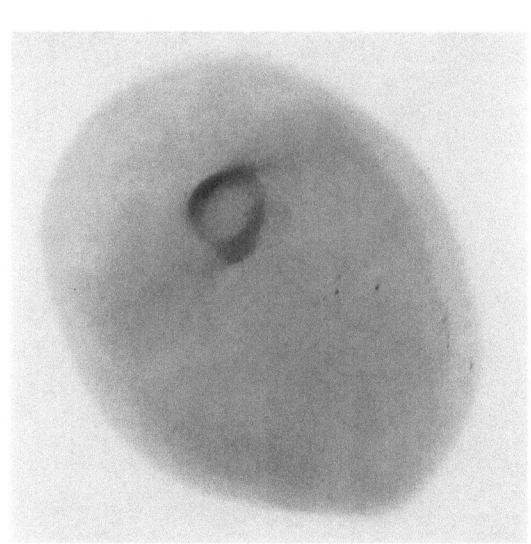

Fig. 486. Axial transverse tomogram

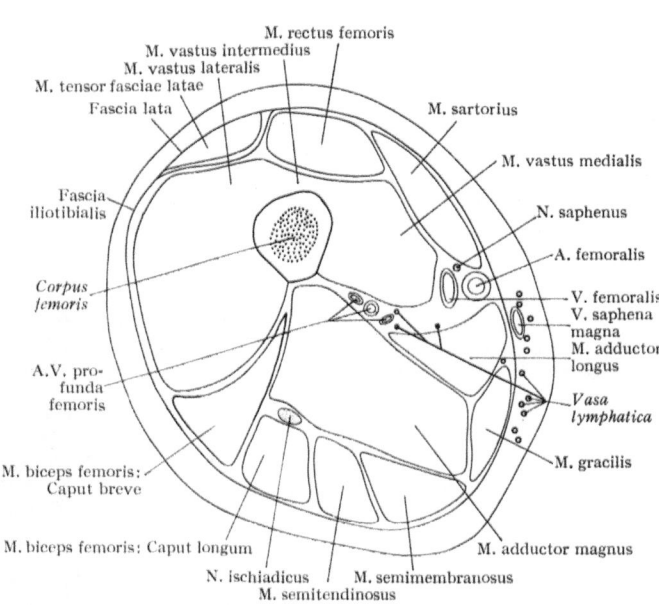

M. rectus femoris
M. vastus intermedius
M. vastus lateralis
M. tensor fasciae latae
Fascia lata
M. sartorius
M. vastus medialis
Fascia iliotibialis
N. saphenus
A. femoralis
Corpus femoris
V. femoralis
V. saphena magna
M. adductor longus
A.V. profunda femoris
Vasa lymphatica
M. gracilis
M. biceps femoris: Caput breve
M. adductor magnus
M. biceps femoris: Caput longum
N. ischiadicus
M. semimembranosus
M. semitendinosus

Fig. 487. Anatomical chart

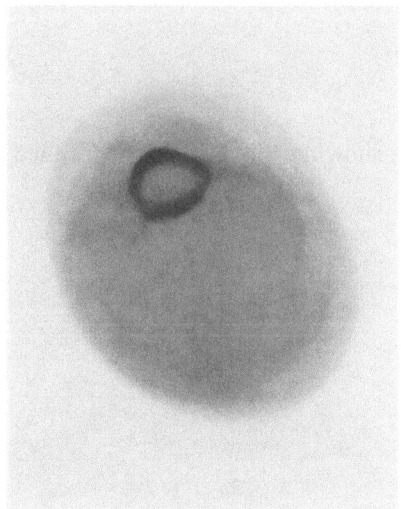

Fig. 488. Axial transverse tomogram

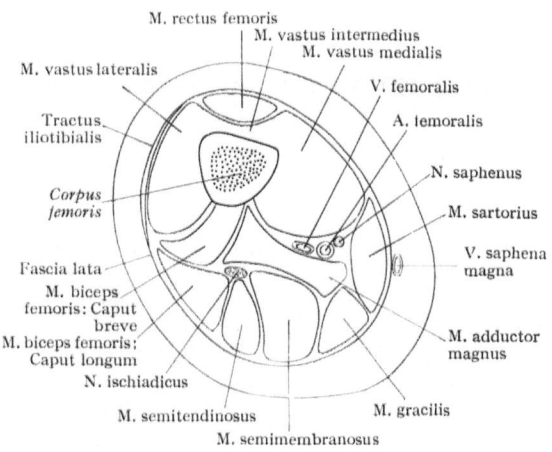

M. rectus femoris
M. vastus intermedius
M. vastus medialis
M. vastus lateralis
V. femoralis
Tractus iliotibialis
A. femoralis
N. saphenus
Corpus femoris
M. sartorius
Fascia lata
V. saphena magna
M. biceps femoris: Caput breve
M. biceps femoris: Caput longum
M. adductor magnus
N. ischiadicus
M. semitendinosus
M. gracilis
M. semimembranosus

Fig. 489. Anatomical chart

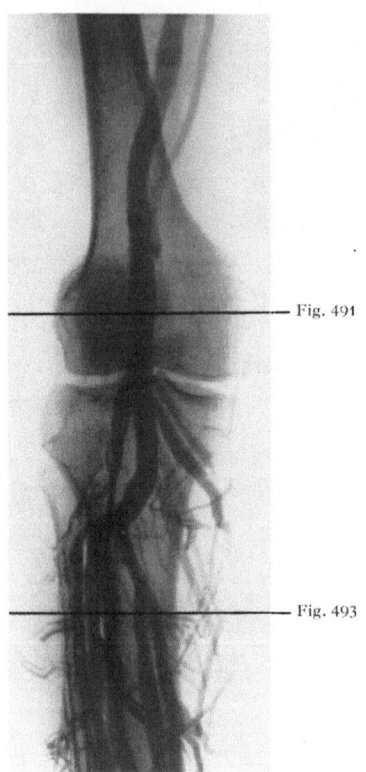

Fig. 491

Fig. 493

Fig. 490. Normal roentgenogram. Horizontal lines showing the levels tomographed

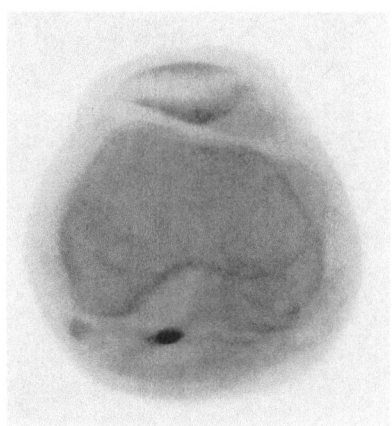

Fig. 491. Axial transverse tomogram

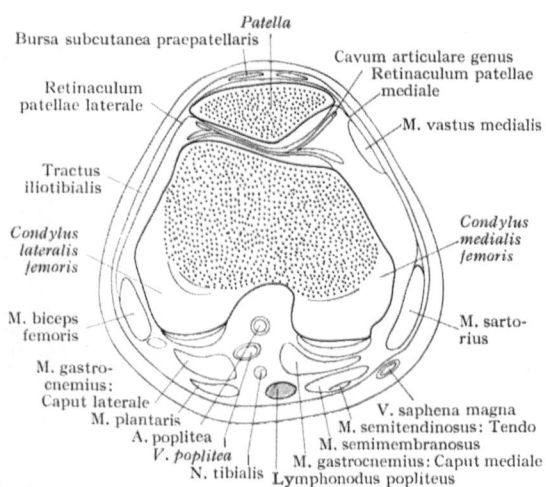

Patella

Bursa subcutanea praepatellaris

Retinaculum
patellae laterale

Cavum articulare genus
Retinaculum patellae
mediale

Tractus
iliotibialis

M. vastus medialis

*Condylus
lateralis
femoris*

*Condylus
medialis
femoris*

M. biceps
femoris

M. sarto-
rius

M. gastro-
cnemius:
Caput laterale

V. saphena magna

M. plantaris

M. semitendinosus: Tendo

A. poplitea

M. semimembranosus

V. poplitea

M. gastrocnemius: Caput mediale

N. tibialis

Lymphonodus popliteus

Fig. 492. Anatomical chart

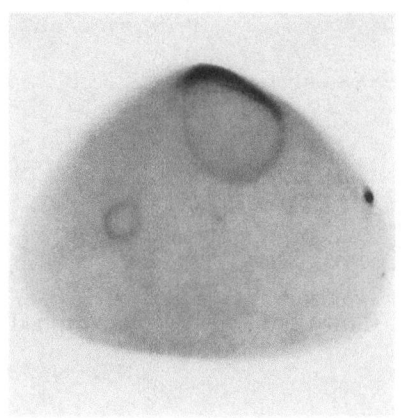

Fig. 493. Axial transverse tomogram

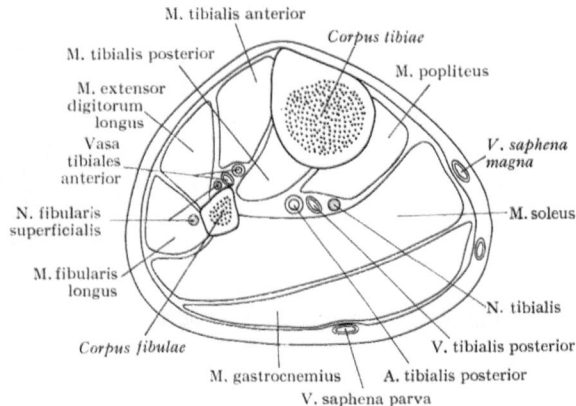

M. tibialis anterior

Corpus tibiae

M. tibialis posterior

M. popliteus

M. extensor
digitorum
longus

*V. saphena
magna*

Vasa
tibiales
anterior

N. fibularis
superficialis

M. soleus

M. fibularis
longus

N. tibialis

Corpus fibulae

V. tibialis posterior

M. gastrocnemius

A. tibialis posterior

V. saphena parva

Fig. 494. Anatomical chart

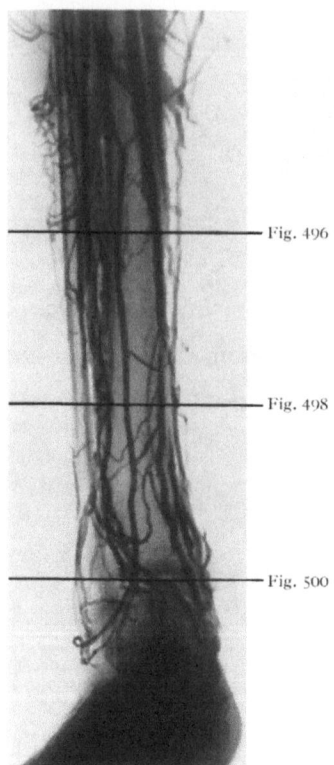

Fig. 495. Normal roentgenogram. Horizontal lines showing the levels tomographed

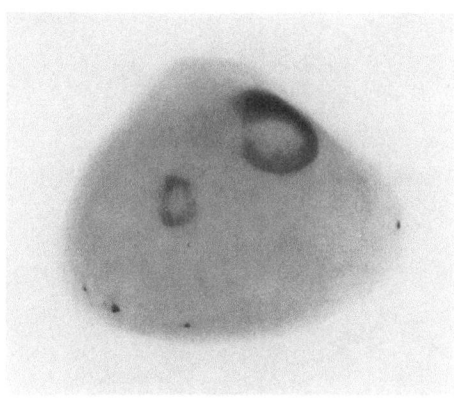

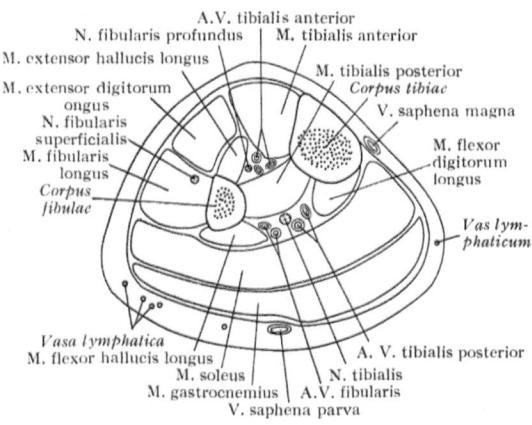

Fig. 496. Axial transverse tomogram

Fig. 497. Anatomical chart

A.V. tibialis anterior
N. fibularis profundus
M. tibialis anterior
M. extensor hallucis longus
M. tibialis posterior
M. extensor digitorum ongus
Corpus tibiae
N. fibularis superficialis
V. saphena magna
M. fibularis longus
M. flexor digitorum longus
Corpus fibulae
Vas lymphaticum
Vasa lymphatica
M. flexor hallucis longus
A. V. tibialis posterior
M. soleus
N. tibialis
M. gastrocnemius
A.V. fibularis
V. saphena parva

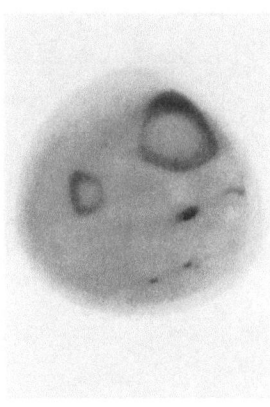

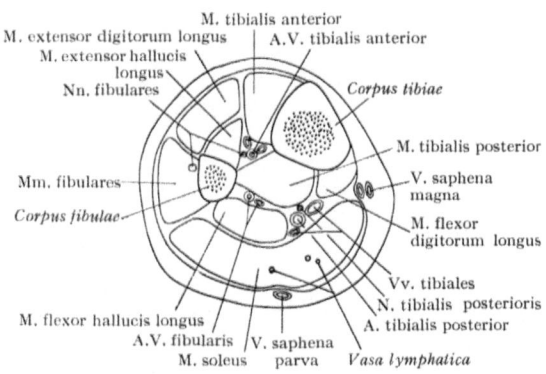

Fig. 498. Axial transverse tomogram

Fig. 499. Anatomical chart

M. tibialis anterior
M. extensor digitorum longus
A.V. tibialis anterior
M. extensor hallucis longus
Nn. fibulares
Corpus tibiae
M. tibialis posterior
Mm. fibulares
V. saphena magna
Corpus fibulae
M. flexor digitorum longus
Vv. tibiales
N. tibialis posterioris
M. flexor hallucis longus
A. tibialis posterior
A.V. fibularis
V. saphena parva
Vasa lymphatica
M. soleus

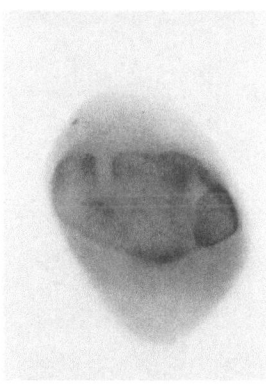

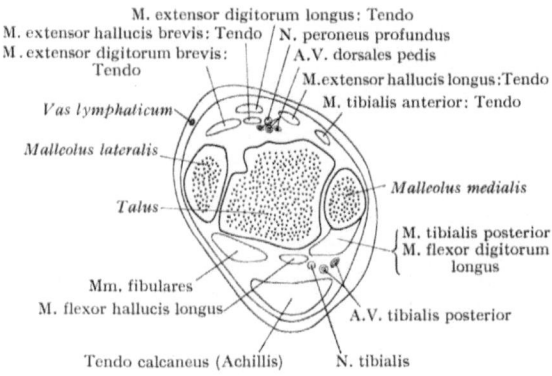

Fig. 500. Axial transverse tomogram

Fig. 501. Anatomical chart

M. extensor digitorum longus: Tendo
M. extensor hallucis brevis: Tendo
N. peroneus profundus
M. extensor digitorum brevis: Tendo
A.V. dorsales pedis
M.extensor hallucis longus:Tendo
M. tibialis anterior: Tendo
Vas lymphaticum
Malleolus lateralis
Malleolus medialis
Talus
M. tibialis posterior
M. flexor digitorum longus
Mm. fibulares
M. flexor hallucis longus
A.V. tibialis posterior
Tendo calcaneus (Achillis)
N. tibialis

231

Part 2

Clinical Applications
of Axial Transverse Tomography

Introduction

Axial transverse tomography applied to clinical practice, especially to diagnosis, has been reported in a number of papers.

The papers I have to hand are as follows:

For axial transverse encephalotomography, papers have appeared by *di Chiro* (16), *Gebauer* (33, 171), *Sansone* et al. (105) while the papers concerning the head were described by *Hammer* (40).

The neck was studied by *Amisano* (5) and the thyroid was examined with insufflation of air into the neck by *Benedetti* (9) and *Farinet* et al. (22).

Pulmonary tuberculosis was dealt with by *Barenbojm* (8), *Kitabatake* (48), *Oliva* (82), *Roussel* et al. (99), *Sharma* et al. (115), *Shimazaki* (118), *Takahashi* (125) and *Voigt* et al. (163), and diagnosis of the tuberculous cavity in the lung by *Matsuda* (65, 67), *Macarini* (56), and *Suchán* (120). Tumor of the lung is discussed by *Balestra* et al. (7) and *Schaudig* et al. (114).

In the diagnosis of the chest the mediastinum is one of the most interesting topics, as the mediastinum is difficult to diagnose by other diagnostic techniques, such as pneumomediastinography, alone; this followed by axial transverse tomography was reported by *Mattine* et al. (76). Mediastinal lesions were examined by *Monod* et al. (78), *Sanquirico* et al. (102), *Sansone* et al. (103), and *Takamatsu* et al. (142). Diagnosis of heart disease was reported by *Bulgarelli* et al. (11—14), *Gremmel* (38), *Ode* et al. (80) and *Vallebona* (155). Aneurysm as well as aortic disease was dealt with by *Alè* et al. (3), *Pompili* et al. (94), *Lodin* (54), *Oliva* (81) and *Thomas* et al. (145, 146). Thymic disease was described by *de Maestri* et al. (61) and *Pompili* et al. (94). Mediastinal lesions were reported by *Buzzi* (15), *Lodin* (53) and *Martin* et al. (62).

The remaining chest diseases were reported by the following: *Fumagalli* et al. (30), *Gebauer* (35, 171, 172), *Hammer* (40), *Kobayashi* et al. (49), *Lodin* (55), *de Maestri* (60), *Matsuda* (64, 69), *Moldenhauer* (77), *Ono* (85, 86), *Ono* et al. (88), *Passeri* (90), *Rollandi* et al. (96), *Sato* (112), *Sharma* et al. (115), *Takahashi* et al. (135), *Vallebona* (153), *de Vulpian* (164) and *Wilk* (168).

As for the diagnosis of the upper abdomen there are very few papers other than those dealing with the pancreas. The pancreas is visualized when air is insufflated into the retroperitoneal space, as was shown by *Clément* (18), *Giraud* et al. (36, 37), *Levrat* et al. (52), *Macarini* et al. (57), *Sansone* et al. (104, 108, 109) and *Wangermez* et al. (165).

The pelvis was studied by *Sansone* et al. (106, 107) for diagnosis of obstetric conditions by *Ono* (84), and congenital luxation of the hip joint by means of a horizontal type unit by *Hachiya* et al. (39).

Recently the method of axial transverse tomography has tended to be applied to radiotherapeutic planning, as it proves useful also to know the bodily extent perpendicular to the body axis.

Nevertheless, axial transverse tomography is not so widely applied to clinical practice as had been expected. One of the reasons could be that interpreters usually have a poor knowledge of the topographical relationship of the organs and tissues arranged in the axial transverse cross section of the body. Moreover, the defect that the existing axial transverse tomograph provides only an indiscernible contour of the axial transverse cross section, due to overexposure at the contour of the body, would make it difficult to apply this method to the planning of radiation therapy. Further, the existing unit of erect type is applied mainly to chest disease but would be difficult to apply to all parts of the body.

Before proceeding to the clinical application of axial transverse tomography either to diagnosis or to therapy, a thorough knowledge of the topographical anatomy of the axial transverse cross section should be obtained, because the establishment of correct roentgen diagnosis and its application to surgical and radiological treatment may be difficult if this knowledge is lacking. This is why this book contains so many normal anatomical illustrations of axial transverse cross section.

In *part two* utilization of axial transverse tomography for diagnostic and therapeutic purposes will be discussed, as the readers are now considered to have obtained from *part one* a sufficient capacity for interpreting normal axial transverse tomograms. The pathological findings of diseased cases are considered to be only deviations from normal cases. With a knowledge of the pathological anatomy as well as of the findings of the axial transverse tomogram of the normal person, the interpretation of the tomographic image of the patient will not be difficult for readers.

I. Application to Diagnosis

Interpretation of findings for the diagnosis of all types of diseases appearing on the axial transverse tomograms will not be described here in order to make the book as simple as possible. It will be dealt with mainly from the theoretical and clinical points of view explaining why and in what points axial transverse tomography is superior to existing methods of roentgenological examination, such as normal roentgenography, conventional tomography and others.

1. Features of Axial Transverse Tomography

Axial transverse tomography is defined as two-dimensional comprehension of the axial transverse cross section of the human body in roentgenological examination. There are two features.

The first is to know the extent of disease in axial transverse cross section by means of a one- shot procedure of roentgenography, and the second is to establish the diagnosis of the disease in one layer of the body by removing shadows of overlapping organs and tissues.

For examining a lesion in the body, normal roentgenography is the most popular type of roentgen examination. In normal roentgenography, conducted by roentgen tube A, however, the three-dimensional body structure is projected on to the two-dimensional roentgen film A', where the concept of depth in the body, dimension X, is lost (Fig. 502).

In order to know the three-dimensional structure of the body, roentgenography conducted by roentgen rays from two directions, A and B, is widely practised.

Findings on a normal roentgenogram A consist of overlapping images of everything contained in the pyramid AA' with its top at focal spot A and its base at roentgen film A'. As in the normal roentgenogram A' the dimension X of the pyramid is lost, the actual construction of the body is not revealed by the roentgen image. In addition to that, the lesions L overlapped by the other tissues T, lacking contrast, would not be discernible and so their existence would be missed. When a normal roentgenogram B is taken in order to avoid these drawbacks, the findings of the pyramid BB' are also examined now. Much more information is obtained thus than from one single normal roentgenogram AA'. The roentgenogram B' newly reveals lesion L free from overlap with tissue T, which in the case of normal roentgenography A alone would be missed.

However, even when these two roentgenograms A' and B' are examined together, the body is still misrepresented as a square pillar rather than a cylinder.

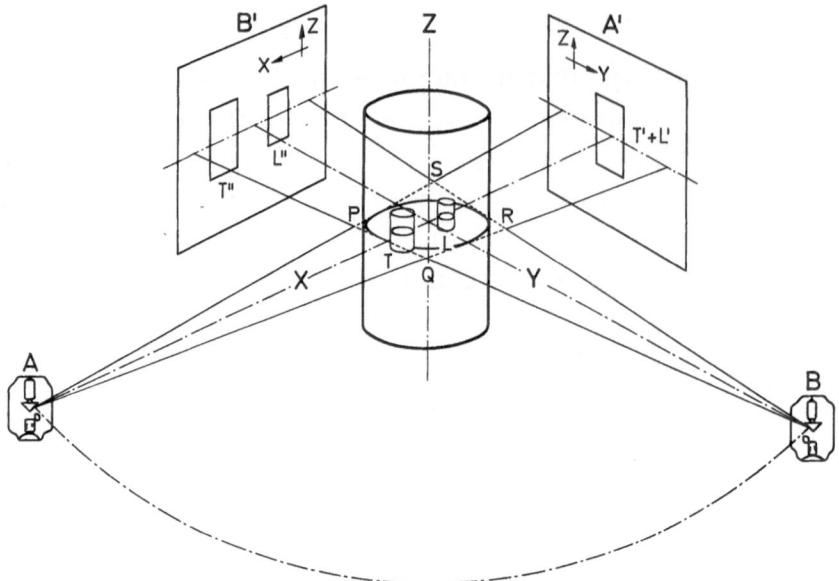

Fig. 502. Schematic drawing of normal roentgenography conducted with two projections. Limited knowledge of three-dimensional structure of the body is obtained. A, B: Roentgen tube. A', B': Film. On the film A' the dimension X is not imaged. T and L are not imaged on film A', but imaged on film B'. Comparative study of film A' and B' does not provide the correct knowledge of the cylinder but misleading knowledge of the square pillar having the rectangular cross-section PQRS

In spite of this fact, it has been generally considered beyond question that a three-dimensional knowledge of the body is obtained if saggital and lateral roentgenograms are taken and examined together.

The femur, for instance, is not regarded as a square pillar, but as a cylinder, when two such roentgenograms are taken and examined.

This is only due to our anatomical knowledge, learned beforehand. As a matter of fact, such a conclusion is theoretically incorrect or, at least, unfounded.

Further, the diagnosis of disease falls outside the normal anatomical field. Lesions take on abnormal position, shape and size in the body and this cannot be concluded from our knowledge of normal anatomy. From this point of view, roentgenograms taken from two directions have essentially weak points for correct diagnosis.

Indeed, roentgenograms taken from many different directions provide more information than those taken from two directions, but the disadvantage still remains that the conclusion obtained from these procedures deviates from the actual construction of the body. Moreover, interpretation becomes a much more troublesome and time-consuming procedure, because the three-dimensional construction of the body is concluded only by integration of these two-dimensional roentgen images.

Even by such an effort, however, the axial transverse cross-section of the body is by no means obtained (Fig. 503).

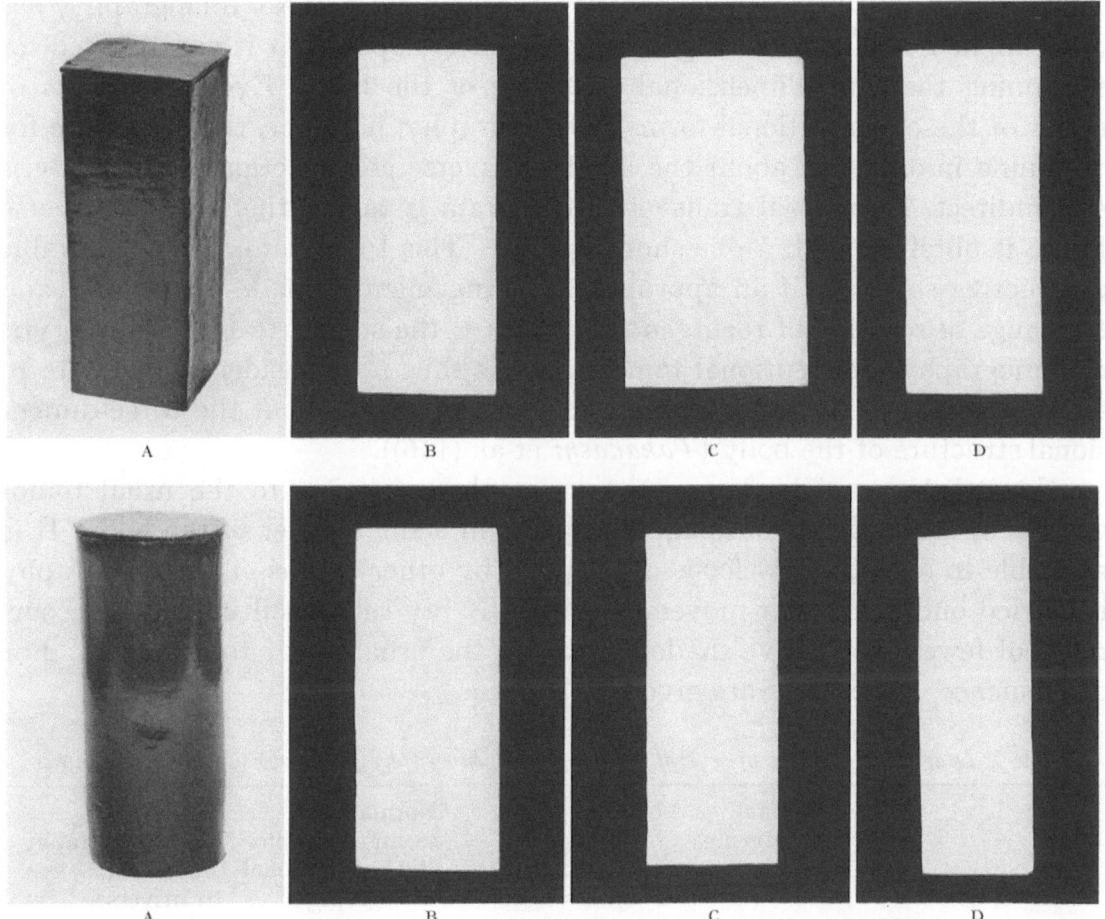

Fig. 503. Three-dimensional knowledge not obtainable by normal roentgenography. Top: Normal photo of a square pillar (A), normal roentgenography in PA view (B), in oblique view (C) and in lateral view (D). Bottom: Normal photo of an elliptic cylinder (A), normal roentgenography in PA view (B), in oblique view (C) and in lateral view (D).
Correct identification of pillar and cylinder is difficult

Axial transverse tomography is thus superior to the examination of normal roentgenograms taken from many directions, in that the dimensions of X and Y can be obtained accurately and concretely with a simple one-shot procedure.

There is another roentgenographic method which provides the information of the dimension of depth and permits the detection of new foci. By means of multisection radiography it may become possible for us to know the three-dimensional structure of the body. Actually, however, multisection radiography is not usually used for such a purpose, because the body structure is not clearly seen because of disturbance by obstructive shadows, especially when the linear tomograph is used. Recently, multidirectional tomography, which is characterised by creating fewer obstructive shadows than linear tomography, has been applied to clinical roentgenology and it is hoped that it can be used for examining the three-dimensional structure of the body. Even by means of either of these conventional forms of tomography, however, the procedure for obtaining information about the axial transverse cross section of the body is still indirect. If an axial transverse tomogram is taken, the axial transverse figure is obtained with a one-shot exposure. This tomogram shows negligible obstructive shadows, if an appropriate arrangement is made of the unit and the range of rotation of roentgen tube. This is the special feature of this type of tomography. Conventional tomography is thus not considered adequate to supply the knowledge of axial transverse cross section or of the three-dimensional structure of the body (*Takahashi* et al. (136)).

Nevertheless, axial transverse tomography is similar to the usual tomography in the principle of image formation in a single layer of the body. It is also able to detect a new focus overlapped by other organs. This tomography is carried out by circular movement of the X-ray tube resulting in the occurrence of fewer obstructive shadows than in the usual linear tomography. For convenience, its features are given in Table 2.

Table 2. *Diagnostic features of several types of roentgenography for establishment of diagnosis*

	Normal roentgenography	Normal roentgenographs taken from two directions	Normal roentgenography and conventional tomography	Normal roentgenography and axial transverse tomography
Detection of lesions	+	++	+++	+++
Comprehension of axial transverse layer	−	+ (indirectly)	+ (indirectly)	+++
Three-dimensional comprehension of the body	−	++	++ or +++	+++

− difficult; + good; ++ better; +++ excellent.

2. Establishment of Diagnosis for Clinical Cases

As the lesions are imaged on the normal roentgenogram, with overlap of shadows of various tissues and organs in the body, the level of the body to be transversely tomographed is determined by observation of the normal roentgenogram. The level to be cross-sectioned is selected and marked in ink on the corresponding portion of the patient's skin. The patient is laid on the roentgenographic table of the horizontal type unit. Normal roentgenography in which the wire representing the level to be tomographed is imaged on the roentgenogram is conducted as described on p. 6.

If there is no gross difference between the location of the expected level and that actually tomographed, axial transverse tomography is then carried out. Otherwise, the position of the patient is adjusted and axial transverse tomography is conducted. Such readjustment will be simple and precise, if an image intensifier or roentgen television is placed under the tomographic table and examined.

At clinical interpretation the findings appearing on the axial transverse tomograms of the patient are compared with those of the normal persons illustrated in the Atlas.

For this, first of all the axial transverse tomogram of the patient is taken in the same position as that of the normal person of the Atlas. When taking the tomogram of a cancer of the maxillary sinus, for instance, the patient is laid supine on the tomographic table, either with his orbitomeatal line or with his acanthiomeatal line vertical, and the axial transverse tomogram is taken.

The standards for positioning are the orbitomeatal line or acanthiomeatal line for the head; the level of the spine for the neck, the chest and the upper abdomen; the pubic bone or pelvic cavity for the lower abdomen. Only when such a procedure of positioning is made can the findings of the axial transverse tomogram be referred to those of the Atlas and the interpretation carried out easily and correctly.

Although with the standard level the positioning of the patient is made the same as that of the normal person of the Atlas, it will be found at times that the figure of the axial transverse tomogram of the patient does not coincide with that of the Atlas. This is frequently the case in diagnosis of the viscera.

In such a case the Atlas is searched for suitable illustrations of the similar part of the body to the figure of the tomogram.

For interpretation of hilum of the lung, for instance, the level tomographed is shown as a transverse line on the normal roentgenogram. The illustration of the Atlas in which the hilum is shown should be adopted. It is advisable not to refer only to the spine as a guide.

For interpretation it is also essential first of all to refer to the original normal roentgenogram. Abnormalities in findings seen or suspected on the normal roentgenogram, which reveals it just on the image of level tomographed, are usually shown on the axial transverse tomogram.

By comparing the normal roentgenogram with the tomogram, the correct diagnosis will be established.

The level of the normal roentgenogram is thus essential for determining the need for tomography, performance of correct positioning and as a guide for interpretation. Without reference to the normal roentgenogram taken with the patient laid on the tomographic table and the Atlas, the application of axial transverse tomography to clinical practice will be limited.

Now, in order to explain how this type of tomography contributes to clinical practice, cases will be shown below.

There is a fear, however, that the number of illustrations could run up to tremendous amount, as this type of radiography has the unique feature of being exclusively capable of imaging axial transverse cross sections of lesions in the body. Yet the space assigned is limited.

Thus, cases are shown here in a rather limited number of presentations, but with examples of every part of the body. The main reasons for this are, first: the illustrations of normal persons which will contribute to the diagnosis are already supplied in the Atlas and, second: no book containing cases of every part of the body has been published before.

In our description we have tried especially to show the unique features of axial transverse tomography in contributing to diagnosis better than or as well as conventional tomography for detecting new lesions, or contributing better to diagnosis than normal roentgenography or conventional tomography, in that axial transverse tomography makes clear with a one-shot procedure the size, shape and location of the lesions in axial transverse cross section of the body.

Cases will be shown with the diagnosis and the history of the patient. Prior to the description of the findings of the axial transverse tomogram concerned, the normal roentgenograms or tomograms will be interpreted.

Diagnosis: Cancer of the right maxillary sinus.

Case: T. O., age 65, female.

History: The patient complains of slight but gradually increasing swelling of the face on the right side and rhinorrhea. Exophthalmus developed in the right side recently.

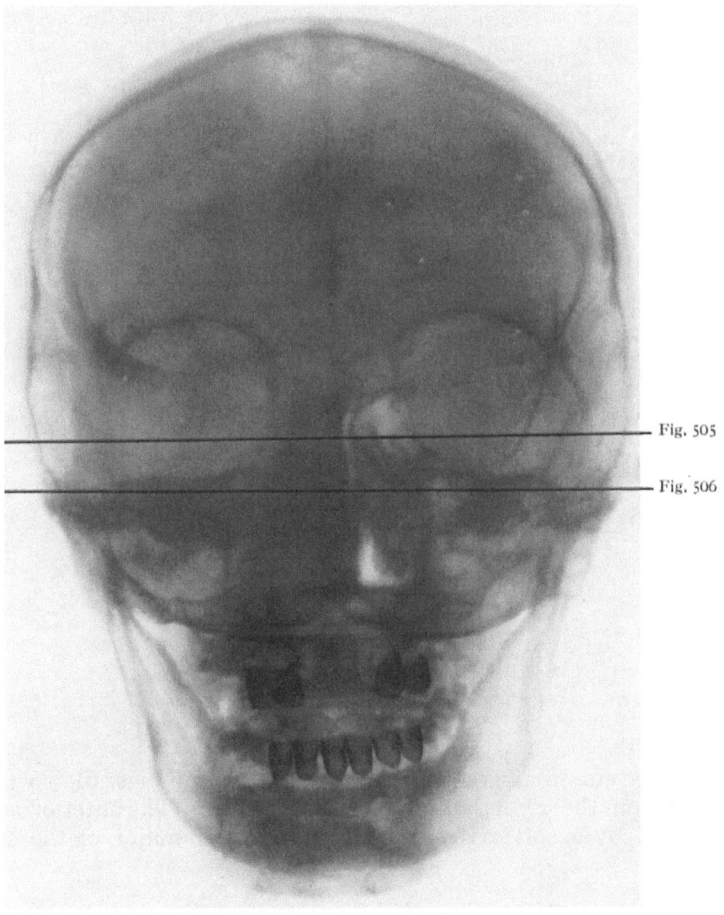

Fig. 504. Normal roentgenogram. Horizontal line showing the level tomographed. There is homogeneous density in the right inferior nasal cavity and ethmoid sinus. The lateral wall of the right maxillary sinus is slightly destroyed

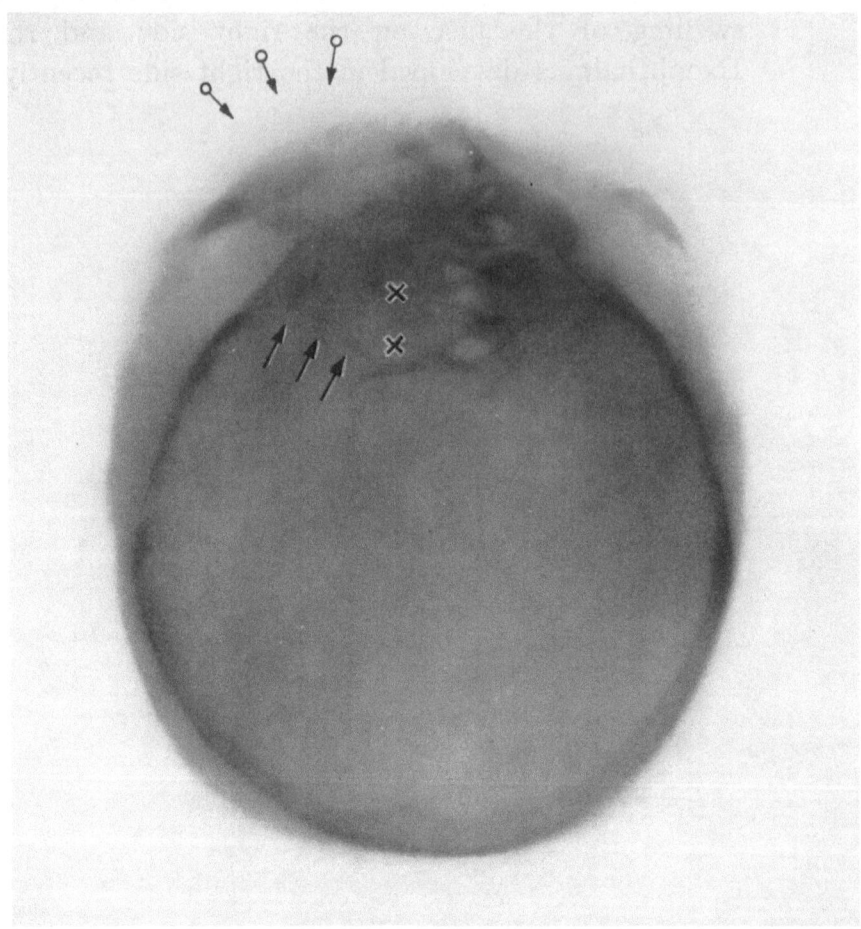

Fig. 505. Axial transverse tomogram. Refer to the normal Figs. 61—65, p. 38. There is soft tissue swelling (⟋) on the right lateral aspect of the face. The anterior and posterior ethmoid sinuses are occupied by a soft tissue mass (✗). The ala major of the sphenoid bone shows destruction (⟋)

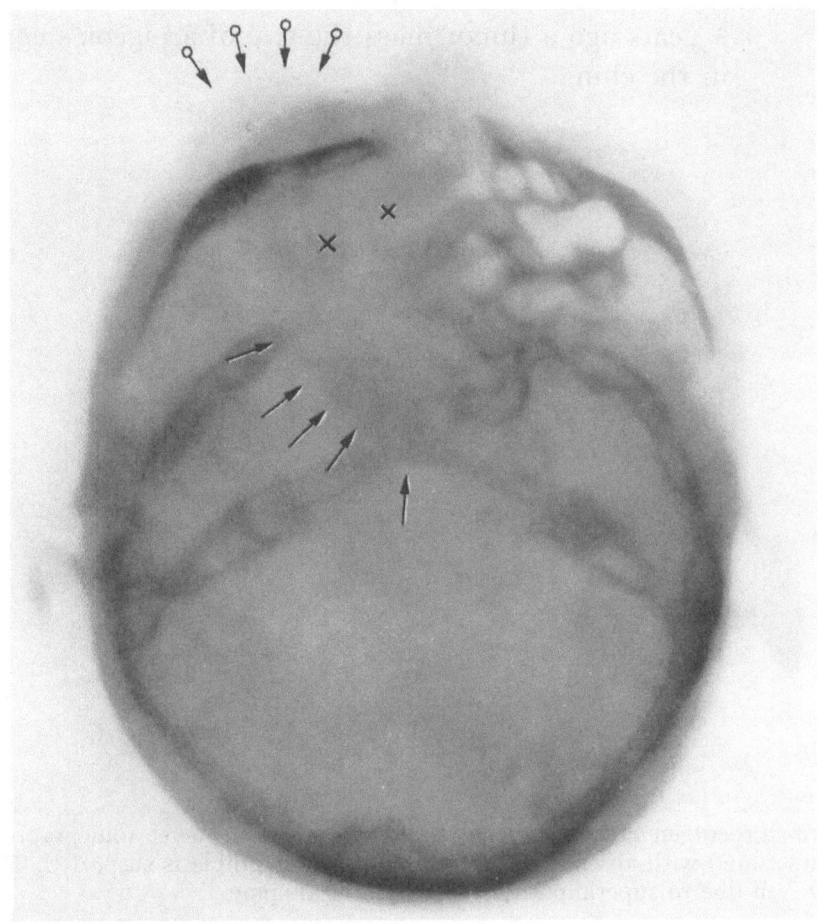

Fig. 506. Axial transverse tomogram. Refer to the normal Figs. 71—75, p. 42. There is soft tissue swelling (↗) noted on the anterior and lateral aspect of the maxillary sinus. The maxillary sinus and nasal cavity on the right side are hazy but no translucency is noted (×). The posterior wall of the maxillary sinus as well as processus coronoideus are indistinctly seen (↗). The anterior wall of the maxillary sinus is partially destroyed

Diagnosis: Metastatic cancer of the mandible.

Case: M. S., age 30, male.

History: After the removal of the cancer from the base of the tongue 3 years ago a tumor mass the size of a pigeon's egg appeared in the chin.

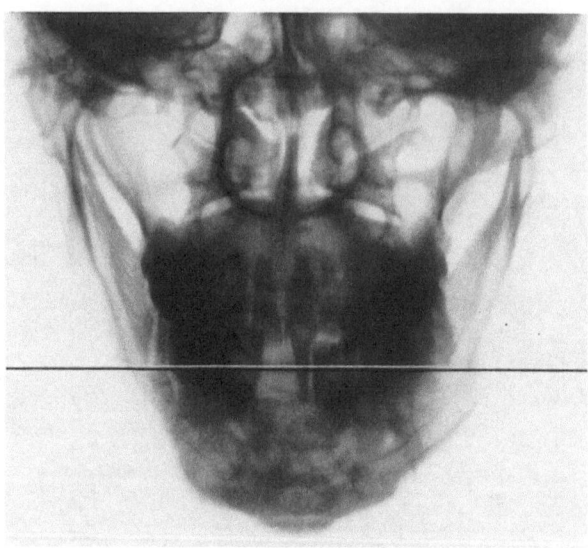

Fig. 507. Normal roentgenogram. Horizontal line showing the level tomographed. Irregular bony defect associated with absence of the incisor in the mandible is suspected. These findings are not easily seen due to superimposition of the cervical spine

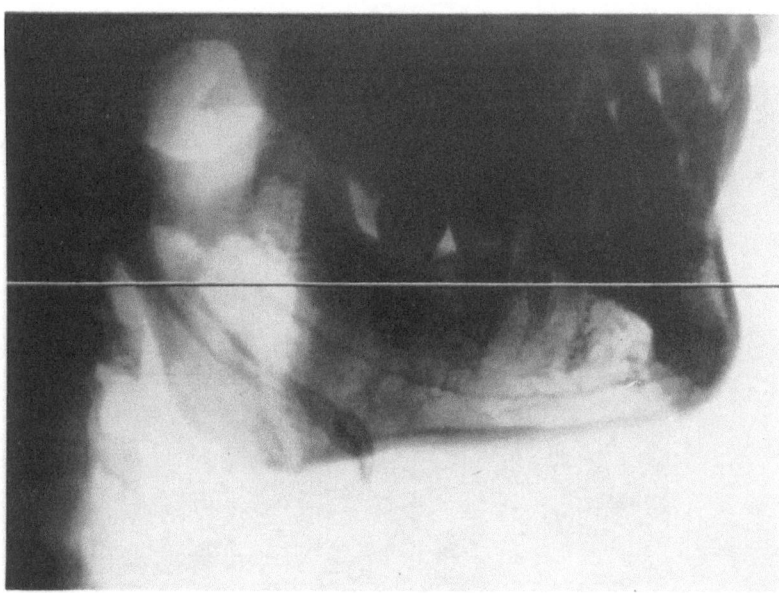

Fig. 508. Normal roentgenogram. Horizontal line showing the level tomographed. In the oblique view, there is a small defect in the anterior portion of the mandible. In the lateral view of the mandible, no evidence of bony defect is noted

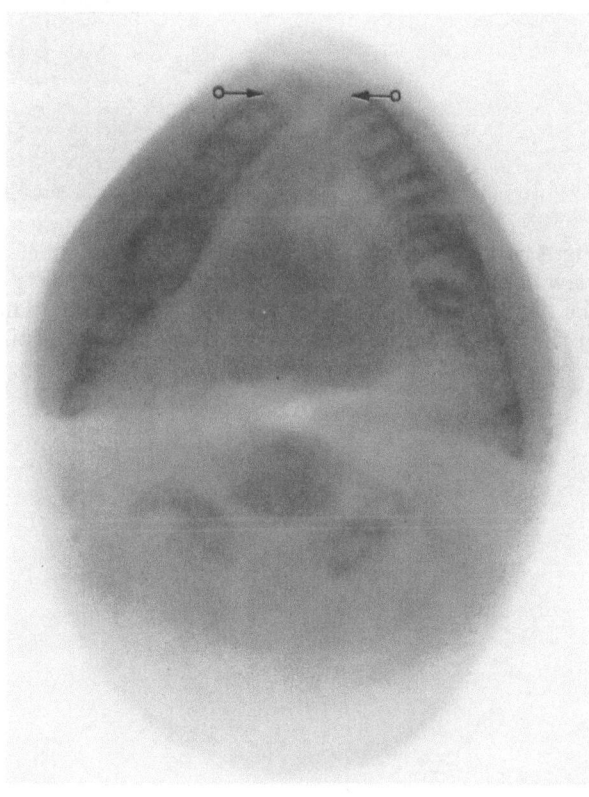

Fig. 509. Axial transverse tomogram. See Figs. 101—105, p. 56, for normal axial transverse tomogram of this level. Axial transverse tomogram shows a defect (✓) measuring 20 mm in length in the mid-portion of the mandibular body. No other abnormality is seen

Diagnosis: Suspected myositis ossificans.

Case: S. H., age 54, male.

History: Numbness of the extremities and difficulty in walking for
                 7 to 8 years.

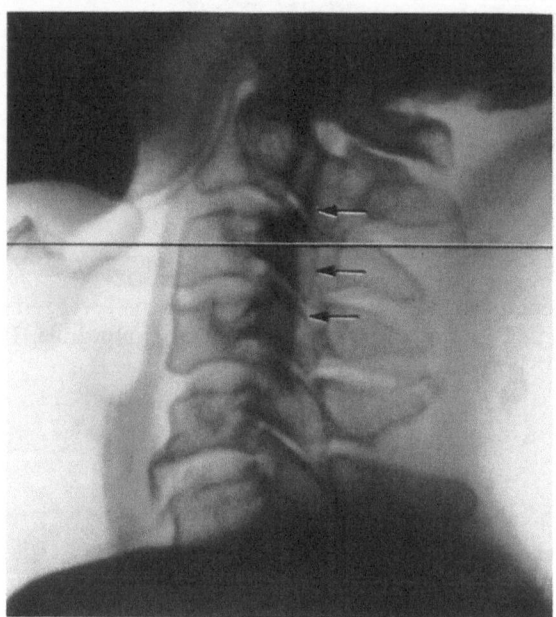

Fig. 510. Normal roentgenogram. Horizontal line showing the level tomographed. The lateral
view of the cervical spine shows a tape-like calcific density (↗) superimposed on the laminae of
the second, third and fourth cervical vertebrae. There is a calcific plaque of 7 × 10 mm in size
in the soft tissues in the posterior aspect of the spine (ligamentum nuchae)

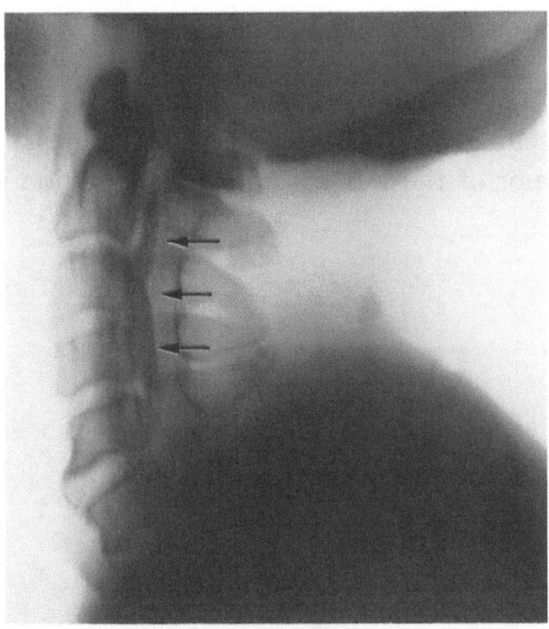

Fig. 511. Conventional tomogram. The lateral view reveals a tape-like calcific density (∕) along the posterior aspect of the vertebral bodies of C_2, C_3, C_4, C_5

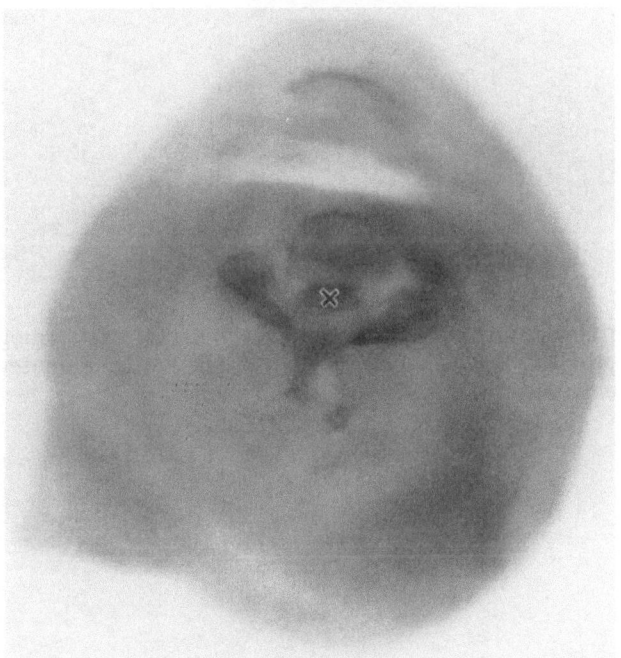

Fig. 512. Axial transverse tomogram. See Figs. 121—125, p. 64, for normal axial transverse tomogram at this level. In the normal neck no calcification is noted in the spine space. The axial transverse tomogram shows the cross-section of the vertebral body, spinal process and other structures of the spine. There is an oval-shaped calcific thickening (✗) in the cervical spinal canal which in view of its position and shape is considered to be calcified posterior longitudinal ligament

Diagnosis: Tumor of the left thyroideal lobe

Case: K. S., age 36, female

History: Swelling of the neck and hoarseness for two years. The tumor of the left thyroideal lobe region is noted.

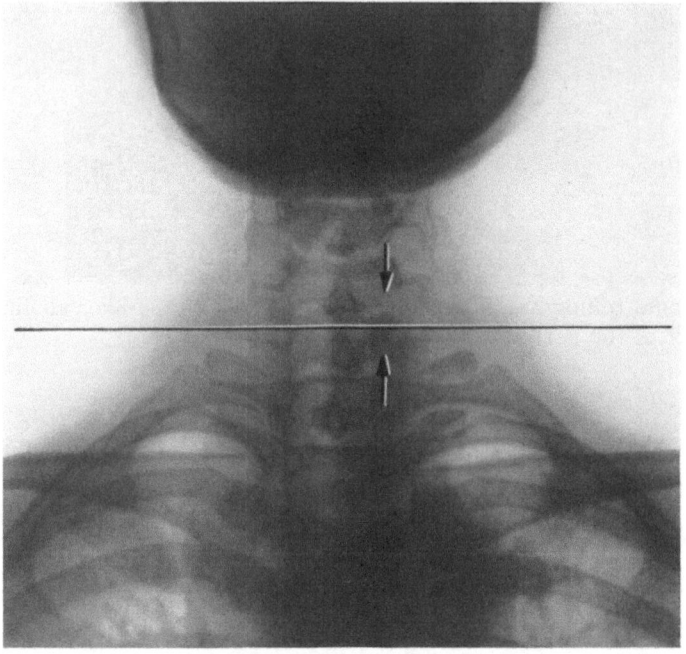

Fig. 513. Normal roentgenogram. Horizontal line showing the level tomographed. The cervical trachea is deviated to the right. A calcified body (✗), one cm in diameter, is seen to be superimposed upon the seventh cervical vertebral body on the left

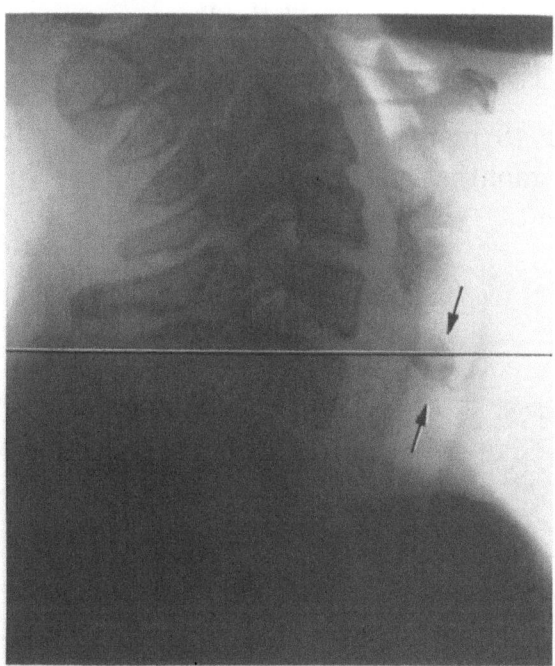

Fig. 514. Normal roentgenogram. Horizontal line showing the level tomographed. Lateral view of the neck shows the body (✗) superimposed on the trachea

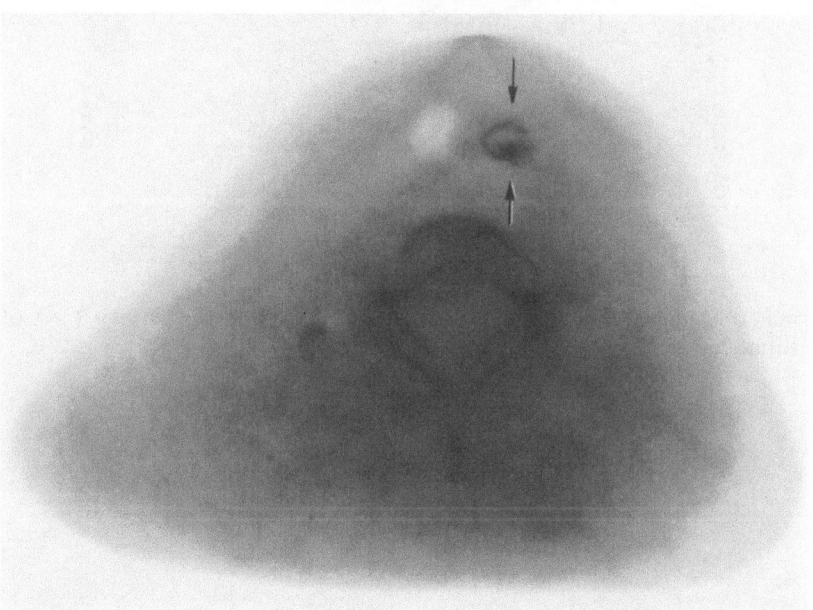

Fig. 515. Axial transverse tomogram. See Figs. 141—145, p. 72 for normal axial transverse tomogram at this level. A light swelling of soft tissue is seen in the left anterior neck. The trachea, whose left side wall is compressed by the tumor, is deviated to the right. A ring shadow with irregular contour of high density is seen in the tumor (✗). In view of the position, the calcification seems to be in the struma

Diagnosis: Tuberculous cavity of the lung.

Case: K. T., age 28, male.

History: For 18 months productive cough and fatigue. For the last 10 months he has been treated with an antituberculous agent.

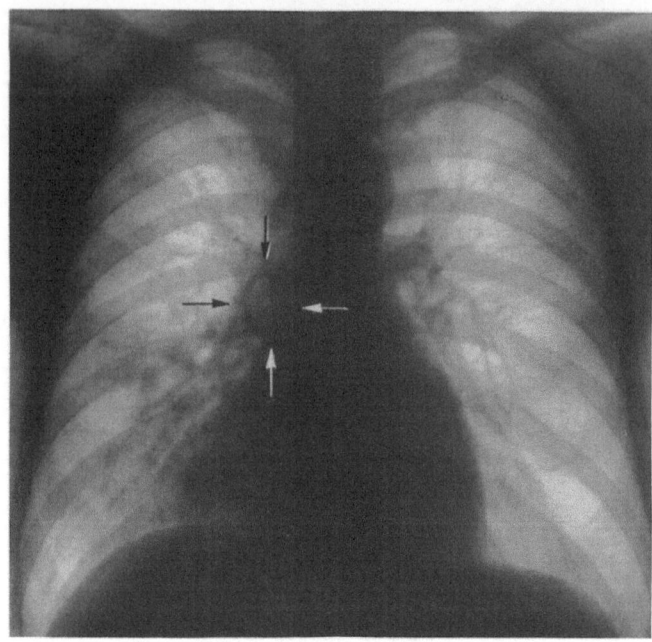

Fig. 516. Normal roentgenogram taken 10 months ago reveals the cavity (⟋) of 3.0 × 2.5 cm in size at the hilum

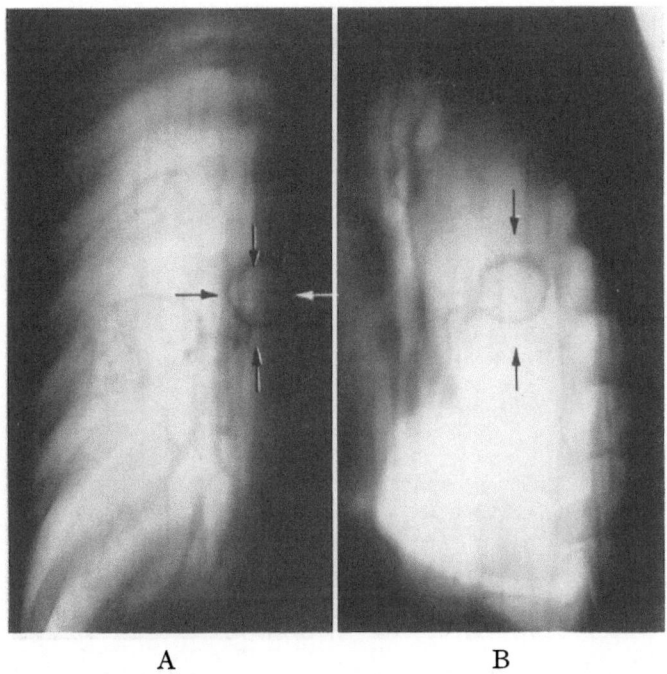

Fig. 517 A and B. Conventional tomograms taken at that time show clearly the location and size of the cavity (↗) in a.p. and lateral view

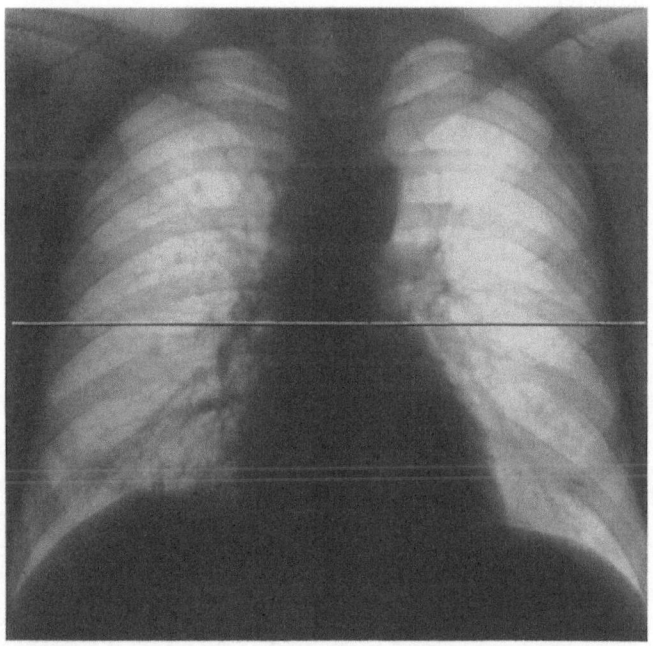

Fig. 518. In the normal roentgenogram taken very recently, nodular lesions are seen to be scattered in the right lower lung field. No evidence of cavity. Horizontal line showing the level tomographed

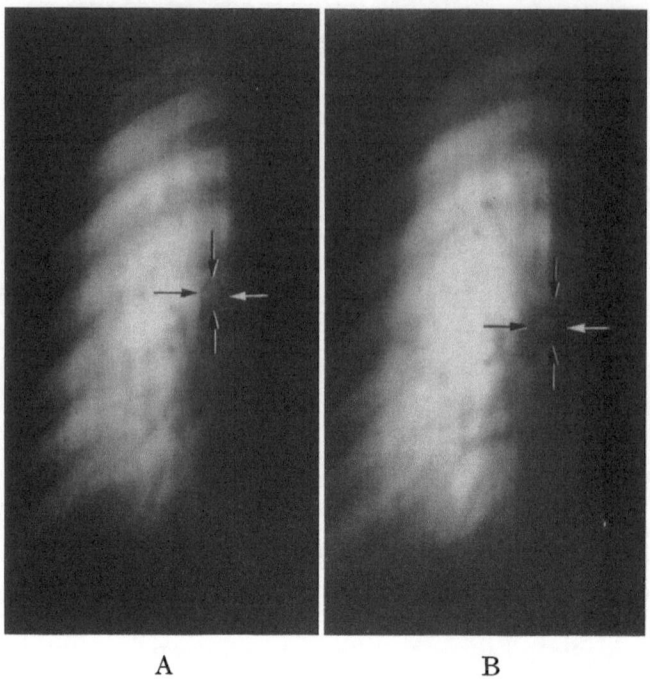

A B

Fig. 519A and B. The conventional tomogram at 5 cm level from posterior chest wall, A, reveals a small thin-walled cavity (↗) medially measuring 8 mm in diameter, while at 6 cm, B, the cavity is 12 mm in diameter

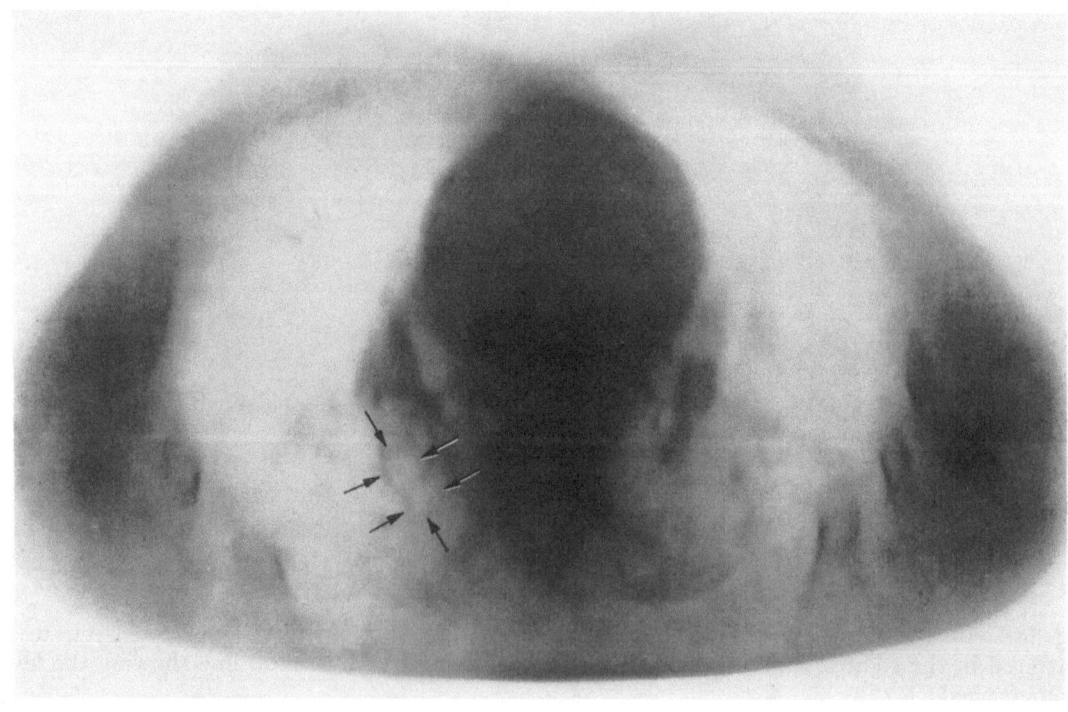

Diagnosis: Foreign body.

Case: T. K., age 35, male.

History: The patient swallowed a nail three months ago accidentally. Right chest pain, cough and expectoration were noted recently.

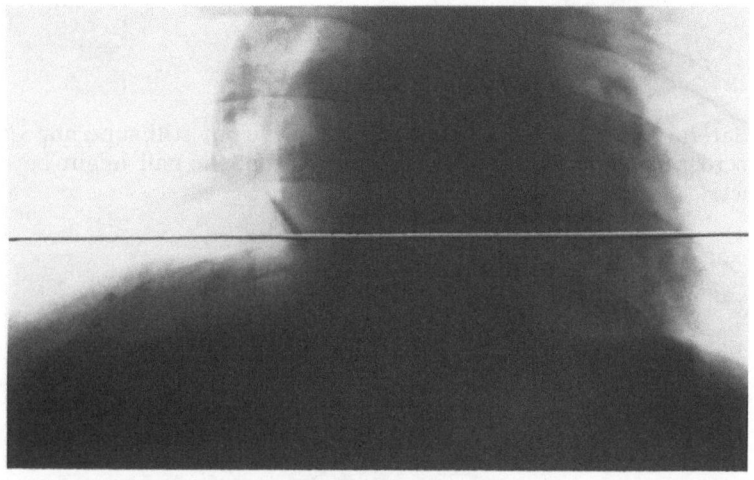

Fig. 521. Normal roentgenogram. Horizontal line showing the level tomographed. In the a.p. view a small nail is seen at the right base medially superimposed on the shadow of the heart

Fig. 520. Axial transverse tomogram. See the normal Figs. 223—227, p. 108. A dumb-bell-shaped radiolucent shadow (↗) is seen in the area of pulmonary infiltration in the right posterior lung field. The location of the cavity coincides with the cavity of the normal roentgenogram taken before chemotherapy and with that of the conventional tomogram taken at the same time as this examination. The anterior part of the cavity is 15 mm in diameter, while the posterior part is 10 mm in diameter. The cavitation is surrounded by the infiltration, and is seen at the postero-median region of the right lung field

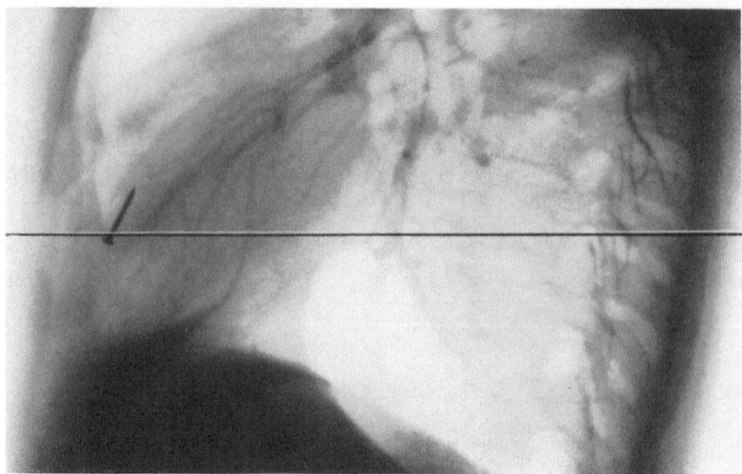

Fig. 522. In the lateral view, the nail is located anteriorly, but still superimposed on the heart. If only these two roentgenograms are used for examination, the nail might be concluded to be in the heart muscle

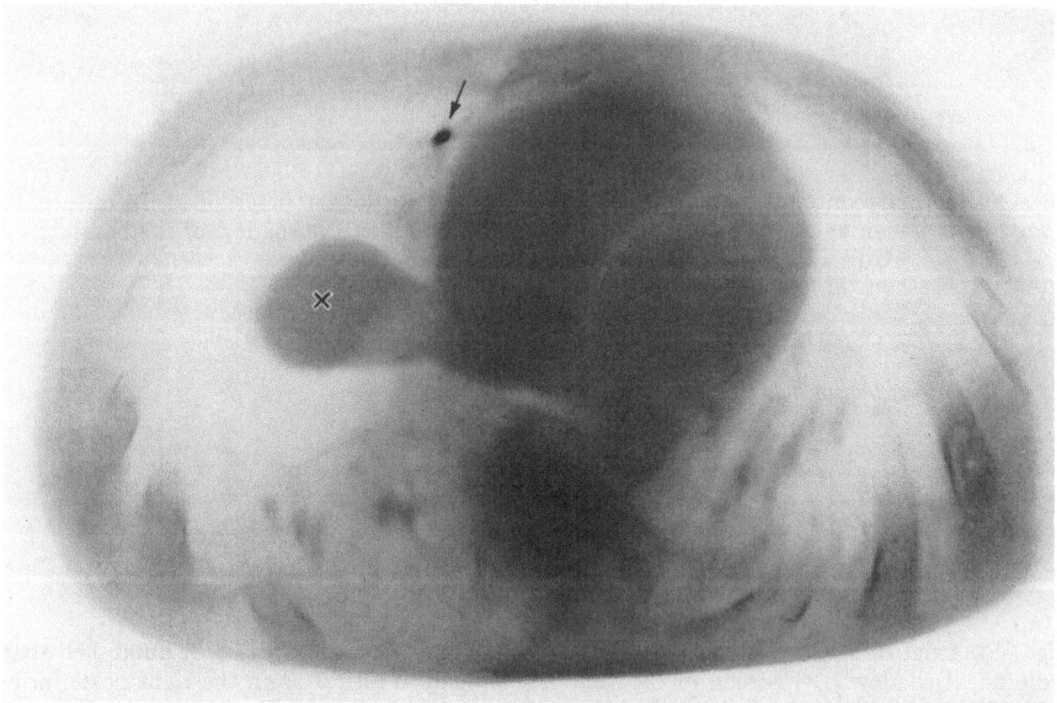

Fig. 523. Axial transverse tomogram. See Figs. 248—252, p. 118, for normal axial transverse tomogram at this level. It is clear from the axial transverse tomogram that the nail (✓) is located definitely in the lung. After establishment of the diagnosis, transbronchial removal of the nail was tried but failed. The foreign body was removed by thoracotomy. Diaphragm (×)

Diagnosis: Malignant lymphoma.

Case: M. A., age 42, male.

History: The patient complains of general fatigue and swelling of the
               lymph nodes in the various parts of the body.

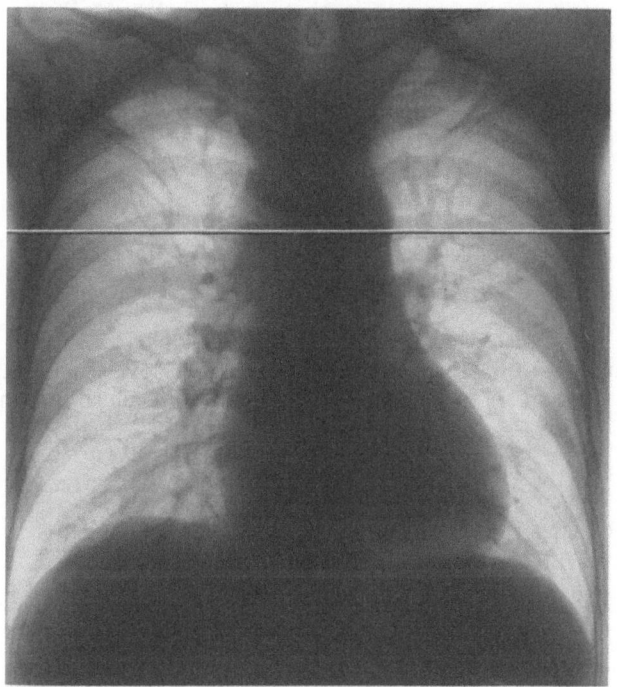

Fig. 524. Normal roentgenogram. Horizontal line showing the level tomographed. The p.a. view
reveals slight widening of the superior mediastinum on the right side but nothing on the left.
Both lung fields are clear

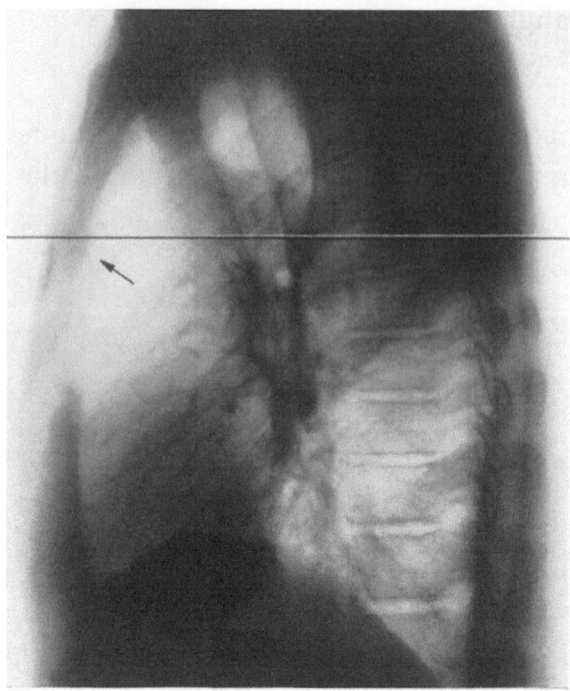

Fig. 525. Normal roentgenogram. Horizontal line showing the level tomographed. Lateral view of the chest, a soft tissue mass (↗) is suspected substernally, measuring about 5 cm in length and 0.5 cm in width

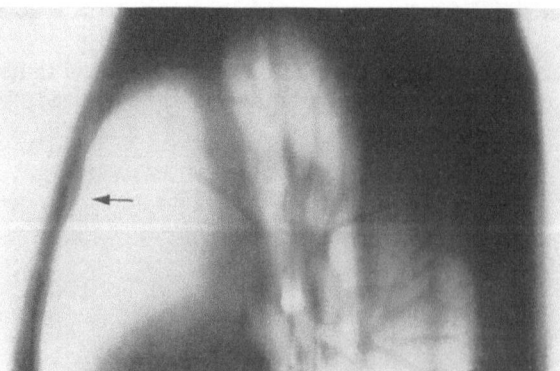

Fig. 526. Conventional tomogram. When the conventional lateral tomogram of this part of the chest is taken (2 cm left of median), a homogeneous, thin crescent-shaped shadow (↗) is seen substernally

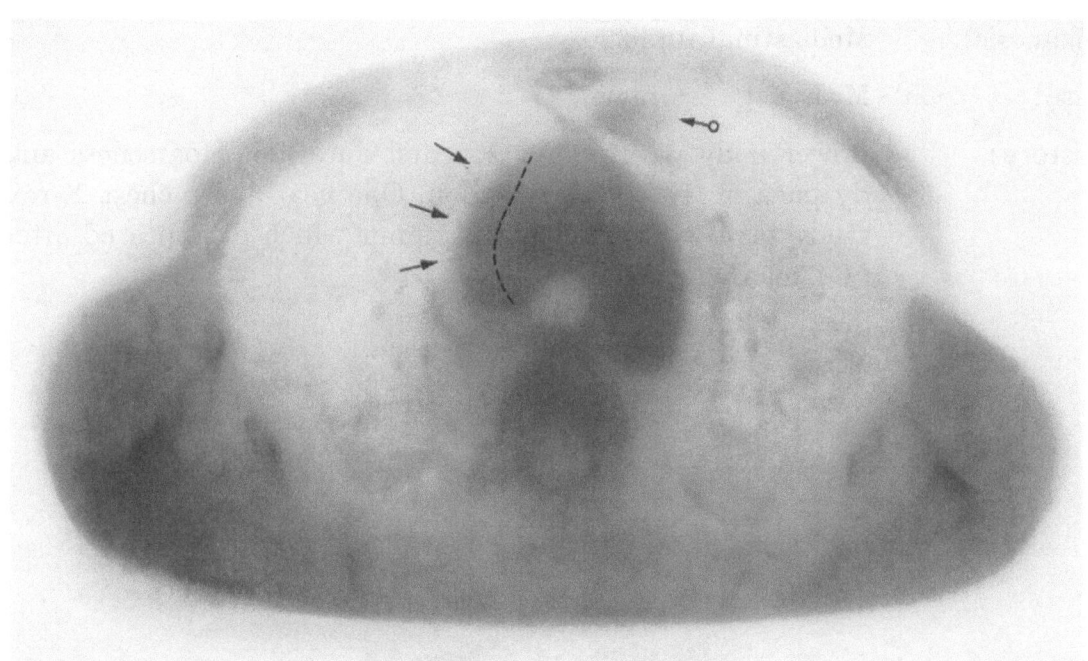

Fig. 527. Axial transverse tomogram. See Figs. 193—202, p. 96, for normal axial transverse tomogram at this level. There is a triangular opacity (↗) substernally on the left side, just anterior to the aortic arch, which is not seen on the normal roentgenogram. The increasing area of homogeneous shadow (↗) adjacent to the ascending aorta is manifested by broadening of its width which corresponds to the shadow noted on the normal roentgenogram

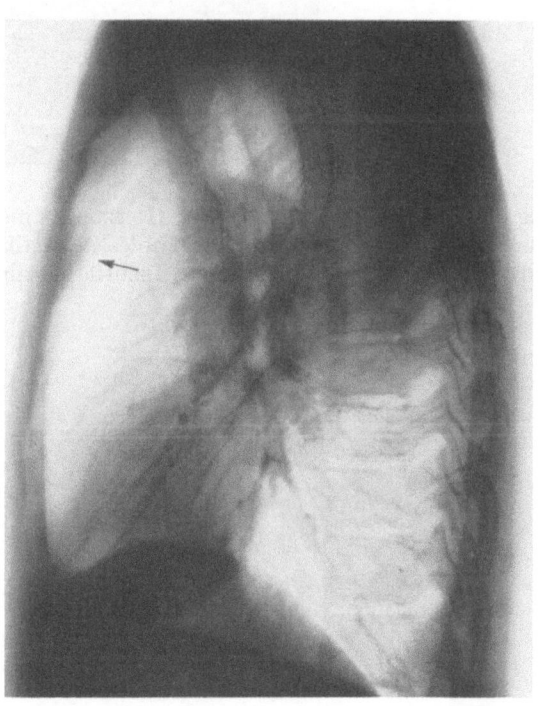

Fig. 528. Normal roentgenogram taken 3 months later reveals the marked crescent-shaped homogeneous shadow (↗) which is considered to be due to the swelling of the lymph nodes along the internal mammary artery

Diagnosis: Mediastinal tumor.

Case: M. K., age 52, male.

History: Lower body paralysis of 2 years' duration. Hoarseness and dyspnea of one year's duration. One year ago a chest X-ray study revealed a mediastinal tumor which disappeared after ^{60}Co teletherapy.

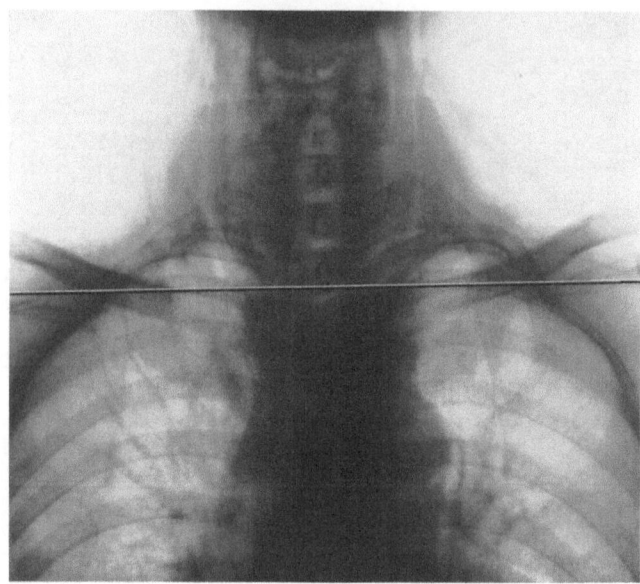

Fig. 529. Normal roentgenogram. Horizontal line showing the level tomographed. The p.a. view of the chest reveals nothing remarkable. A small calcification in the right pulmonary apex but with right clavicle superimposed. Insufflated air is imaged in the mediastinum and in the neck

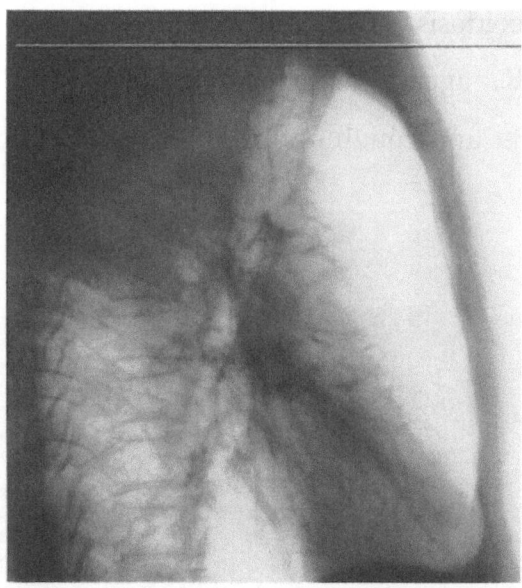

Fig. 530. Normal roentgenogram. Horizontal line showing the level tomographed. A soft tissue mass is suspected in the superior mediastinum posteriorly in the lateral view

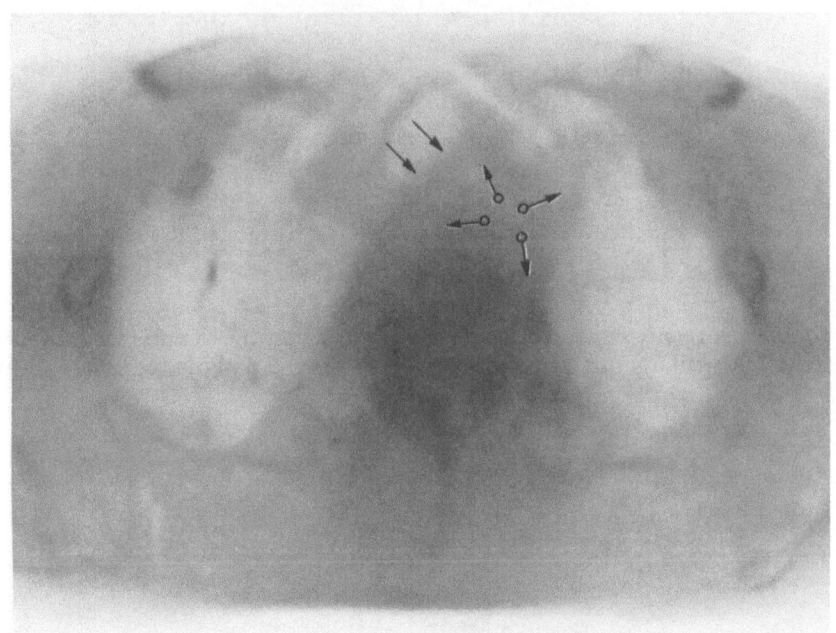

Fig. 531. Axial transverse tomogram. See Figs. 168—172, p. 86, for normal axial transverse tomogram at this level. A soft tissue mass about 3 × 3 cm is seen in the superior mediastinum on the left side, compressing the trachea slightly anteriorly to the right (↗). The cross-section of the trachea is not circular but semilunar. Increase of shadow (↗) at the anterior mediastinum especially sinistrally. Small opaque spot in the right lung field is the shadow of calcification seen on the pulmonary apex of the normal roentgenogram

Diagnosis: Sarcoidosis.

Case: K. K., age 10, male.

History: Fever and cough of two months' duration.

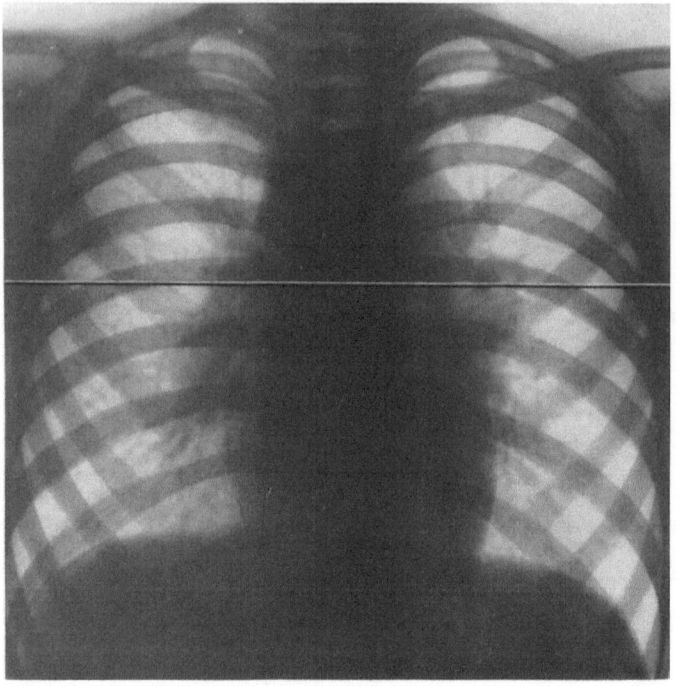

Fig. 532. Normal roentgenogram. Horizontal line showing the level tomographed. Bilateral hilar adenopathy with enlargement of mediastinal shadow. The lung fields are clear

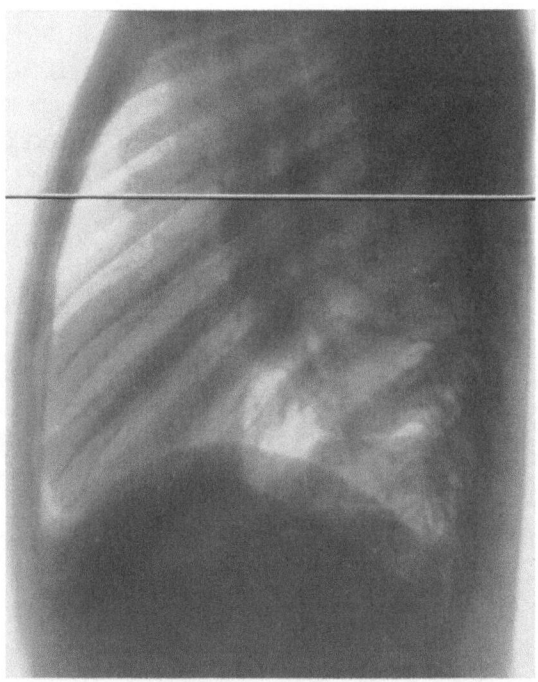

Fig. 533. Normal roentgenogram. Horizontal line showing the level tomographed. Lateral view shows similar findings to Fig. 532

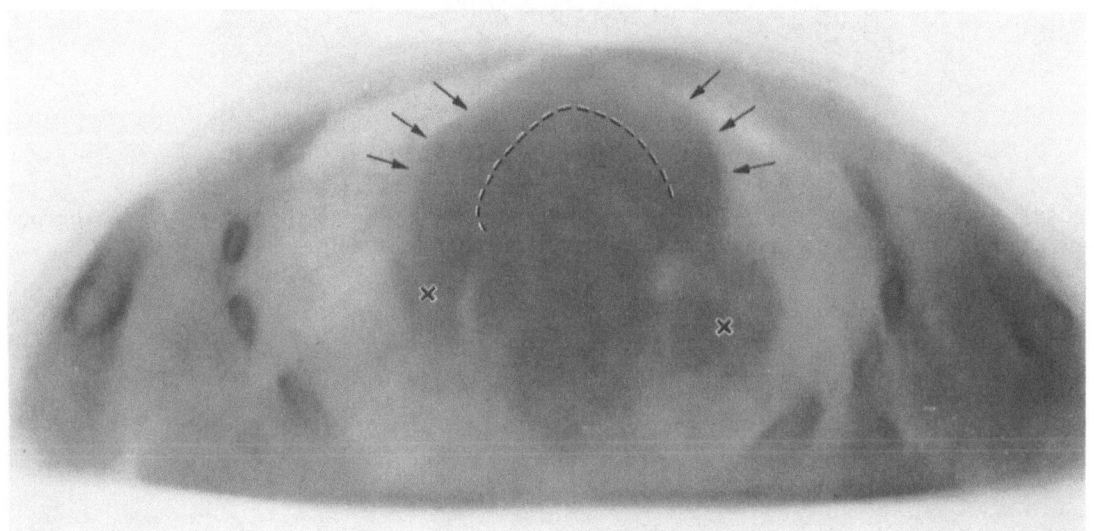

Fig. 534. Axial transverse tomogram. See Figs. 218—222, p. 106, for normal axial transverse tomogram at this level. The axial transverse tomogram reveals a remarkable mediastinal lymphadenopathy. The bronchopulmonary lymph nodes (×) are also markedly enlarged along both sides of the bronchus. The shadow of the anterior mediastinum increases in width, suggesting a marked swelling of the anterior mediastinal lymph nodes (↗)

Diagnosis: Vanishing tumor.

Case: T. M., age 53, female.

History: The patient, who has a history of cured cancer of the uterus, noted low backaches and coughs.

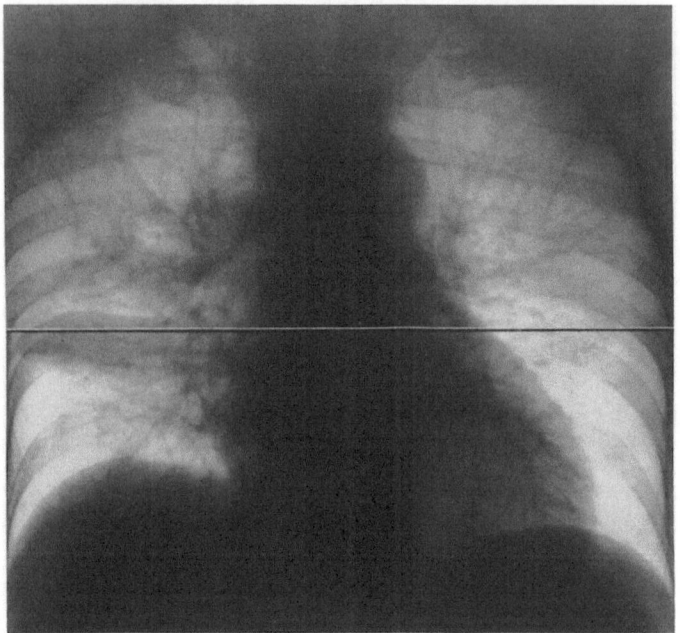

Fig. 535. Normal roentgenogram. Horizontal line showing the level tomographed. In the p.a. view there is an ellipsoid homogeneous shadow in the right horizontal fissure

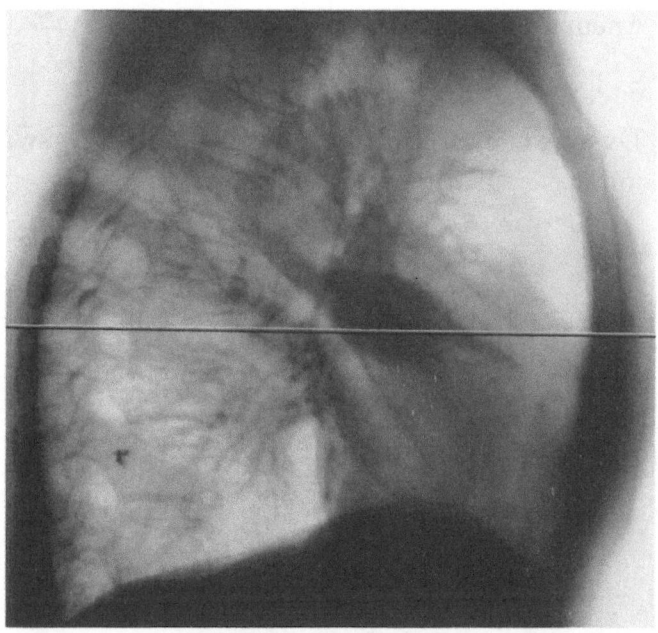

Fig. 536. Normal roentgenogram. Horizontal line showing the level tomographed. The lateral view reveals a round homogeneous shadow with three wings spreading over the main and horizontal fissures

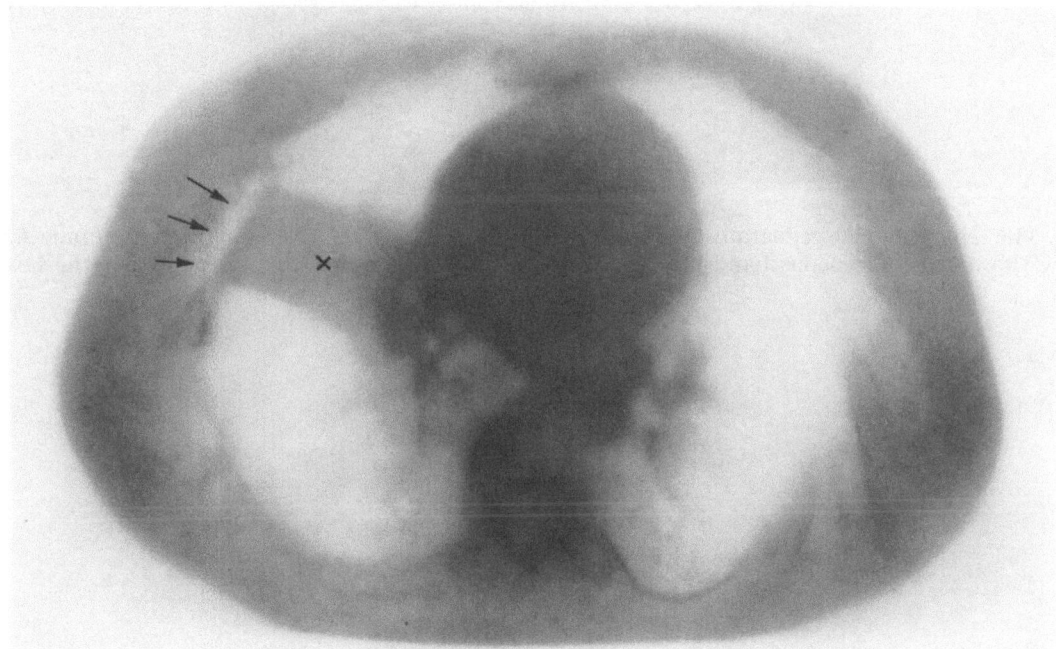

Fig. 537. Axial transverse tomogram. See Figs. 223—227, p. 108, for normal axial transverse tomogram at this level. The axial transverse tomogram reveals a rectangular homogeneous opacity (×) in the middle lobe of the right lung slightly anteriorly. A slit-like radiolucency (╱) is noted between the opacity and the lateral chest wall, revealing the curved downward turn of the horizontal fissure

Diagnosis: Aneurysm of the thoracic aorta.

Case: S. T., age 56, male.

History: Dyspnea, palpitation and difficulty in swallowing of two months' duration.

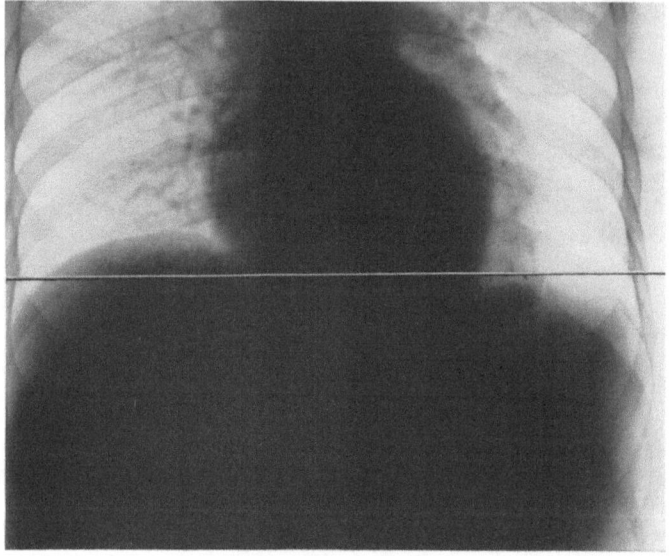

Fig. 538. Normal roentgenogram. Horizontal line showing the level tomographed. Supine a.p. view shows a homogeneous band-like shadow along the left margin of the shadow of the heart

Fig. 540. Axial transverse tomogram. See Figs. 258—267, p. 122, for normal axial transverse tomogram at this level. There is a large aneurysmal dilation (×) of the aorta, about 7 cm in diameter, with semicircular calcification left laterally (╱). The widening of the aorta causes moderate displacement of the fornix of the stomach (S) toward the anterior

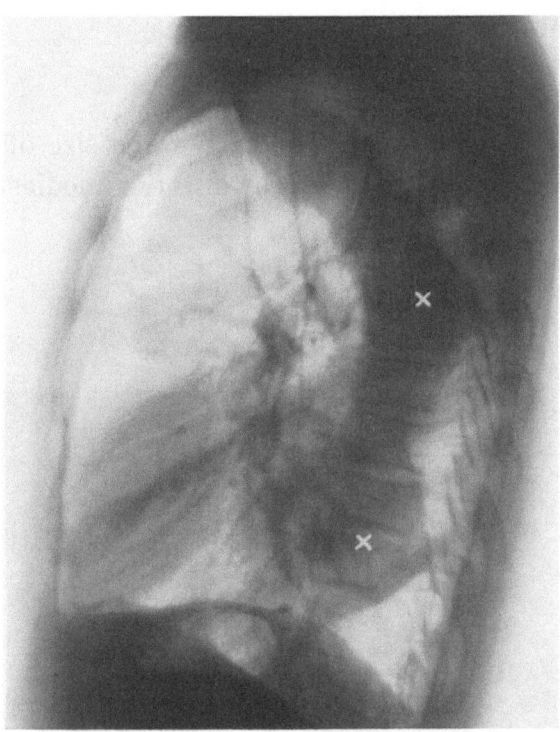

Fig. 539. The lateral view of the chest reveals at least two aneurysmal dilatations (×) of the descending thoracic aorta with calcification of the wall

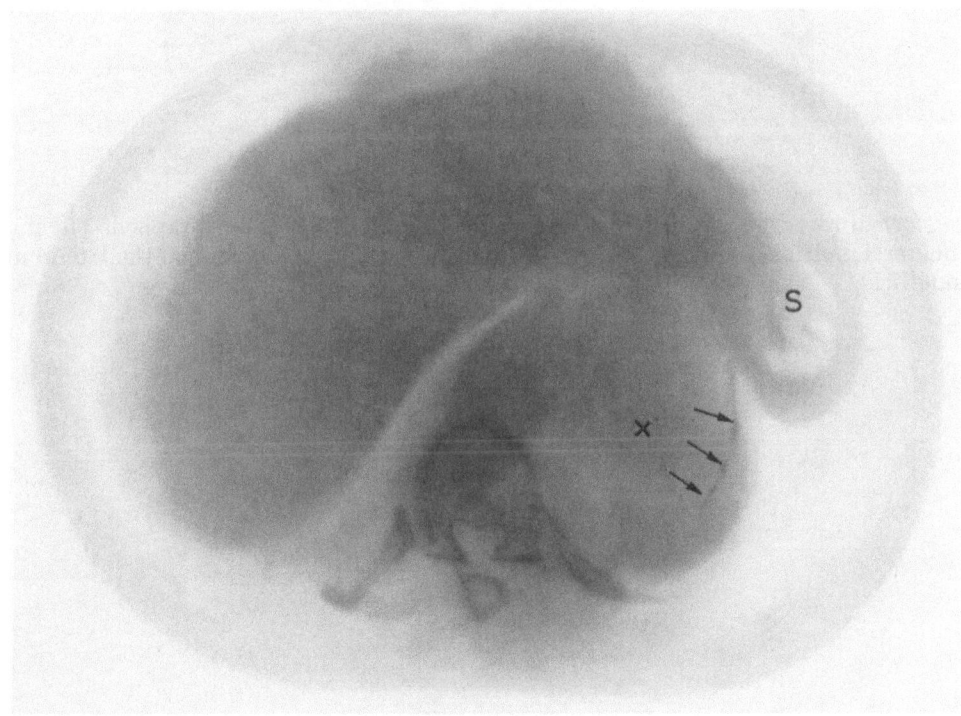

Diagnosis: Metastatic cancer of the pleura.

Case: A. N., age 32, male.

History: About one year ago, a tumor the size of a fist was removed
               surgically from the right anterior mediastinum.

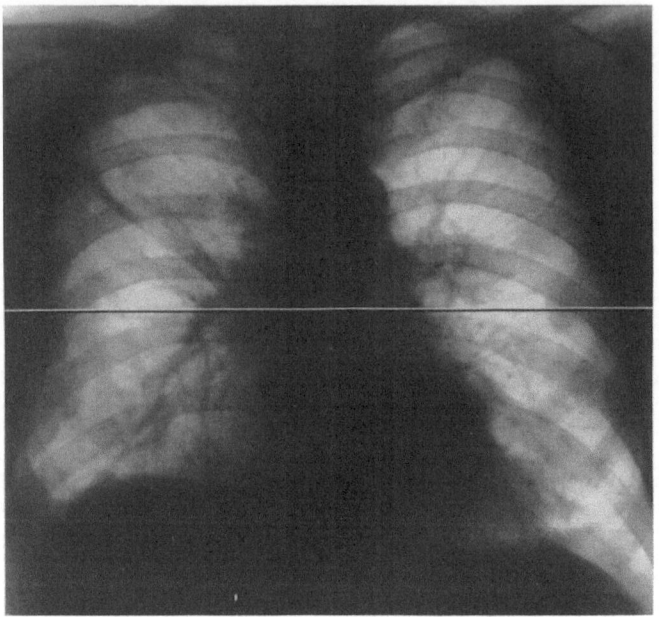

Fig. 541. Normal roentgenogram. Horizontal line showing the level tomographed. The p.a. view reveals bilateral multiple round and crescent-shaped homogeneous shadows in the lateral margins of the lung field

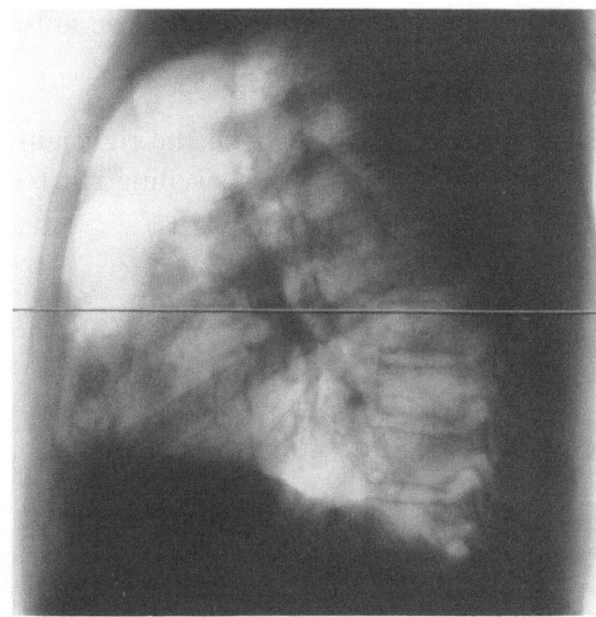

Fig. 542. Normal roentgenogram. Horizontal line showing the level tomographed. In the lateral view the findings are similar to the above. The increased shadows at the hilum are noted

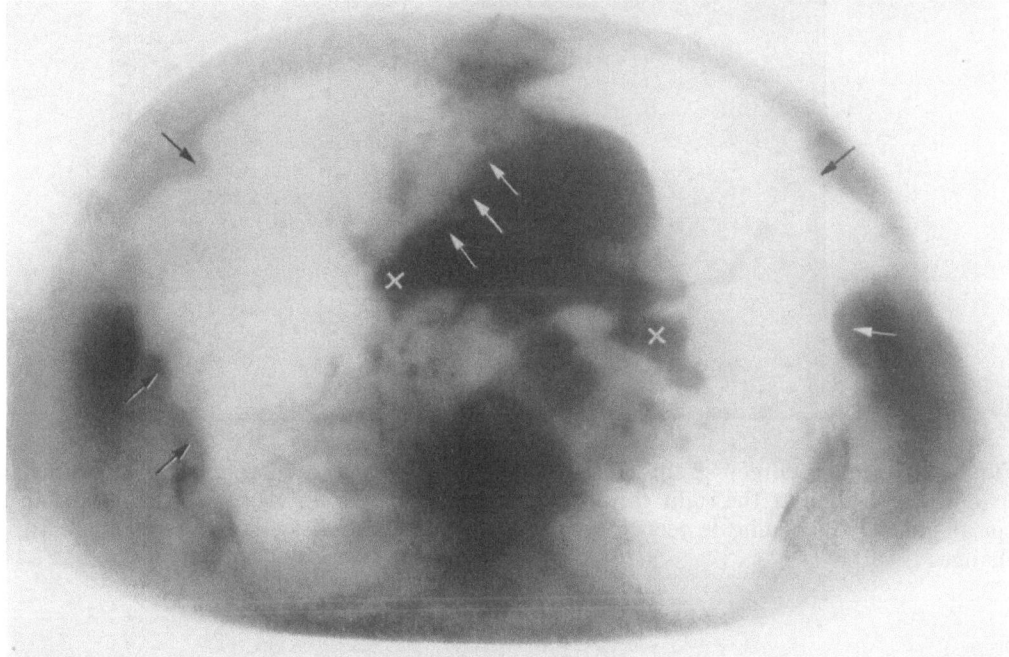

Fig. 543. Axial transverse tomogram. See Figs. 218—222, p. 106, for normal axial transverse tomogram at this level. There are multiple crescent-shaped tumors of homogeneous density ($\nearrow$) on the pleural surface, protruding bilaterally into the lung field. In both hilar regions there are round opacities ($\times$) of various sizes, 2 on the right and 3 on the left. The findings represent pleural, metastasis and hilar lymph node involvement. These changes are also seen in the contour of the anterior mediastinum which is imaged exclusively on the axial transverse tomogram. No evidence of lesions in the lung

Diagnosis: Cold abscess of the anterior chest wall.

Case: M. K., age 51, male.

History: Swelling of the right anterior chest wall was noted five years
                 ago. The swelling started growing in size one year ago. Pain
                 and tenderness.

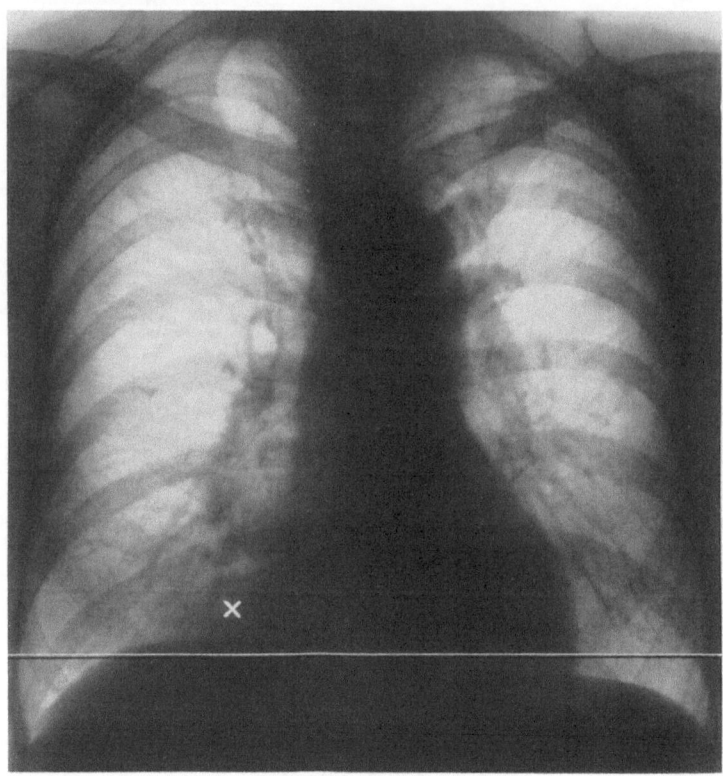

Fig. 544. Normal roentgenogram. Horizontal line showing the level tomographed. Some abnormal
shadow (×) is seen at the right cardiophrenic angle in the p.a. view. Fibronodular and bilateral
apical pleural thickening is seen in the left superior lung field, suggestive of old tuberculous
changes

Fig. 546. Axial transverse tomogram. See Figs. 253—257, p. 120, for normal axial transverse
tomogram of this level. There is a large soft tissue mass of homogeneous density on the right
breast anteriorly. The mass (╱) is protruding anteriorly through the chest wall and is about
8 cm in diameter. The posterior part of the mass (×) is in contact with the right hemidiaphragm
and the heart. The calcification in the central part of the mass probably represents a calcified
cartilaginous rib

Fig. 545. Normal roentgenogram. Horizontal line showing the level tomographed. In the lateral view, a dumb-bell-shaped soft tissue shadow (✕) is noted substernally

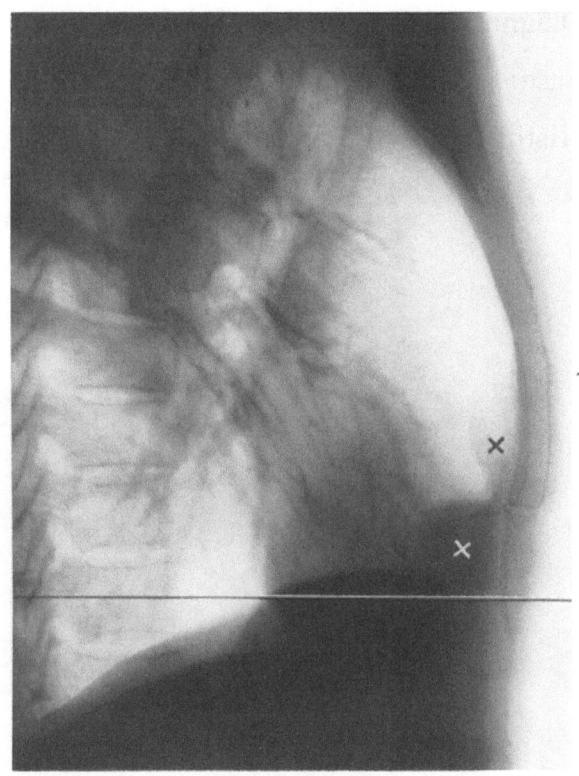

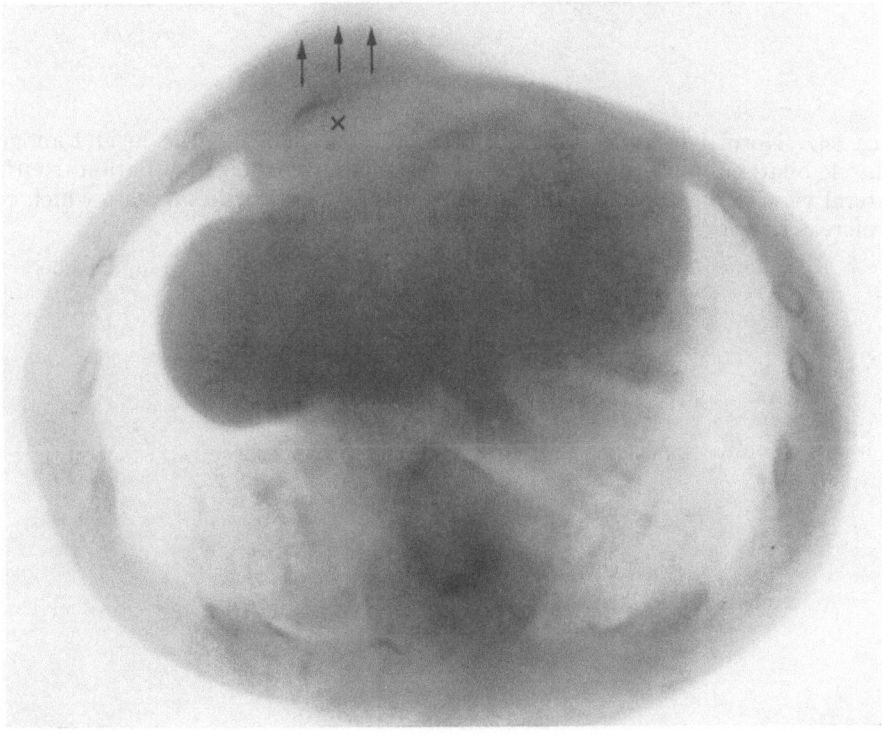

Diagnosis: Cancer of the pancreas.

Case: T. S., age 65, female.

History: Abdominal pain in the left upper abdomen and backaches
                    with anorexia and loss of weight of 6 months' duration.
                    Recently a hard mass was noted in the left hypochondrium.

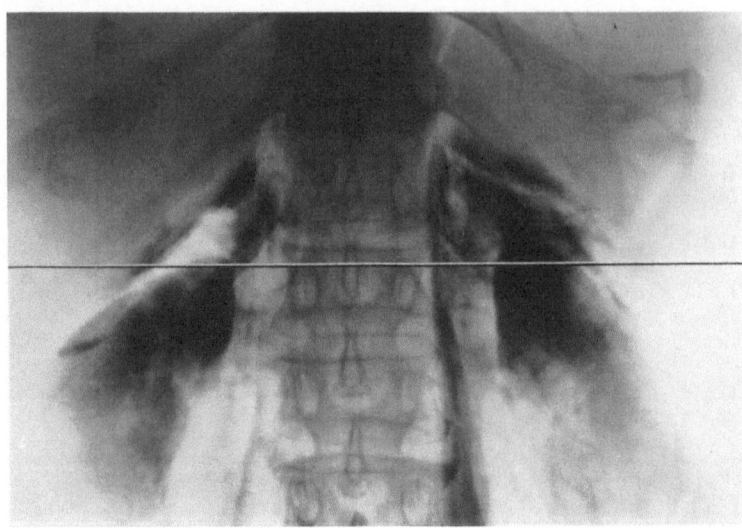

Fig. 547. Normal roentgenogram. Horizontal line showing the level tomographed. The psoas muscle bilaterally well delineated due to retroperitoneal air insufflation. Neither the a.p. nor the lateral view of the normal roentgenogram reveals and identifies a mass which could be a suspected pancreas tumor

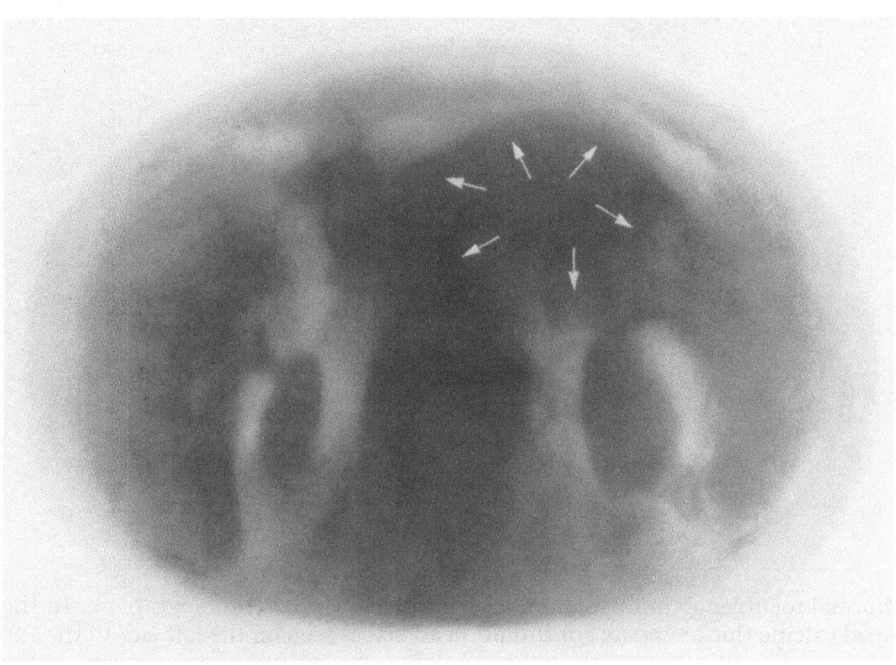

Fig. 548. Axial transverse tomogram. See Figs. 311—315, p. 150, for normal view at this level. There is a large homogeneous opacity (↗) due to compression occupying the position from the vertebral body to the narrowed pylorus. The opacity is surrounded by air sinistrally at the front of the left kidney and dextrally at the right of the vertebral body

Diagnosis: Left suprarenal cyst.

Case: M. N., age 38, female.

History: Epigastric discomfort of two years' duration.

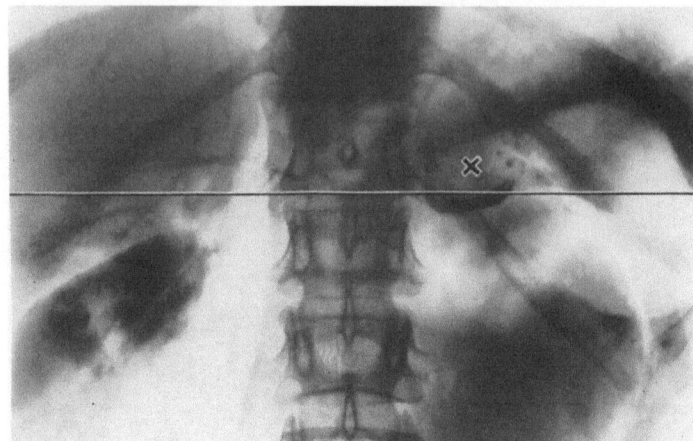

Fig. 549. Normal roentgenogram. Horizontal line showing the level tomographed. In the p.a. view an egg-shaped calcific thickening (✕) of thumb-head size is seen on the left side of the 12th thoracic vertebra

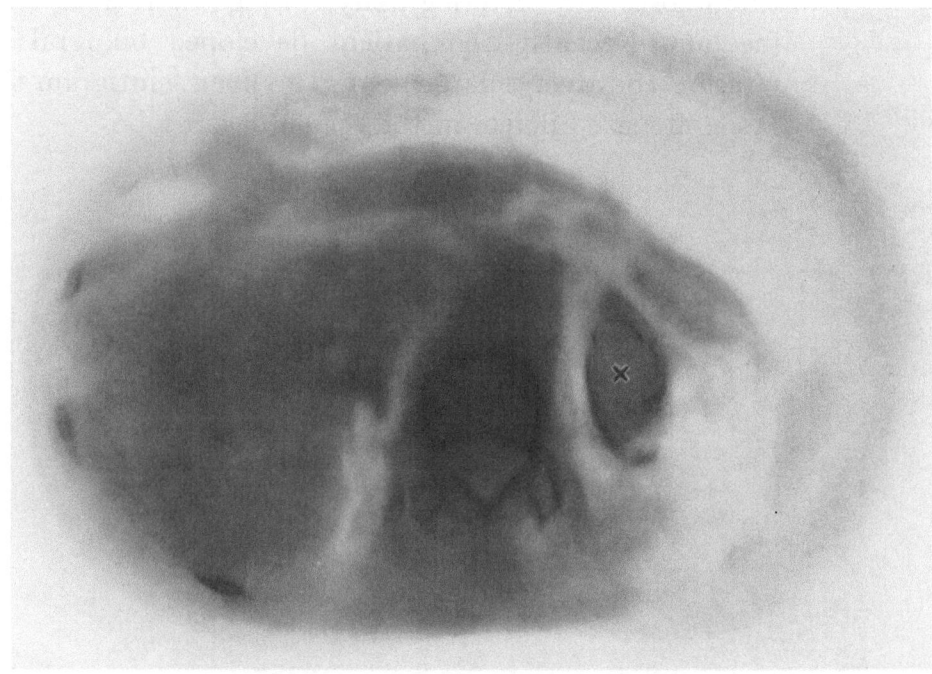

Fig. 550. Axial transverse tomogram. See Figs. 301—305, p. 146, for normal view at this level. An oval soft tissue mass (×) with thin calcific plaque is seen on the outer wall in the left retroperitoneal cavity which is projected just to the left of the vertebral body. In view of its location, it was concluded it could only be a suprarenal tumor. After surgical operation it was histologically proved to be a suprarenal cyst

Diagnosis: Thorotrast liver.

Case: S. T., age 56, male.

History: About 30 years ago the patient was examined for coronary thrombosis by arteriography, using thorotrast contrast medium. Recently the patient developed bilateral pleural effusion and liver enlargement. The liver scintigram shows a moderate sized defect in the region of left lobe.

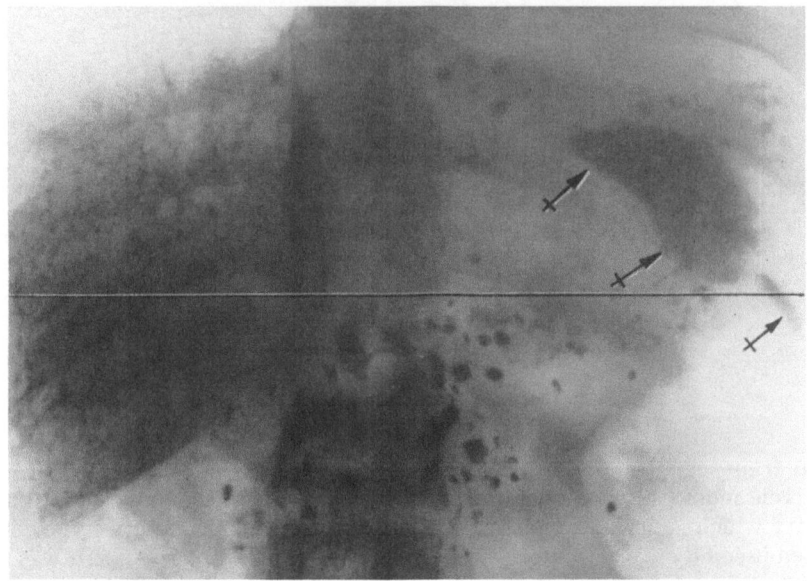

Fig. 551. Normal roentgenogram. Horizontal line showing the level tomographed. The antero-posterior view of the upper abdomen shows diffuse deposition of the thorotrast in the liver in a reticular pattern. The spleen (↗) is smaller than normal with thorotrast deposits. Multiple deposits are noted in the mesenteric lymph nodes

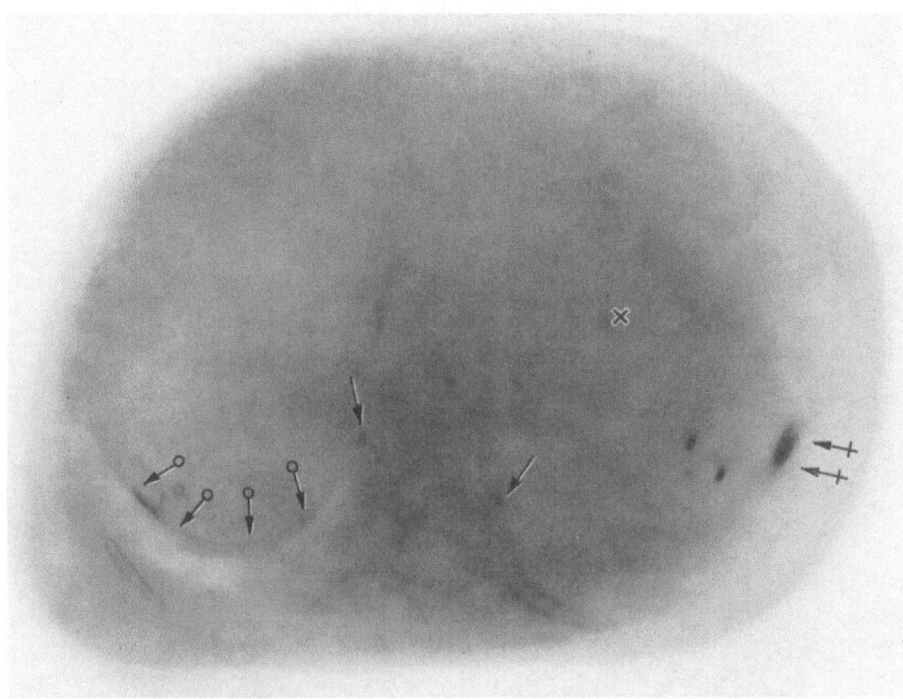

Fig. 552. Axial transverse tomogram. See normal Figs. 296—300, p. 144. A curvilinear density is seen in the posterior margin of the right lobe of the liver (↗), and a few calcific densities in the anterior aspect of the vertebral body due to thorotrast deposits in the mesenteric (×) and retroperitoneal lymph nodes (↗). There is an oval calcific density in the left lateral aspect of the abdomen due to a lower tip of the spleen (↗) with thorotrast deposit

Diagnosis: Tuberculous calcification of the mesenteric lymph nodes.

Case: K. A., age 52, male.

History: He suffered from the tuberculosis of the lung about 25 years
               ago. Backaches for 2 years.

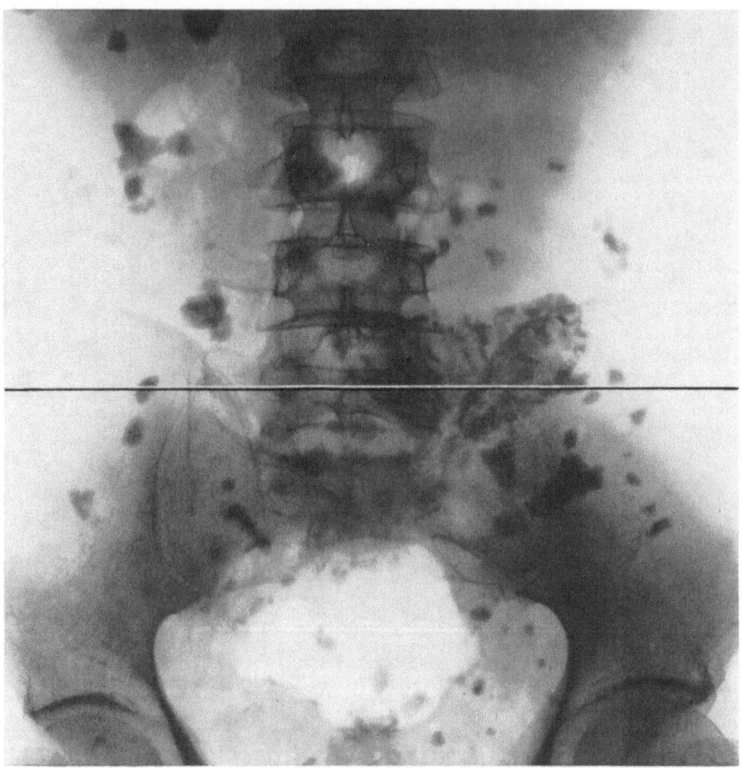

Fig. 553. Normal roentgenogram. Horizontal line showing the level tomographed. Multiple
calcified bodies of various sizes are seen in the abdomen in the p.a. view

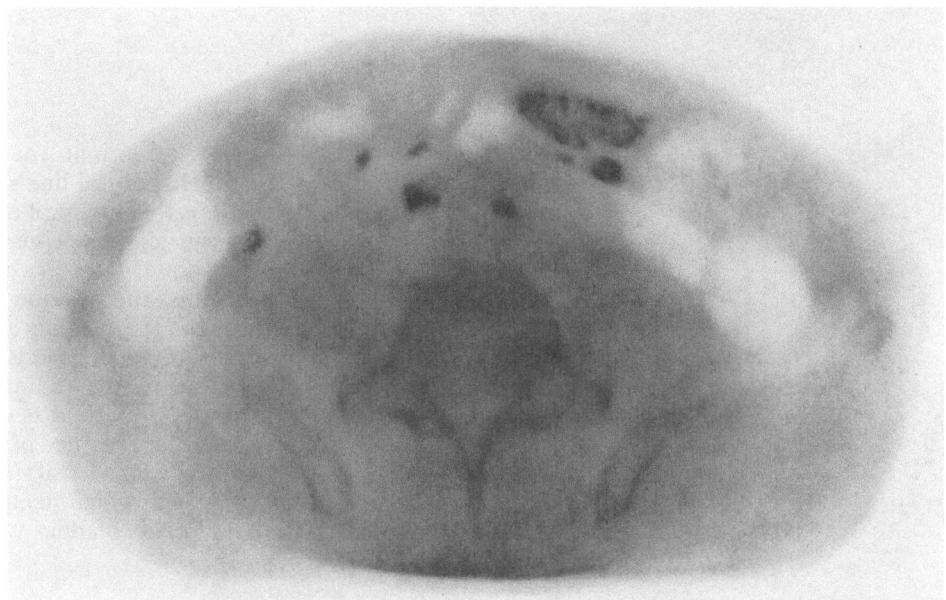

Fig. 554. Axial transverse tomogram. See Figs. 377—381, p. 180, for normal view at this level. The location of the calcified bodies is limited to the anatomical position of the mesenterium, and is distinguishable from intestinal gas patterns

Diagnosis: Myoma uteri.

Case: S. Y., age 42, female.

History: A large pelvic mass was found incidentally. The patient
               had not complained.

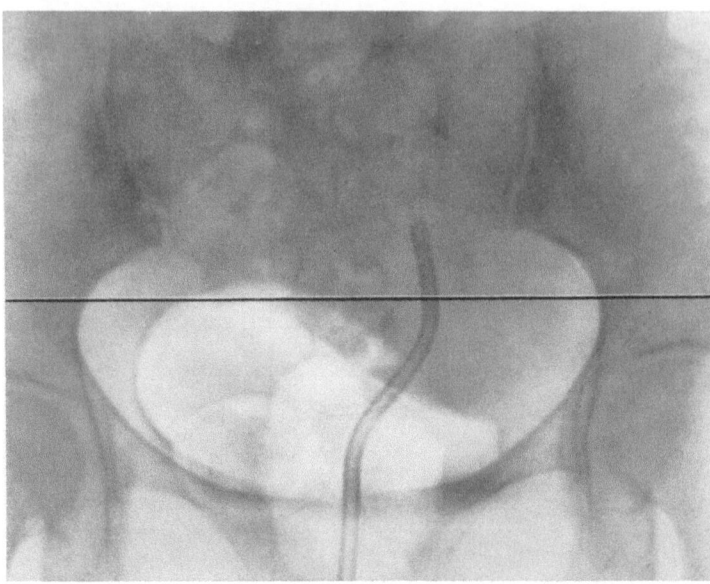

Fig. 555. Normal roentgenogram. Horizontal line showing the level tomographed. The a.p. view of the pelvis with a radiopaque catheter introduced into the uterine cavity through the vagina, air insufflation of the bladder and insertion of the radiotranslucent mass into the vagina reveals the presence of a large homogeneous density in the left pelvis which compresses the superior bladder wall

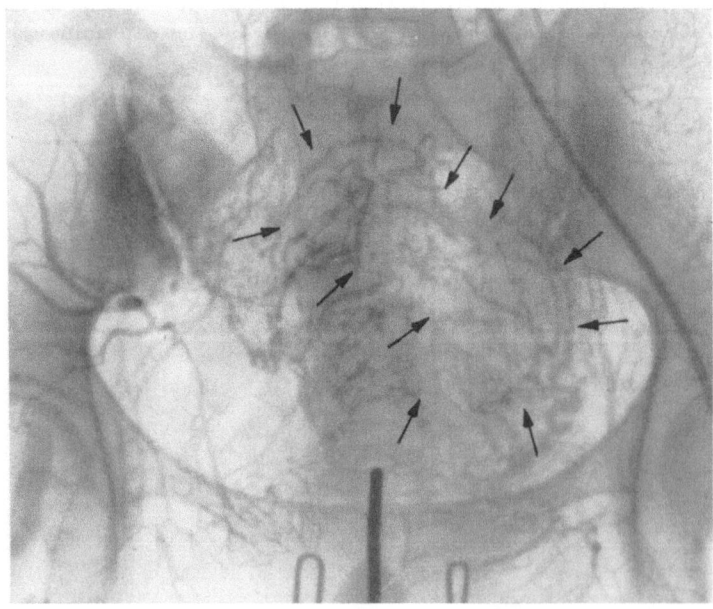

Fig. 556. Angiogram of the pelvis shows the location and the size of the tumor (↗)

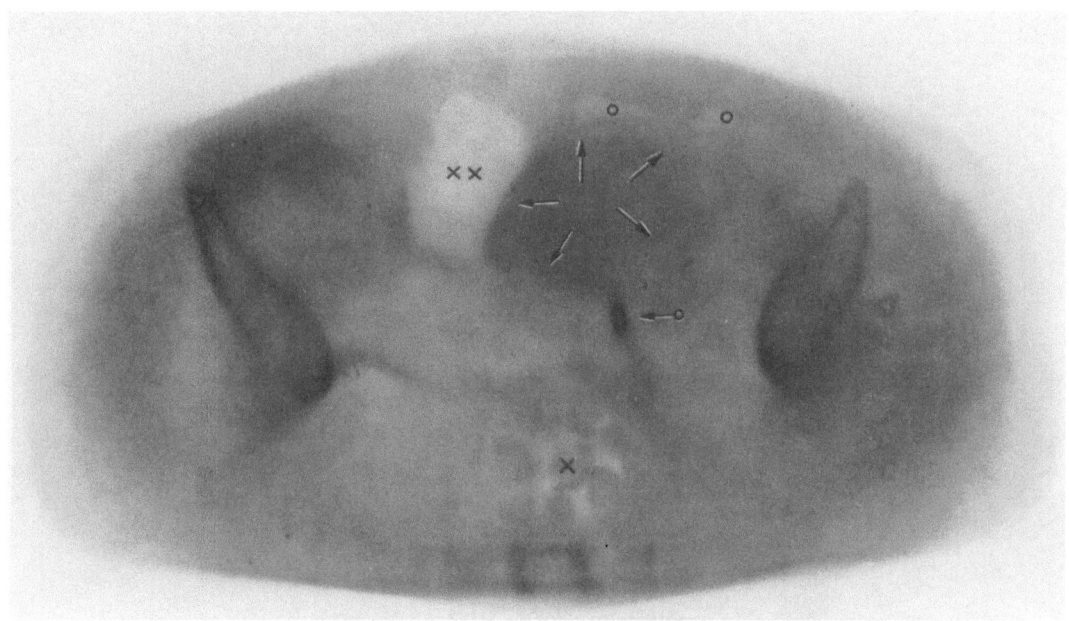

Fig. 557. Axial transverse tomogram. See Figs. 397—401, p. 188, for normal axial transverse tomogram at this level. The cross-section of the catheter (↗) imaged at the center of the tomogram reveals the position of the uterine cavity in the pelvis. Just behind this shadow, there is imaged the rectum (×) filled with feces in heaps mixed with a small amount of gas. At the anterior aspect of the catheter a large homogeneous shadow (↗) of 6 × 7 cm in size is noted suggesting the tumor mass of the anterior wall of the uterus. The left wall of the bladder (××) is compressed and deformed by this shadow. The narrow translucent zone between the tumor shadow and the abdominal skin is concluded to be the small intestine (o) by interpreting the finding of the normal roentgenogram

Diagnosis: Fracture of the left iliac bone.

Case: H. N., age 29, male.

History: Three months ago a heavy iron pillar fell on him and he
                  sustained a bruise on his left hip.

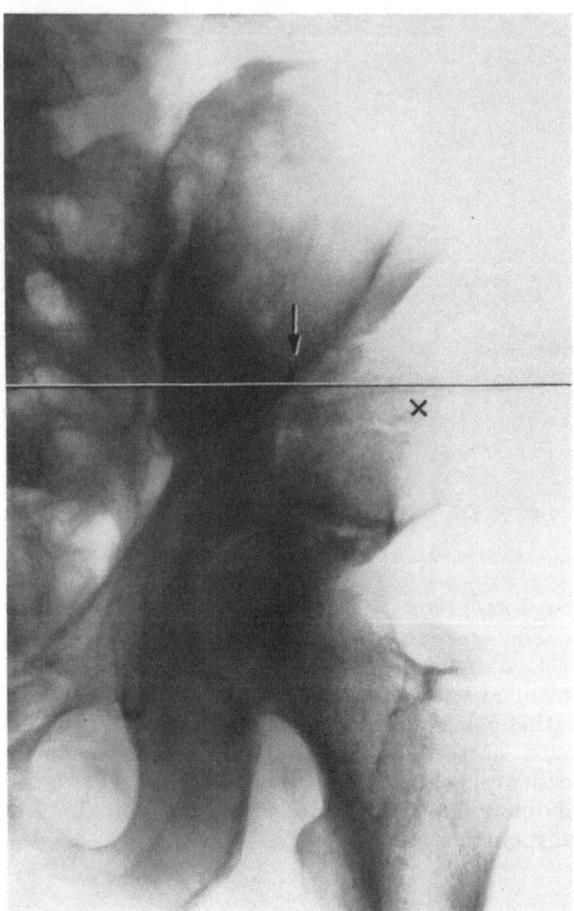

Fig. 558. Normal roentgenogram. Horizontal line showing the level tomographed. Extensive fracture (×) of the left iliac bone. A spindle-shaped opacity (╱) of 1.5 × 0.3 cm in size is seen at the center of the fracture

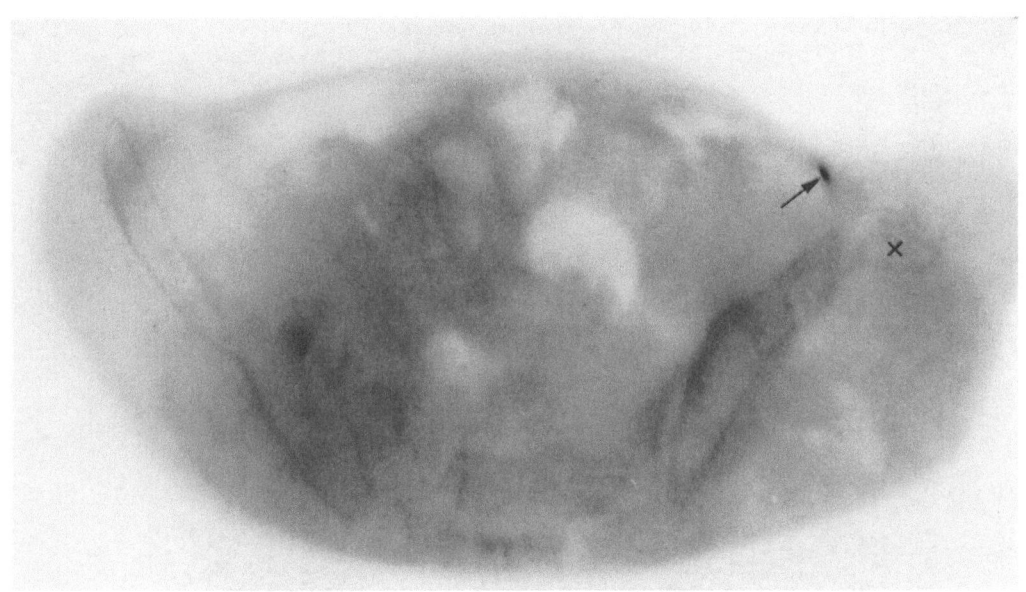

Fig. 559. Axial transverse tomogram. Refer to Figs. 387—391, p. 184. The axial transverse tomogram taken at the level of the opacity reveals the fractured part of the anterior iliac bone (×). The opacity (↗) is located 1 cm below the skin. That is the foreign body which has been pressed into the lower abdomen at the time of the accident

Diagnosis: Thickening of the periosteum.

Case: Ch. I., age 26, female.

History: The patient complains of pain in the right ankle, aggravated
                  by walking. Neurologically negative.

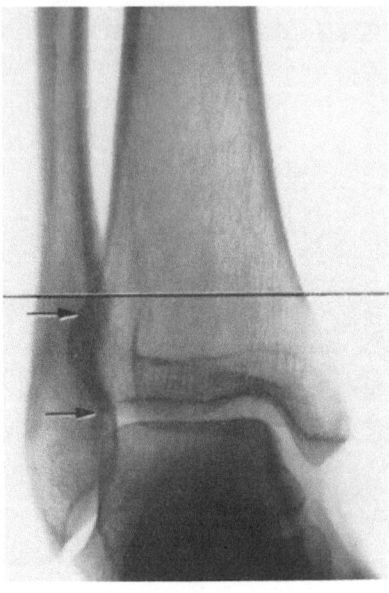
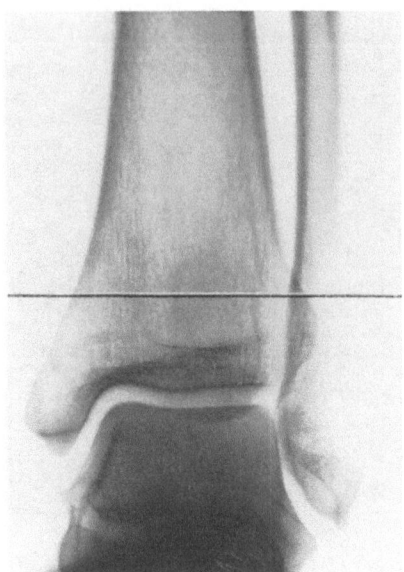

Fig. 560   Fig. 561

Fig. 560. Normal roentgenogram. Horizontal line showing the level tomographed. Right lower leg shows slight thickening (↗) of the periosteum in the distal portion of the fibula about 3 cm in length

Fig. 561. Normal roentgenogram. Horizontal line showing the level tomographed. Healthy fibula; there is an apparent difference in the thickness of the periosteum compared with Fig. 560

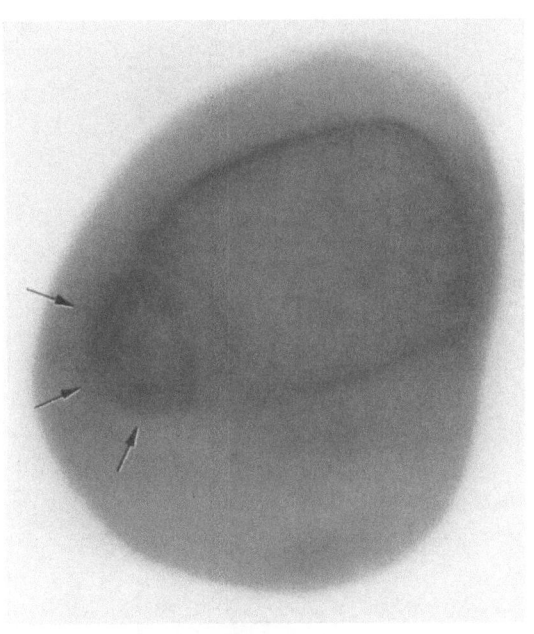 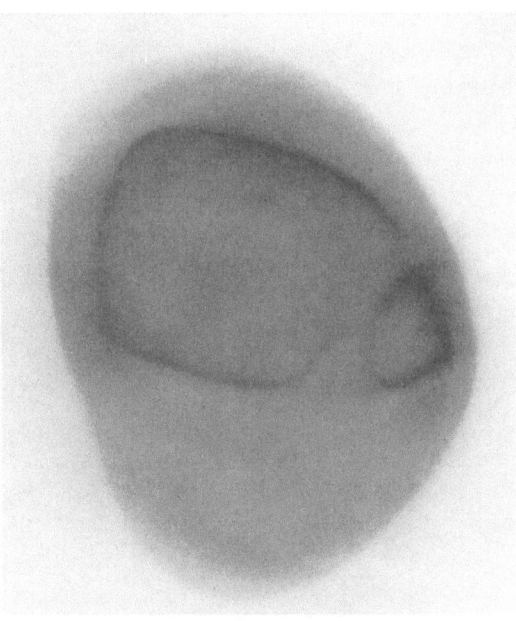

Fig. 562   Fig. 563

Fig. 562. Axial transverse tomogram. The right fibula shows thickening of the periosteum with slight irregular marginal outline (╱). This is clearly demonstrated on the axial transverse tomogram and it is apparent in the difference in thickness of the periosteum when compared with that of the healthy fibula on the axial transverse tomogram

Fig. 563. Axial transverse tomogram of the left leg. Normal

Diagnosis: Fibrosarcoma.

Case: Y. T., age 52, female.

History: For two years she has complained of gradually increasing
                 swelling in her right knee.

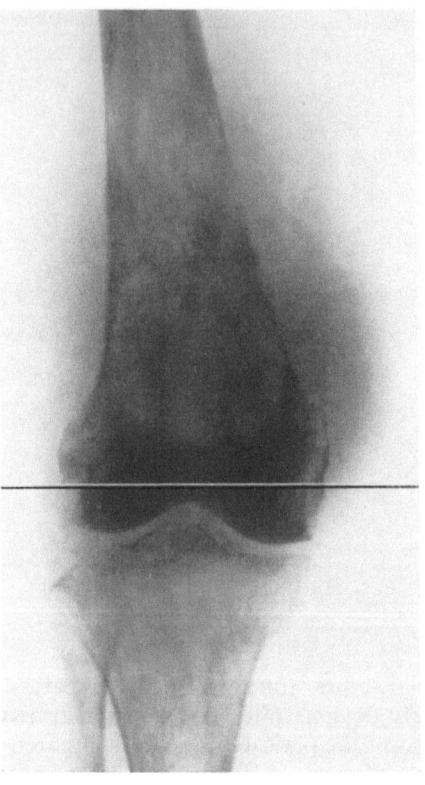
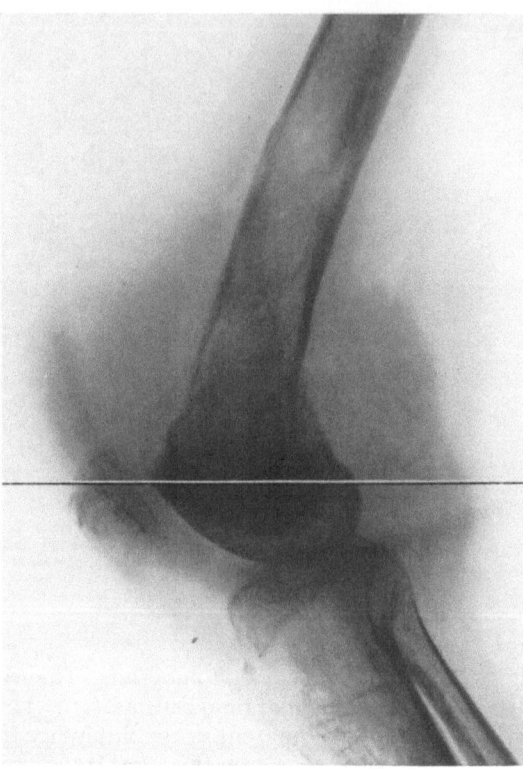

Fig. 564   Fig. 565

Fig. 564. Normal roentgenogram in the a.p. view. Horizontal line showing the level tomographed.
There is bone destruction involving the lower third of the femur, approximately 10 cm in length.
The articular surface of the femur shows moderate increase of bone density, but the joint space is
well preserved

Fig. 565. Normal roentgenogram in the lateral view. There is moderate soft tissue swelling at the
level of the lower third of the femur described above, mainly in the right anterior aspect

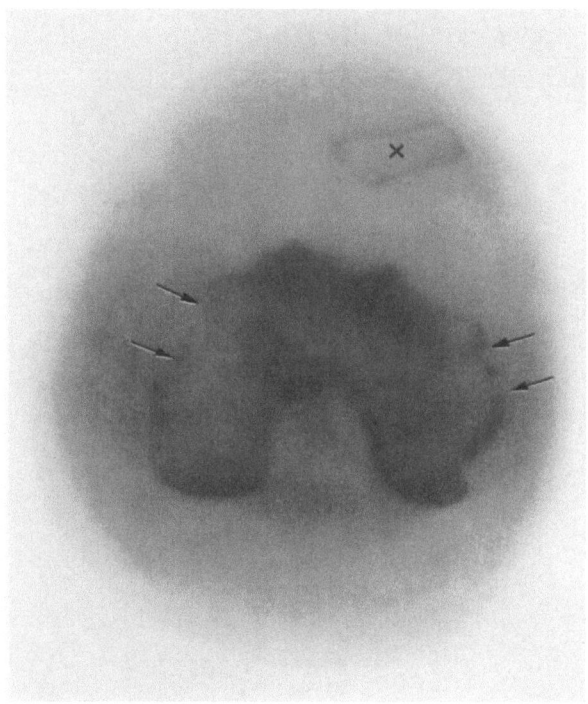

Fig. 566. Axial transverse tomogram. As compared with the normal (Figs. 490—492, p. 228), marked swelling of the anterior and posterior part of the soft tissue in the leg is seen. The patella (×) is shifted to the left and is atrophic. Both sides of the median and lateral condyle (╱) of the femur are destroyed with partial hyperosteosis

II. Application to Pretherapeutic Procedure

For the treatment of disease by means of either irradiation or surgical operation, three-dimensional knowledge of the lesion in the body obtained before the operation will make the procedure easy as well as correct. It will be explained below how and why axial transverse tomography is useful.

1. Radiation Therapy

A basic problem in radiation therapy is to give dense and homogeneous radiation to the tumor alone, while delivering the minimum possible dose to the surrounding normal tissues. This area of high dose is termed by *Takahashi* (175) *beam focus*.

In order to coincide the beam focus with the region to be treated, the first step should be to make the location, size and shape of the region clearly known and determined and to plan the most appropriate technique to produce the beam focus to cover the region to be irradiated. After the consideration of this planning, the actual procedures of the correct positioning of the patient on the treatment table and the correct determination of the direction and the size of radiation beam are performed. Finally, confirmation is needed as to whether this planned treatment has been properly carried out or not. The systematic work for applying the rotation technique to radiation therapy was described by *Takahashi* (175).

Application of axial transverse tomography to the determination of the region to be treated was dealt with by *Pierquin* (93), *Roswit* et al. (98), *Vallebona* (159) and *Watanabe* et al. (166). Its application to the radiation planning was discussed by *Fleischer* et al. (23), *Frain* et al. (28), *Jucker* et al. (46), *Onuma* (89), *Pierquin* et al. (92), *Roswit* et al. (97), *Sannazzari* et al. (101), *Takahashi* et al. (140), *Vallebona* (160) and others, because of its essential value for treatment planning. For positioning of the patient in radiation therapy, *Matsuda* et al. (71) and *Takahashi* et al. (137) described the usefulness of axial transverse tomography. For confirming whether or not correct irradiation was carried out, the contribution of axial transverse tomography was described by *Egan* et al. (21), *Sakuma* et al. (100) and *Takahashi* (141). Actually, however, these procedures have not been much used in the field of radiation therapy up to the present time.

One of the reasons may be that the tomography was usually performed with the unit of the erect type, while the radiotherapy is carried out with the patient in the lying posture. It is the natural conclusion that axial transverse tomography taken by the unit of the erect type is of less value for

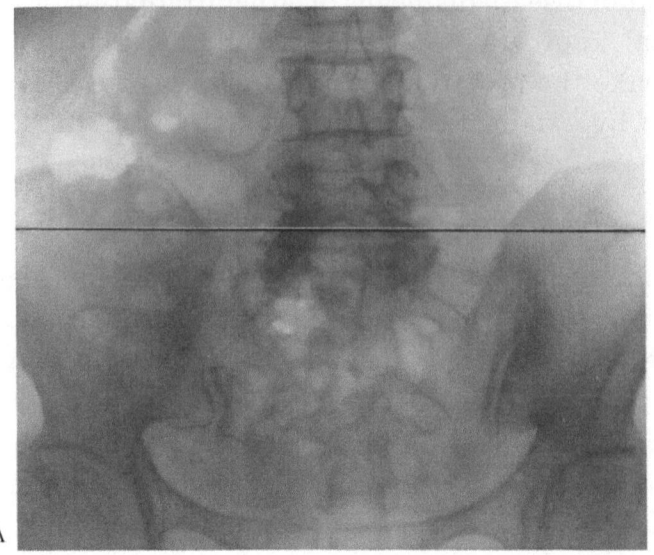

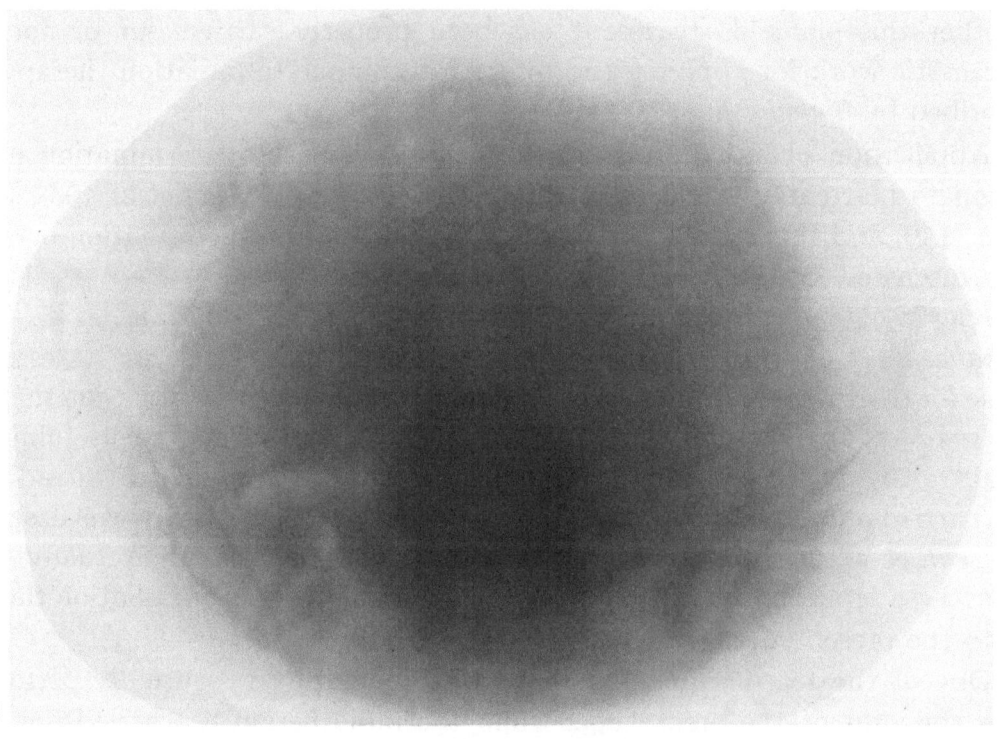

Fig. 567 A and B. Axial transverse tomogram of the lower abdomen of a woman at the level of the anterior superior iliac spine taken by means of the axial transverse tomograph of the erect type

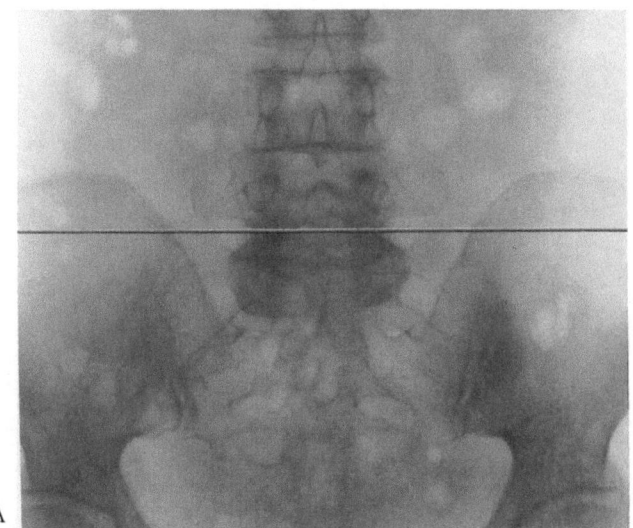

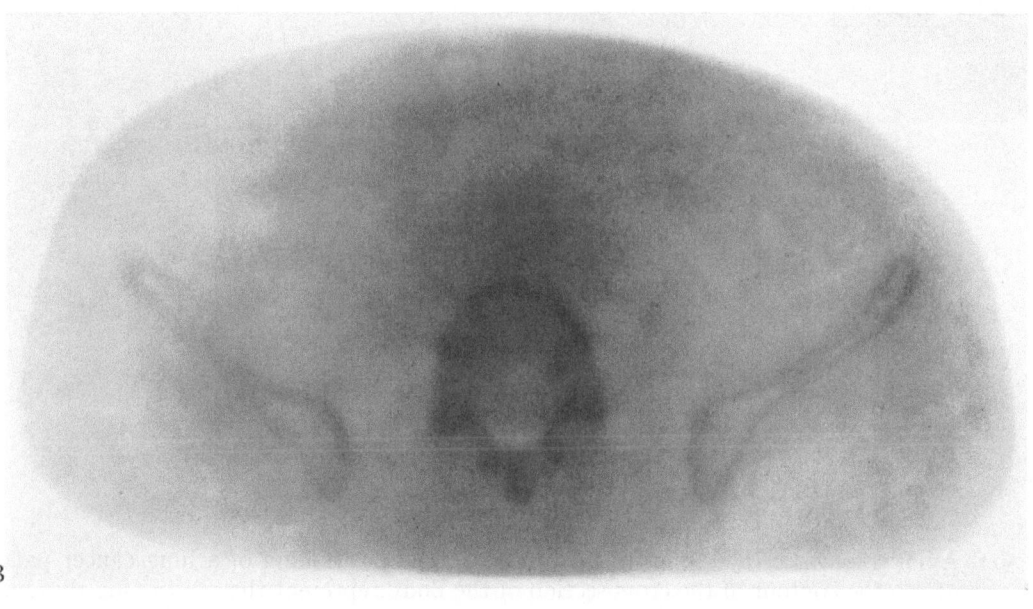

Fig. 568 A and B. Axial transverse tomogram at the same level of the same woman as in Fig. 567. The tomogram is taken by means of the horizontal type of unit. The difference from Fig. 567 is caused by the change in the position of the viscera

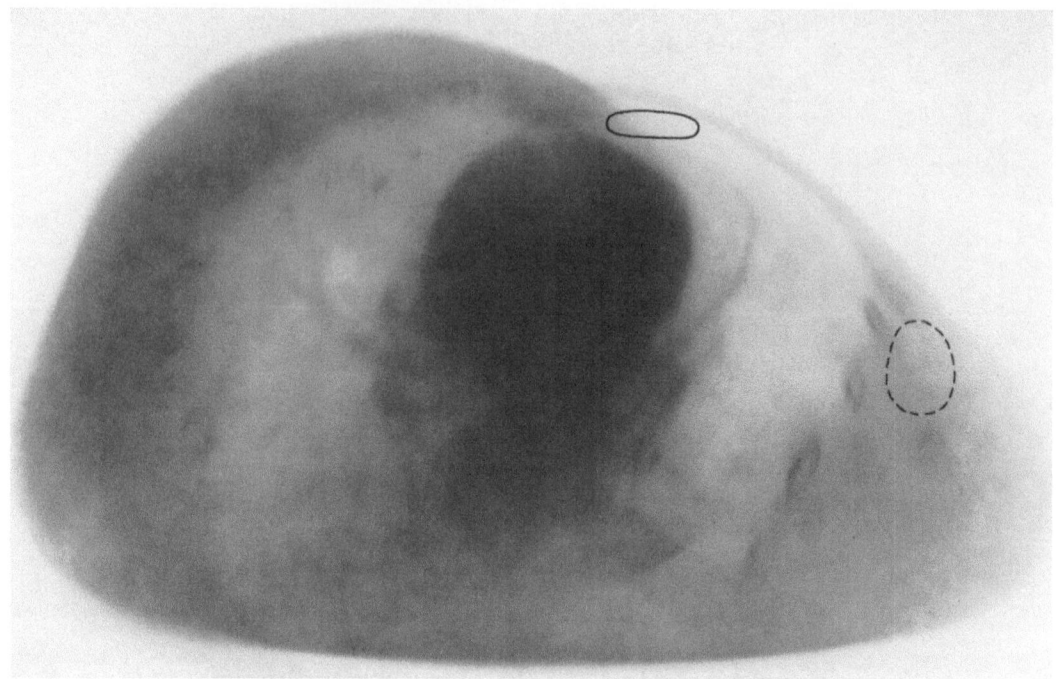

Fig. 569. Region to be treated for irradiation of postoperative breast cancer. The lymph nodes (solid line) along the internal mammary vessels and the axillary lymph nodes (broken line) are determined for irradiation. Operated breast wall is not irradiated, as the operation was radically carried out in this case

Fig. 571. Axial transverse tomogram to be applied to the positioning of a lung cancer patient. Three points on the contour of the cross section of the body represent the positioning skin marks a, b and c. Standard lines (solid lines) are drawn from the center 0 of the region to be treated so that one is parallel to the line b—c (broken line) and the other perpendicular to it. By extending these two lines to the contour of the cross section of the body, the centering skin marks A, B and C are obtained

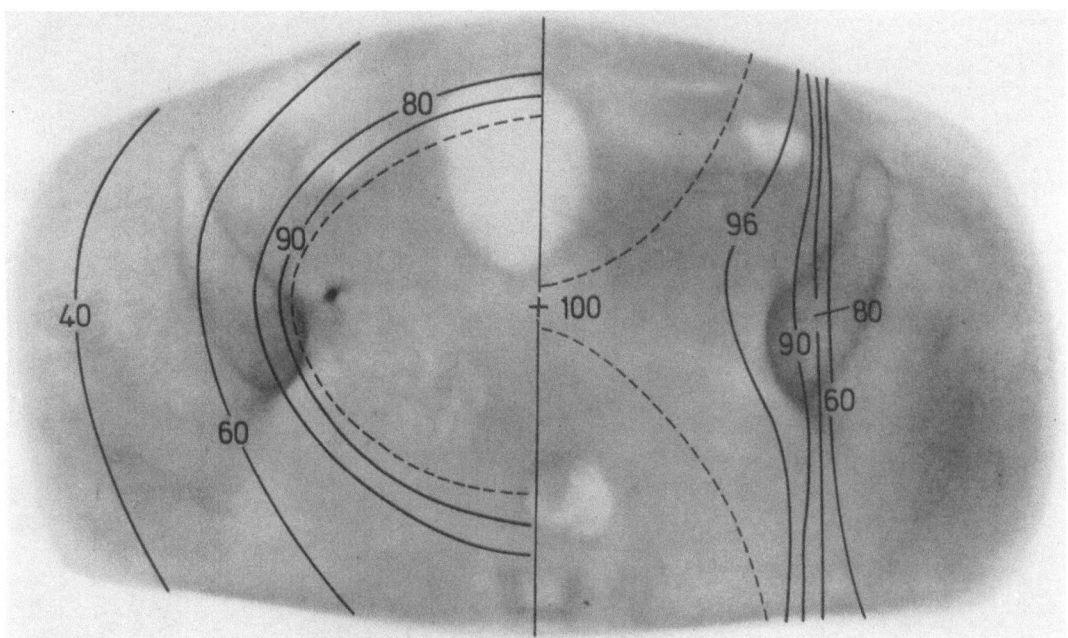

Fig. 570. Isodose curves for irradiation of cancer of the uterus by ⁶⁰Co conformation radiotherapy (left) and ⁶⁰Co radiotherapy through two portals (right). Region to be irradiated is shown by the broken line (left). The conformation radiation technique provides better dose distribution than the two-portal stationary irradiation

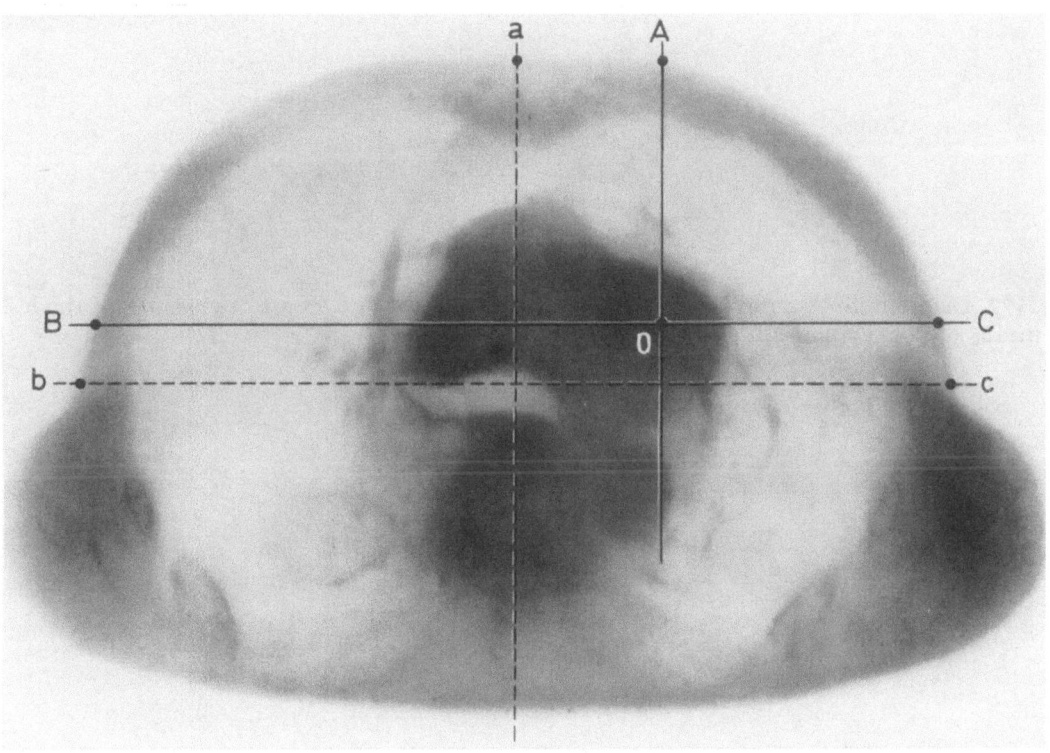

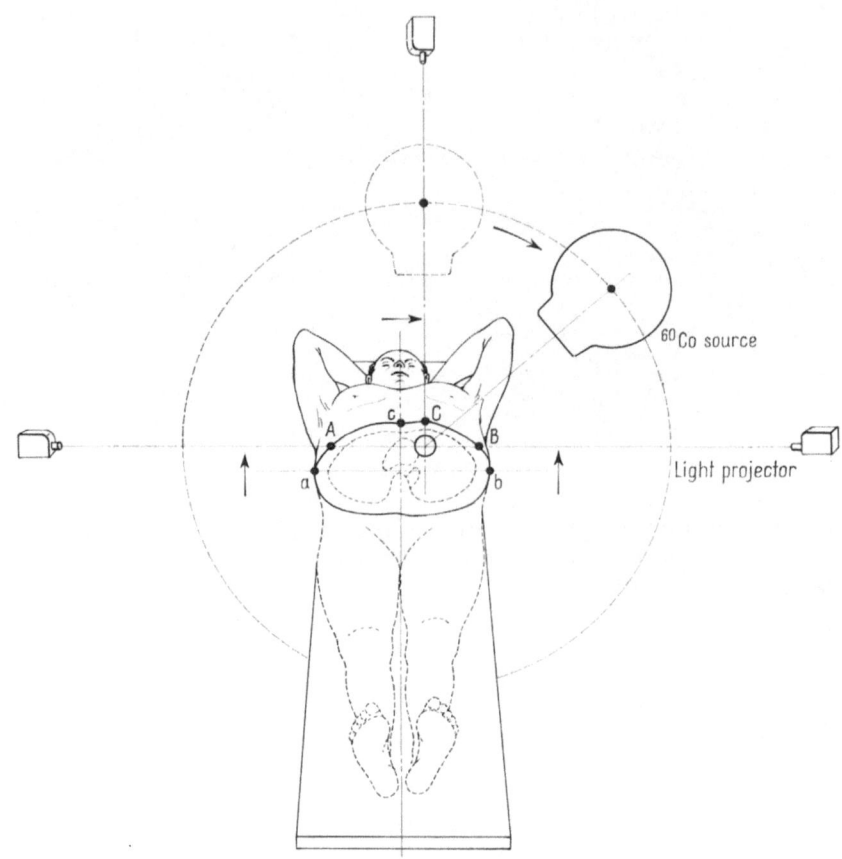

Fig. 572. Diagram illustrating adjustment of the central γ-ray of ^{60}Co to the center of the lesion by means of positioning skin marks and centering skin marks

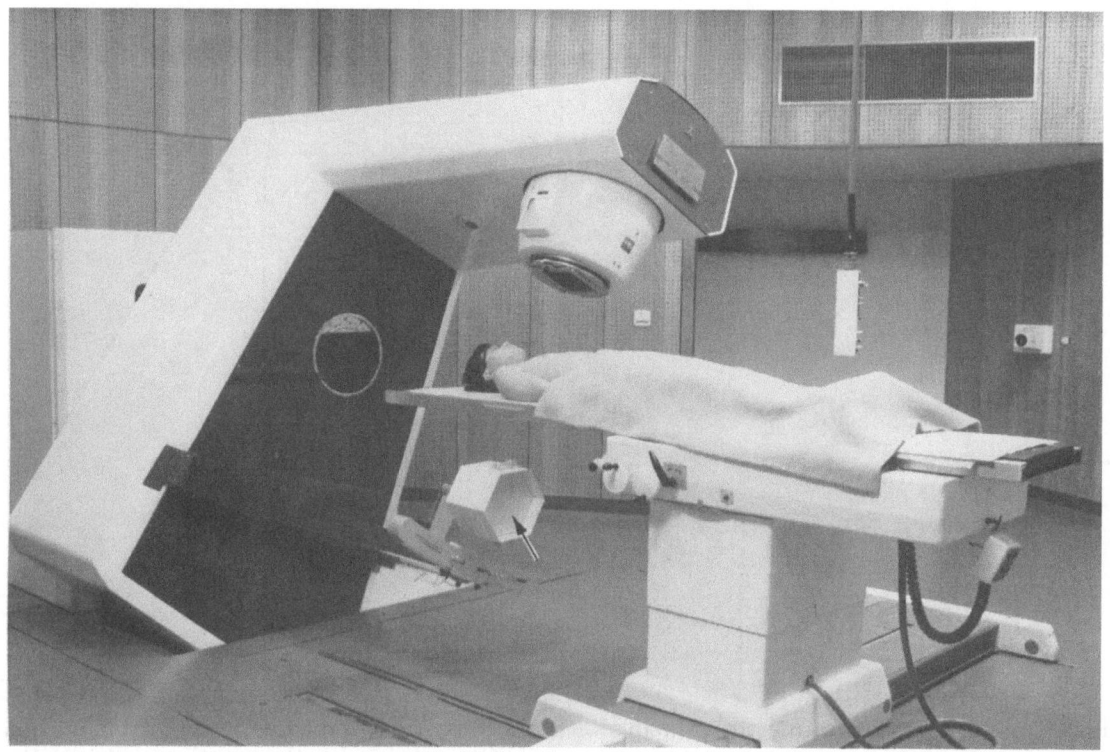

Fig. 573. Beam focus radiography in action. Beam focus radiograph (⟋) is attached to the rotational accelerator therapy unit (Mitsubishi)

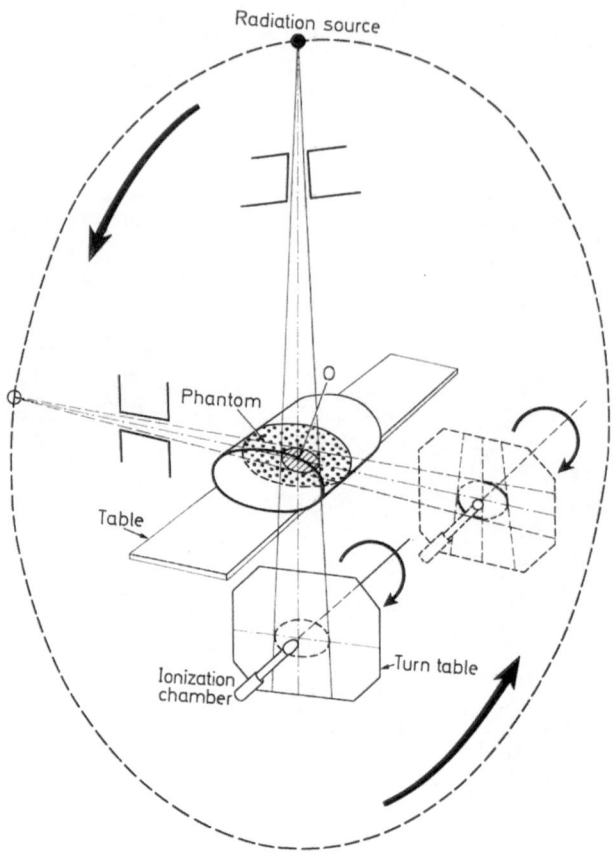

Fig. 574. Diagram illustrating the principle of beam focus radiography. The center of rotation of the film is arranged on the line joining the radiation source with the rotation center of the unit (0). With counter-clockwise rotation of the radiation source, the cassette keeping definite direction by clockwise rotation rotates around the patient

Fig. 576. Axial transverse tomogram applied to needle puncture for biopsy. a, b and c: positioning skin marks. P: point to be punctured

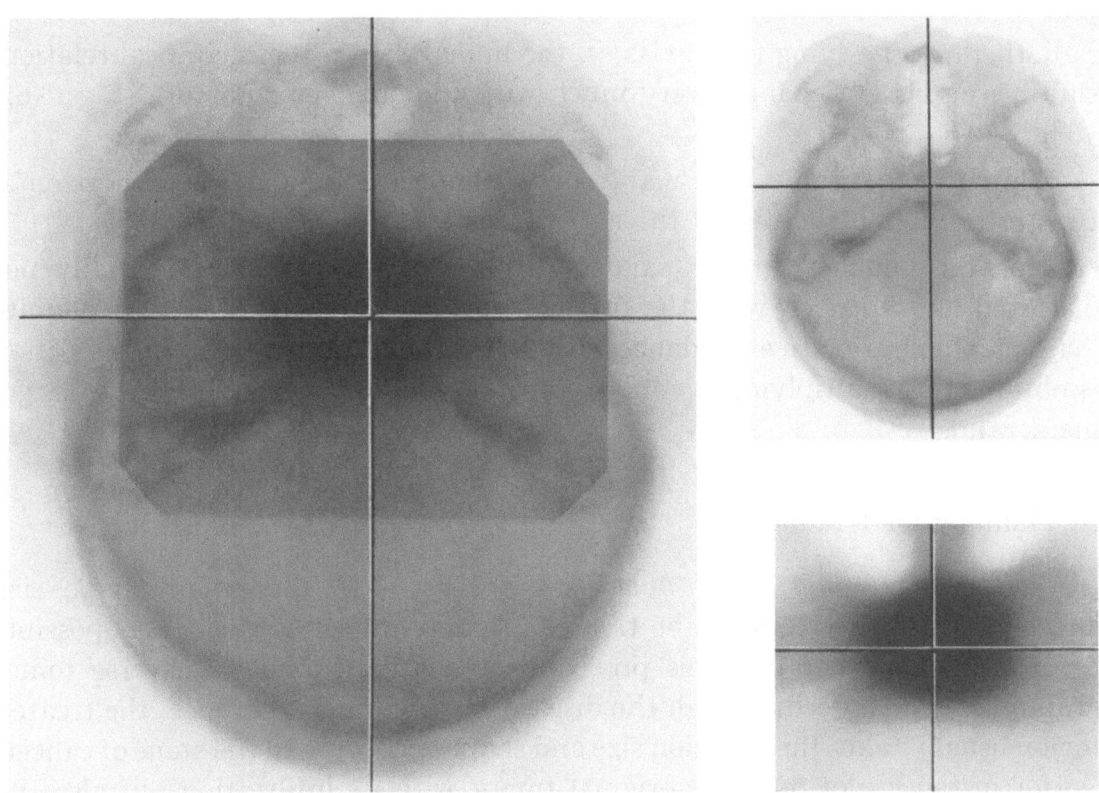

Fig. 575. Confirmation of coverage of the correct beam focus in radiation therapy. Beam focus in axial transverse cross section of the head at the level of the pituitary tumor. The large image on the left shows the overlapping of the axial transverse tomogram (top right) and the beam focus radiogram (bottom right)

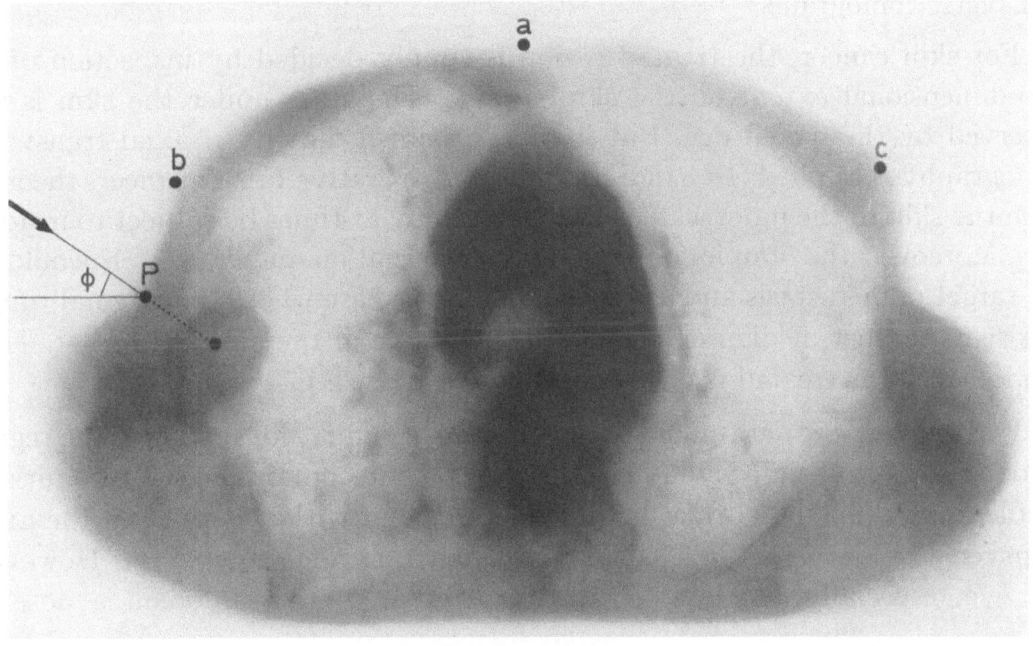

radiotherapy of a lying patient as, in the human body, the reciprocal relationship of the viscera changes very much with the change of posture (Figs. 567, 568).

Thus it is desirable to use the axial transverse tomograph of horizontal type for radiation therapy of the lying patient.

Roentgen images on the axial transverse tomogram are essentially not distorted as compared with the original figure, but enlarged with a definite magnification ratio. In accordance with this, the actual size of the cross-section is obtained by multiplying the image of the tomogram by the inverse enlargement ratio.

A. Planning for Irradiation

1. Determination of Region to be Treated. First of all the extent, shape, size and location of the region to be treated are determined as exactly as possible before radiation therapy. This procedure is simple if axial transverse tomography is used. Indeed, though the disease is varied in appearance, the treated region usually takes the common size and shape according to the stage of cancer, as, for instance, not only the original tumor with its infiltration but also the primary lymph nodes of the lesion are included in the region to be treated.

In order to obtain three-dimensional knowledge of the region there arises the need for comparative examination of normal roentgenograms with axial transverse tomograms.

For skin cancer, the treated region is simply decided by inspection of its two-dimensional extent on the skin surface. The state under the skin is not observed by the naked eye. But it can be known directly if axial transverse tomography is applied. In irradiation for postoperative breast cancer, the area from the skin to the inner wall of the thorax may at times be subject to irradiation. Moreover, the lymph nodes along the internal mammary vessels would be the target of metastasis and are irradiated in the case where the original tumor was seated upper median or median of the nipple of the affected breast. Thus the region to be treated is considered to be as shown in Fig. 569.

For the deep-seated tumor, the hypophyseal tumor, for instance, the region to be treated will be a cylinder, with the height containing the full turkish saddle imaged on the normal roentgenograms and with the circle in the axial transverse cross-section imaged on the axial transverse tomogram. However, the eye, especially the lens, should be irradiated with as small a dose as possible (Fig. 575). At any rate, by means of the tomogram the location of the eye or the distance between the tumor and the skin becomes clear.

2. Selection of Irradiation Technique. It is the purpose of irradiation planning to select the appropriate technique of irradiation on the basis of the axial transverse tomogram.

The actual procedure is to place an axial transverse tomogram on the viewing box. The isodose chart, in which the isodose curves are drawn on the translucent film with the same magnification ratio as that of the axial transverse tomogram, is placed over the axial transverse tomogram (Fig. 570). If the tumor is considered to be localized in the superficial part of the body, electron beam therapy of adequate MeV would be suitable. If stationary radiation technique is considered appropriate, the number of the radiation fields, and the direction and size of the cross-section of the beam are determined to meet effective radiation planning. When the number of portals of the radiation field is increased, that will be regarded as the irradiation technique of moving field therapy. The dose distribution in the lesion as well as in the normal region is given on the isodose chart prepared by previous measurement of the dose by phantom experiment.

Indeed, there are various types of irradiation technique such as rotational, arc or conformation therapy. If moving field therapy is considered adequate for the case, the merits and defects of the rotational, arc or conformation radiation techniques are compared with each other and the most suitable one is adopted. In our opinion, the conformation irradiation technique, though not yet widely used, generally provides the ideal dose distribution.

Without axial transverse tomography, such precise determination of the region and planning of irradiation could not be realized.

B. Positioning of Patient

The next problem is to conduct irradiation with the correct positioning of the patient. With inadequate or wrong positioning, the radiation beam will stray away from the region to be treated, resulting in partial coverage of the beam focus to the treated region, which will cause recurrence. The effort to make the correct irradiation planning to produce the minimum beam focus is more likely to be harmful.

The positioning of the patient in connection with the correct planning is carried out by means of axial transverse tomography as follows:

The patient is laid supine or in a relaxed posture on the tomographic table. The body level where the region to be treated exists on the normal roentgenogram is adjusted to the plane g of the unit. The light spots are projected on to the plane g of the patient from the light projectors attached to the walls and ceilings of the tomography room (see p. 12). The light beams are contained in a vertical plane of the isocenter of the axial transverse tomograph.

The light spot projected on the anterior part of the skin of the patient is termed point a, that on the right b and that on the left c. These points marked in ink on the skin are termed positioning skin marks a, b and c (Fig. 571).

Lead wires 0.5 mm in diameter of the cross section and 1 cm long are placed at the points a, b and c respectively with the arrangement parallel to the axis of the body.

The axial transverse tomogram is taken. On the tomogram there are imaged three points on the contour of the body, corresponding to positioning skin marks a, b and c.

The line joining the points b and c is termed the horizontal line and the line which forms a perpendicular from a to this line is termed the vertical line.

By interpreting the axial transverse tomogram, the region to be treated is determined and the center 0 of this region is selected.

From this center 0 lines are drawn parallel and perpendicular to the horizontal line bc.

These new lines are termed the horizontal and vertical standard lines of the axial transverse tomogram. The crossing points of these lines and the contour of the skin on the tomogram are termed centering skin marks B, C and A.

In the rotational therapy unit three light projectors are also attached to the walls and ceiling, their light spots being adjusted to cross at the isocenter of the rotational therapy unit (Fig. 572). The patient is laid on the therapy table in the same posture as on the tomographic table. By shifting the therapy table to and fro, or right or left, the light spots are made to coincide with each of the positioning skin marks a, b and c which are drawn in ink on the skin.

Then the distances between the horizontal and vertical lines of the positioning skin marks and those of the centering skin marks on the axial transverse tomogram are measured and their values divided by the magnification ratio of the axial transverse tomogram. The therapy table is then shifted exactly up or down, right or left in accordance with the value of the distance thus obtained.

The light projectors in the radiation therapy room thus serve for the correct positioning of the patient on the therapy table.

The final position of the light spots on the skin is on the centering skin marks of the patient which correspond to the points A, B and C of the axial transverse tomogram.

After this procedure the isocenter of the rotational unit is located at the center of the region to be treated. This means that the central radiation ray will hit the center of the region to be treated irrespective of the direction of the radiation beam. If the cross-section of the radiation beam is selected by reference to the size of the lesion, the region to be treated will be covered correctly whatever the direction of the beam. Thus, both stationary radiation therapy and moving field therapy can be performed by a simple but exact procedure, with the centering skin marks contributing to the correct conduct of radiation therapy. For conducting either multiportal or moving field therapy, the rotational teleradiation therapy unit is thus recommended.

Even when the stationary teleradiation unit is used with multiportal irradiation, the procedure of planning and positioning of patients is similar to the above. The patient is laid on the therapy table in the same posture as on the tomographic table and the same procedure is followed as in the case of the rotational therapy unit. The size of the radiation beam is adjusted to that of the radiation field, and the central ray is focused with the same direction as the planning on the axial transverse tomogram.

These processes will be carried out by means of the usual light beam localizer.

C. Confirmation of Correct Positioning

Where axial transverse tomography is applied to radiation therapy, it is possible to confirm whether the radiation has been correctly planned during the actual procedure of the radiation therapy. This is the device of beam focus radiography (Fig. 573).

Under the therapy table a rotating disc having a cassette holder is attached, the center of which is located on the extension of the straight line joining the radiation source and the center of the rotational radiation therapy unit. Although the disc rotates around the patient on the therapy table simultaneously with the rotation of the radiation source, the disc itself rotates in inverse direction to the rotation of the radiation source (Fig. 574). As a result, the disc maintains its position relative to the radiation source as it rotates. Thus, the side of the cassette attached to the disc holder stays at right angles to the direction of the radiation beam. 10×12 inch industrial film, is used.

Inside the front cover of the cassette there are horizontal and vertical lines of 0.5 mm lead wire in place of the intensifying screens. The crossing point is adjusted so as to be located at the rotation center of the disc. The image of the lead wire is recorded on the film with the electron rays emitted during exposure of supervoltage rays.

The crossing lines imaged on the film are termed horizontal and vertical standard lines (Fig. 575 c).

In conducting multiportal radiation therapy or moving field therapy, the radiation beam passes through the body and images dense radiation figure of beam focus on the center of this film. This image represents the figure of the treated region. The radiographic method is thus termed beam focus radiography.

The beam focus radiogram is enlarged with the magnification ratio of β.

$$\beta = \frac{A' + B'}{A'}$$

where A' is the distance between the radiation source and the rotation center of the therapy unit and B' is that between the rotation center of the unit and that of the disc.

The axial transverse tomography is not actual size but enlarged with a certain magnification ratio, say α. To get the actual size of the tomogram (Fig. 575 b) and the beam focus radiogram (Fig. 575 c), the radiograms are reduced by multiplying the reciprocal value of the magnification ratio.

When the figures in actual size are obtained, the two radiograms are overlapped by placing the centering vertical and horizontal standard lines of the axial transverse tomogram over those of the beam focus radiogram (Fig. 575 a). The actual location, size and shape of the beam focus within the body is obtained. This procedure enables the confirmation to be made, whether the beam focus correctly covers the region to be treated or not.

In practice, it is troublesome and time-consuming to reduce the tomogram and beam focus radiogram to actual size. Thus the overlapping viewing box is used instead.

The construction of the viewing box is such that there is the following relation between the position of the eye, the axial transverse tomogram and the beam focus radiogram:

$$b = a\left(\frac{\beta}{\alpha} - 1\right)$$

where b is the distance between the beam focus radiogram and the axial transverse tomogram, a is that between the eye and the axial transverse tomogram, α the magnification ratio of the axial transverse tomogram, and β that of the beam focus radiogram.

Taking 50 cm as the distance between the eye and the axial transverse tomogram, the adequate value of b will be given, as α and β are constant in accordance with the distances between the radiation source the rotation center of the unit and that of the films for the axial transverse tomography or for the beam focus radiography.

By arranging the distances between these three points accordingly, the magnification ratio of the beam focus radiogram to the eye becomes the same as that of the axial transverse tomogram. When this viewing box technique is used, the result is effectively similar to reduction of the two radiograms to the actual size.

When the radiation technique is proved to be correct by means of beam focus radiography, the centering skin marks are tattooed intracutaneously with sterilized Indian ink.

After this procedure the positioning of the patient on the therapy table becomes simple, as the centering skin marks are merely made to coincide with the light spots of the projectors.

Usually, in order to confirm the correct coverage of the radiation beam on the treated region, radiograms are taken with the direct beam, such as ^{60}Co γ-ray, and examined. However, the radiogram taken for cancer of the esophagus, for instance, reveals the image of the esophagus with difficulty, due to lack of contrast between the bone, barium and soft tissue and so this method is of limited application.

The method of applying the beam focus radiogram to confirm the correct coverage of the tumor by the radiation beam is considered superior to the method of ^{60}Co γ-ray radiography in that the confirmation is achieved directly and it is known how the beam focus covers the lesion and whether the planning was carried out correctly or not.

The simulator on the other hand is also considered useful for correct positioning and its confirmation. Nevertheless, the whole task of determining the region to be treated, planning by using the isodose chart, positioning and confirmation may be limited when conducted only by means of the simulator.

2. Surgical Operation

According to *Iglauer* (42), *Monod* et al. (79) or *Piazza* (91) axial transverse tomography has contributed to the determination of operability. *Benedetti* (10) studied the chest after operation. *Imaoka* (43) applied rotation radiography to the removal of a foreign body in the thigh.

From the practical point of view, it is not always necessary to know thoroughly the state of lesion before the surgical operation, as more information about the lesion is usually obtainable in the course of the operation than by means of radiological examination. Moreover, trouble arises from the easy change of the relation between the tissue and organs during the operation. Nevertheless, for the puncture or the small incision of a lesion located deep in the body, it will be better to establish the size, location and shape of the lesion before operation. In order to remove a foreign body, determination of its location is also most essential.

Axial transverse tomography will contribute much to the surgical planning of the operation.

Normal radiography will, of course, inform us whether or not the lesion exists, and in what level of the body it is located.

If this lesion cannot be inspected or palpated because of its deep seated location and is considered suitable for treatment by puncture or small excision, the patient is laid on the tomographic table in the position convenient for surgical operation. The level of the lesion on the axial transverse cross section is made to coincide with plane g. For this, fluoroscopic examination or roentgenography with small-sized film will be sometimes useful.

The skin of the patient is illuminated by the three light projectors and the positioning skin marks are determined in the way described on p. 300.

The axial transverse tomogram is made and examined. The tomogram reveals the location, size and shape of the lesion. After that procedure the surgical technique is selected. The patient is laid on the table of the surgical room where the light projectors are set in the walls and ceiling in the same way as in the tomography room.

When performing a biopsy puncture, the location of the point for puncture is selected and called point P (Fig. 576). Next, the angle of the needle of the syringe to the horizontal level and the distance from the tip of the needle of the syringe to the lesion are measured by examining the axial transverse tomogram, bearing in mind what procedure will avoid injury to the critical tissue.

The distance between the point P and the lesion is deduced by multiplying the magnification ratio of the tomogram. The point P which is obtained as the point with the above distance nearest one of the positioning skin marks is marked in ink on the skin of the patient. From this point P the needle is introduced into the skin at the definite angle Φ and depth planned with the axial transverse tomogram.

References

1. Papers on Axial Transverse Tomography

1. *Abreau, de:* Tomografia horizontal do torax. Radiologia (B. Aires) **7**, 223 (1944). Reported by title only in J. Radiol. Électrol. **28**, 10 (1947).

2. *Albertis, P. de:* Contributo della stratigrafia assiale trasversa associata al retro-pneumoperitoneo e alla insufflazione gastrica nello studio della masse abdominali. Minerva med. **50**, 3 (1959).

3. *Alè, G.*, e *L. Macchi:* Studio morfologico e topografico degli aneurismi dell'aorta toracica mediante la tomografia assiale trasversa. Ann. Radiol. diagn. (Bologna) **36**, 303 (1963).

4. *Amisano, P.:* La stratigrafia toracica a strato trasverso. Radiol. med. (Torino) **32**, 418 (1946).

5. — La stratigrafia assiale trasversa nell'età pediatrica. Policlin. infant., Suppl. al fascicolo di Gennaio, 1947.

6. — Three dimensional stratigraphic examination; axial transverse stratigraphy. Part II. Amer. J. Roentgenol. **74**, 777 (1955).

7. *Balestra, Passeri* et *Macarini:* La stratigraphie axiale transversale dans la pathologie de l'appareil pulmonaire. J. Radiol. Électrol. **31**, 462 (1950).

8. *Barenbojm, A. M.:* Die Transversaltomographie als Ergänzungsmethode für die topographische Erfassung hilusnaher Kavernen. Rozhl. Tuberk. **18**, 735 (1958).

9. *Benedetti, G.:* Studio stratigrafico assiale della regione cervicale. Radiol. sperimentale **2**, 110 (1948).

10. — Studio stratigrafico del pneumotorace extrapleurico chirurgico. Minerva med. **2**, 543 (1951).

11. *Bulgarelli, R.*, e *L. Oliva:* Su di un caso di doppio arco aortico associato a probabile morbo di Roger e su due casi accertati di morbo di Roger studiati mediante la stratigrafia assiale trasversa e la stratigrafia frontale. Minerva pediat. **3**, 1 (1951).

12. — — Prime ricerche sulla stratigrafia assiale trasversa associata alla stratigrafia frontale con o senza pneumomediastino anteriore nella tetralogia di Fallot prima e dopo intervento alla Blalock-Taussig e nella sindrome di Eisenmenger. Minerva pediat. **3**, 275 (1951).

13. *Bulgarelli, R.*, e *L. Oliva:* Prime ricerche sulla stratigrafia assiale trasversa associata alla stratigrafia frontale nelle cardiopatie acquisite reumatiche. Minerva pediat. **3**, 311 (1951).

14. — — Prime ricerche sulla stratigrafia assiale trasversa associata alla stratigrafia frontale nella pervietà del dotto di Botallo. Minerva pediat. **3**, 259 (1951).

15. *Buzzi, G.:* La stratigraphie axiale transversale dans la pathologie du médiastin. J. Radiol. Électrol. **31**, 146 (1950).

16. *Chiro, G. di:* Axial transverse encephalography. Amer. J. Roentgenol. **92**, 441 (1964).

17. — Axial transverse encephalography with the radiotome. Medica Mundi **10**, 92 (1965).

18. *Clément, J. P.:* Contribution à l'exploration radiologique de la région pancréatique par la stratigraphie axiale transverse. J. belge Radiol. **48**, 151 (1965).

19. *Duhamel, J.*, e *P. L. Martin:* Considerazioni sulla esatta determinazione del piano dei punti fissi in stratigrafia assiale trasversa. Radiol. med. (Torino) **39**, 1014 (1953).

20. — —, et *J.-C. Roques:* Théorie élémentaire des images induites thoraciques en tomographie axiale transversale. J. Radiol. Électrol. **42**, 470 (1961).

21. *Egan, R.*, and *G. C. Johnson:* Multisection transverse tomography in radium implant calculations. Radiology **74**, 407 (1960).

22. *Farinet, G., G. L. Sannazzari* e *A. Torretta:* La stratigrafia assiale trasversa quale esame complementare della radioisotopografia nello studio degli strumi benigni e maligni. Minerva fisioter radiobiol. **4**, 291 (1959).

23. *Fleischer, H., A. Gebauer* u. *F. Wachsmann:* Verwendung transversaler Schichtaufnahmen bei der Festlegung des Bestrahlungsplanes intrathorakaler Tumoren. Fortschr. Röntgenstr. **76**, 52 (1952).

24. *Frain, C.*, et *F. Lacroix:* Effet stratigraphique et coupes horizontales. C.R. Acad. Sci. (Paris) **224**, 973 (1947).

25. — — Étude expérimentale sur l'obtention de coupes horizontales. Paris méd. **37**, 94 (1947).

26. — — Courbe-enveloppe et coupes horizontales. J. Radiol. Électrol. **28**, 142 (1947).

27. — — De l'obtention de coupes horizontales. J. Radiol. Électrol. **29**, 256 (1948).

28. —, *J. Surmont, M. Tubiana, B. Pierquin, R. Marlois, J. Abbatucci* et *A. Dutreix:* Intéret de la tomographie transversale (coupes horizontales) dans le repérage, le centrage et al dosimétrie des tumeurs thoraciques traitées par radiothérapie transcutanée. J. Radiol. Électrol. **38**, 792 (1955).

29. *Frik, W., C. E. Buchheim* u. *H. Jupitz:* Der Einfluß von Rotationswinkel, Strahleneinfallswinkel und Objektlage auf die Qualität transversaler Schichtaufnahmen. Fortschr. Röntgenstr. **97**, 94 (1962).

30. *Fumagalli, G., A. Passeri* e *D. Vallebona:* Stratigrafia assiale trasversa e spirometria nella valutazione delle alterazioni ventilatorie. Contributo del singolo polmone. Minerva med. **52**, 2731 (1961).

31. *Gardella, G.:* La stratigrafia assiale dell'ilo polmonare. La stratigrafia assiale trasversa, Genova, p. 20 (1947).

32. *Gebauer, A.,* u. *F. Wachsmann:* Geometrische Betrachtungen und technische Fragen zur Herstellung transversaler (horizontaler) Körperschichtaufnahmen. Röntgen-Bl. **2**, 215 (1949).

33. — Körperschichtaufnahmen in transversalen (horizontalen) Ebenen. Fortschr. Röntgenstr. **71**, 669 (1949).

34. — Das transversale Schichtbild des normalen Thorax, ein Beitrag zur topographischen Anatomie am lebenden Menschen. Fortschr. Röntgenstr. **74**, 14 (1951).

35. — Diagnostische Vorteile und Indikationsstellung der Körperschichtaufnahmen in transversalen Ebenen gegenüber denen in vertikalen. Fortschr. Röntgenstr. **75**, 9 (1951).

36. *Giraud, M., Ch. Gros, J. P. Walter, P. Bloch* et *Y. Grumbach:* Exploration du pancréas par la tomographie axiale transverse. J. Radiol. Électrol. **46**, 863 (1965).

37. *Giraud, M., P. Bret, M. Levrat, M. Croisille* et *G. Bousquet:* Exploration radiologique du pancréas par stratigraphie axiale transverse. Bilan de dix années d'expérience. Ann. Radiol. **9**, 563 (1966).

38. *Gremmel, H.:* Die Transversalschichtuntersuchung des Herzens und der großen Gefäße. Fortschr. Röntgenstr. **96**, 3 (1962).

39. *Hachiya, H.,* and *H. Ito:* The rotatory cross-section radiography of hip joint, especially of measuring antetorsion. Centr. Jap. J. orthop. traum. Surg. **2**, 51 (1958) [Japanese].

40. *Hammer, G.:* Quere Schichtaufnahmen mit dem „Transversotom". Wien. med. Wschr. **103**, 464 (1953).

41. *Hartley, J. B.:* Localization by transverse tomography. Brit. J. Radiol. **34**, 550 (1961).

42. *Iglauer, E.:* Das transversale Schichtverfahren und das Pneumomediastinum in der Thoraxchirurgie. Kongreßber. 2. Tagg Med.-Wiss. Ges. Röntgenol. DDR, p. 208 (1958).

43. *Imaoka, M.:* Application of the discontinuous rotatography to the removal of the foreign body. Nippon Acta radiol. **10** (7), 5 (1950) [Japanese].

44. — Rotatory cross section radiography of the gall bladder. Nippon Acta radiol. **12** (8), 32 (1952) [Japanese].

45. *Janker, R.:* Ein Universal-Schichtaufnahmegerät. Fortschr. Röntgenstr. **73**, 253 (1950).

46. *Jucker, C.,* e *B. Pierquin:* Utilità della stratigrafia assiale trasversa nella radioterapia delle neoplasie endotoraciche. Radiol. med. (Torino) **48**, 740 (1962).

47. *Jusztusz, Gy.:* Transversalis rétegfelvételekröl. Magy. Radiol. **3**, 84 (1951).

48. *Kitabatake, T.:* Frequency of tuberculous lesions in the mediastinal lung field. Nagoya J. med. Sci. **18**, 35 (1955).

49. *Kobayashi, T., S. Nitta, S. Kaii,* and *H. Takamura:* Rotatory cross section radiography of chest. J. Juzen med. Soc. **57**, 759 (1955) [Japanese].

50. *Kubota, Y., Y. Sato,* and *M. Yoshida:* Rotatory crossgraphy of pelvis. Hirosaki med. J. **4**, 11 (1953) [Japanese].

51. *Lacroix, F.:* I. Tomographie axiale transverse du membre inférieur. II. De l'importance du role joué en tomographie axiale par le couvercle de la cassette. J. Radiol. Électrol. **40**, 91 (1959).

52. *Levrat, M., P. Mallet-Guy, P. Bret, P. Grandmottet* et *J. Michoulier:* Le diagnostic radiologique des tumeurs endocriniennes du pancréas par la stratigraphie axiale transverse. A propos de deux observations: volumineux épithélioma, petit adénome langheransien kystique. Presse méd. **70**, 679 (1962).

53. *Lodin, H.:* Mediastinal herniation and displacement studied by transversal tomography. Acta radiol. (Stockh.) **48**, 337 (1957).

54. — Transversal tomography of the descending aorta. Acta radiol. (Stockh.) **56**, 251 (1961).

55. — Transversal tomography in the examination of thoracic deformities (Funnel chest and kyphoscoliosis). Acta radiol. (Stockh.) **57**, 49 (1962).

56. *Macarini, N.:* La stratigrafia nello studio dell'ascesso pulmonare, delle cisti da echinococco e delle pneumopatie cistiche. Lezioni del Primo Corse Internaz. Teorico-Pratico di Aggiornamento e Perfezionamento sulla Stratigrafia, 431 (1950).

57. —, e *L. Oliva:* La dimostrazione radiologica diretta del pancreas. Radiol. med. (Torino) **37** (12), 1 (1951).

58. — — Sur l'insufflation retroperitoneale associée a la stratigraphie tridimensionelle. J. belge Radiol. **34**, 281 (1951).

59. *Maestri, A. de:* Metodo di riconoscimento dello strato fisso nella stratigrafia assiale trasversa. Radiol. sperimentale **2**, 118 (1948).

60. — La stratigraphie transversale du thorax en pédiatrie. J. Radiol. Électrol. **31**, 464 (1950).

61. —, e *C. Lombroso:* Studio stratigrafico trasverso nelle iperplasie timiche. Minerva pediat. **3**, 255 (1951).

62. *Martin-Lalande, J.,* et *Y. T. Jean Lo:* Radiotomographie transverse de la trachée dans le médiastin supérieur: Quelques aspects et rapports normaux et pathologiques. Bronches **11**, 209 (1961).

63. *Matsuda, T.:* Rotatory cross section radiography of the chest. Nippon Acta radiol. **12** (2), 14 (1952) [Japanese].

64. — Evaluation of the rotatory cross section radiography applied to chest diseases. Nippon Acta radiol. **12** (10), 31 (1953) [Japanese].

65. — Position of the tuberculous cavity in the thoracs. Nippon Acta radiol. **13**, 485 (1953) [Japanese].

66. —, and *H. Yaguchi:* Rotatory cross section radiography of the upper abdomen insufflated air extraperitoneally. Jap. J. Urol. **45**, 673 (1954) [Japanese].

67. —, and *Y. Sato:* Tomography and rotatory cross section radiography of pulmonary tuberculous cavity. Nippon Acta radiol. **13**, 674 (1954) [Japanese].

68. — Rotatory cross section radiography of the stomach and the duodenum. Nippon Acta radiol. **14**, 197 (1954) [Japanese].

69. — Rotatory cross section radiography of the chest disease. Curr. Med. **5**, 121 (1957) [Japanese].

70. —, *Y. Kubota,* and *M. Yoshida:* High voltage radiographic technique applied to rotatory cross section radiography. Nippon Acta radiol. **16**, 1104 (1957) [Japanese].

71. —, and *T. Watanabe:* Rotatory cross section radiography applied to coverage of radiation beam to malignant tumor. Nippon Acta radiol. **18**, 1584 (1959) [Japanese].

72. —, *K. Ban,* and *S. Endo:* The compensating filter applied to rotatory cross section radiography. Nippon Acta radiol. **26**, 273 (1966) [Japanese].

73. — Moving filter applied to axial transverse tomography. Tohoku J. exp. Med. **94**, 163 (1968).

74. — Adjustment of axial transverse tomograph. Tohoku J. exp. Med. **95**, 331 (1968).

75. — Wedge grid applied to axial transverse tomography. Tohoku J. exp. Med. (in press).

76. *Mattina, M., G. Curiale* e *A. Cricchio:* La tomografia trasversale nello studio del mediastino. Radiol. prat. **14**, 93 (1964).

77. *Moldenhauer, W.:* Indikationen zur Transversaltomographie der Thoraxorgane. Radiol. diagn. (Berl.) **3**, 151 (1962).

References

78. *Monod, R., Ch. Frain* et *P. Court:* L'association tomographie transversale et pneumomédiastin. J. franç. Méd. Chir. thor. **9**, 389 (1955).

79. —, *Roche* et *Parent:* De l'intérêt des tomographies transversales en chirurgie thoracique. Lyon chir. **48**, 897 (1953).

80. *Ode, R.,* and *I. Miura:* Axial transverse tomography of the heart diseases. Therapeutics (Tokyo) **11**, 472 (1957) [Japanese].

81. *Oliva, L.:* Lo studio stratigrafico assiale trasverso dell'aorta toracica patologica. Radiologia (Roma) **6**, 649 (1950).

82. — La stratigrafia assiale trasversa nello studio delle caverne polmonari. Arch. Tisiol. **5**, 292 (1950).

83. — Le possibilità della stratigrafia assiale trasversa a giro parziale. Radiol. med. (Torino) **37**, 433 (1951).

84. *Ono, T.:* The application of the rotatory cross-section radiographing to obstetrics. Nippon Acta radiol. **13**, 141 (1953) [Japanese].

85. — The application of the rotatory cross section radiography to the diagnosis of chest diseases. Nippon Acta radiol. **13**, 469 (1953) [Japanese].

86. — An application to artificial pneumothorax of the rotatory cross-section radiography. Nippon Acta radiol. **13**, 568 (1953) [Japanese].

87. — On the rotatory cross section radiography of lower abdomen. Nippon Acta radiol. **14**, 711 (1955) [Japanese].

88. —, and *T. Sotani:* On the rotatory cross section radiogram of extrapleural thoracoplastic chest. Nippon Acta radiol. **19**, 655 (1959) [Japanese].

89. *Onuma, I.:* Conformation radiotherapy by means of stereosynthesis obtained by the axial transverse multisection radiography. Nippon Acta radiol. **26**, 201 (1966) [Japanese].

90. *Passeri, A.:* La stratigrafia assiale trasversa nella patologia polmonare. Radiol. sperimentale **2**, 122 (1948).

91. *Piazza, A.:* La stratigrafia nello studio delle indicazioni e degli esiti degli interventi chirurgici polmonari collasso-terapici. Lezioni del Primo Corso Internaz. Teorico-Pratico di Aggiornamento e Perfezionamento sulla Stratigrafia, 365—390 (1950).

92. *Pierquin, B., D. Chassagne* et *M. Gasiorowski:* Technique de dosimetrie en curietherapie interstitielle par tomographie transversale. Acta radiol. (Stockh.) **53**, 314 (1960).

93. — La tomographie transversale: Technique de routine en radiothérapie. J. Radiol. Électrol. **42**, 131 (1961).

94. *Pompili, G.,* e *G. Alè:* Molfologia degli strumi tiroidei cervico-toracici ed endotoracici in stratigrafia assiale trasversa. Ann. Radiol. diagn. (Bologna) **34**, 191 (1961).

95. *Retzepis, G.:* La tomographie transversale combinée avec bronchographie zonaire dans l'étude anatomo-radiologique de certaines zônes pulmonaires (Etude expérimentale sur des pièces anatomiques des poumons humains). Rev. Tuberc. (Paris) **17**, 1080 (1953).

96. *Rollandi, A.,* e *G. Reggiani:* Ilo del pulmone e stratigrafia assiale trasversa. Radiol. med. (Torino) **41**, 1087 (1955).

97. *Roswit, B., S. M. Unger, J. Stein, S. J. Malsky,* and *C. B. Reid:* Transverse laminagraphy: the third dimension in body section roentgenography: applications in radiation therapy. Amer. J. Roentgenol. **81**, 130 (1959).

98. — — Tumor localization with transverse tomography: diagnostic and therapeutic applications. Radiology **74**, 705 (1960).

99. *Roussel, J., P. Schoumacher, Pernot, A. Gaucher* et *R. Poire:* Intérêt de la tomographie axiale transversale dans l'étude des tumeurs bronchopulmonaires. Rev. méd. Nancy **83**, 55 (1958).

100. *Sakuma, S.,* and *S. Takahashi:* Beam focus radiography for taking the radiogram of the axial transverse cross section of the treated region in high density of dose. Tohoku J. exp. Med. **87**, 244 (1965).

101. *Sannazzari, G. L.,* e *A. Torretta:* La stratigrafia assiale trasversa nella preparazione die piani di cura radioterapici della neoplasie endotoraciche. Radiol. med. (Torino) **45**, 1 (1959).

102. *Sanquirico, G., R. Cignolini* et *F. Perassi:* La stratigraphie axiale transversale dans l'étude des organes médiastinaux. J. Radiol. Électrol. **31**, 463 (1950).

103. *Sansone, G.,* e *A. de Maestri:* Visualizzazione simultanea del mediastino posteriore ed anteriore dopo insufflazione per vis peridurale. Studio stratigrafico tridimensionale. Minerva pediat. **3**, 332 (1951).

104. — — Ulteriori ricerche sulla visualizzazione degli organi addominali dopo insufflazione retroperitoneale e stratigrafia assiale e trasversa. Minerva pediat. **3**, 328 (1951).

105. — —, *P. Durand* e *N. Macarini:* Pneumoencefalografia e stratigrafia assiale trasversa nel bambino. Minerva pediat. **3**, 358 (1951).

106. —, *N. Macarini* e *G. Corradi:* Studio stratigrafico tridimensionale della vascica dopo insufflazione extraperitoneale. Minerva pediat. **3**, 365 (1951).

107. —, e *A. de Maestri:* Stratigrafia assiale trasversa per lo studio degli organi addominali dopo insufflazione retroperitoneale nel bambino. Minerva med. **137** (1951).

108. —, *N. Macarini* e *L. Oliva:* La visualizzazione del pancreas nel bambino per mezzo della stratigrafia e della insufflazione retroperitoneale. Minerva pediat. **3**, 343 (1951).

109. — — — Nouvelle méthode d'exploration radiologique du pancréas chez l'enfant. J. Radiol. Électrol. **32**, 726 (1951).

110. *Sasaki, T.:* Rotatory cross section radiographic examination of stomach and duodenum of healthy adults in erect and supine position. Nippon Acta radiol. **19**, 1402 (1959) [Japanese].

111. — Axial transverse tomography applied to pancreas. Clin. All-round (Osaka) **14**, 1757 (1965) [Japanese].

112. *Sato, Y.:* Study on deformity of thorax and displacement of mediastinum after thoracoplasty. Observed by the rotatory cross section radiography. Therapeutics (Tokyo) **7** (11), 9 (1953) [Japanese].

113. *Sato, Y.:* Rotatory cross section radiography and artificial pneumoperitoneum. Therapeutics (Tokyo) **8**, 395 (1954) [Japanese].

114. *Schaudig, E.,* u. *J. Kirst:* Das Transversalschichtbild des Mediastinum beim Bronchialkarzinom. Radiol. diagn. (Berl.) **1**, 404 (1960).

115. *Sharma, S. R.,* and *N. G. Gadekar:* Transverse tomography in diagnosis of intrathoracic lesions. Indian. J. Radiol. **16**, 83 (1962).

116. *Shimazaki, T.:* On rotary cross-section radiography. 2. report. Nippon Acta radiol. **12** (5), 29 (1952) [Japanese].

117. — Rotatory cross section radiography. J. med. Soc. Communic. (Tokyo) **5**, 389 (1953) [Japanese].

118. — Rotatory cross section radiography. Kekkaku-Shinryo **9**, 553 (1955) [Japanese].

119. *Stevenson, J. J.:* Horizontal body section radiography. Brit. J. Radiol. **23**, 319 (1950).

120. *Suchán, M.:* Transversal tomography in the diagnosis of pulmonary tuberculosis. Bratisl. lek. Listy **37**, 346 (1963).

121. *Takahashi, S.:* Study on rotation radiography. Aomori-ken Gakuzyutsu-Shinko Kenkyu-Happyo Hokokusho No. **1** (1948) [Japanese].

122. — Rotation radiography. Jap. med. J. **1313**, 3 (1949) [Japanese].

123. —, *M. Imaoka,* and *T. Shinozaki:* Rotatory cross section radiography. Nippon Acta radiol. **10**, 1 (1950) [Japanese].

124. — — Rotatory cross-section radiography of the living human body. Nippon Acta radiol. **10** (8), 29 (1950) [Japanese].

125. — Rotatory cross section radiography of the pulmonary tuberculosis. Jap. J. clin. Tuberc. **9**, 587 (1950) [Japanese].

126. — A method to take radiograms of the transsection of the body at any inclination and curvature. Prel. report. Tohoku J. exp. Med. **52**, 138 (1950).

127. —, and *T. Nikaido:* A method to take a radiogram of the body in three dimensions. Prel. report. Tohoku J. exp. Med. **52**, 144 (1950).

128. *Takahashi, S.:* Study on rotatography. Hirosaki med. J. **2**, 1 (1951) [Japanese].

129. —, *M. Imaoka*, and *T. Shinozaki:* Rotatory cross-section radiography. Study on the rotatography, 4. report. Tohoku J. exp. Med. **54**, 59 (1951).

130. —, *T. Matsuda*, and *T. Nikaido:* Obstructive shadow superimposed to the pulmonary field of the rotatory cross section radiogram of the chest. Nippon Acta radiol. **12** (7), 10 (1952) [Japanese].

131. — *S. Anzai*, and *J. Obara:* Rotatory crossgraphy (rotatory cross section radiography) of ventricles and subarachnoid cisterns. Tohoku J. exp. Med. **56**, 161 (1952).

132. —, and *J. Obara:* Rotatory crossgraphy (rotatory cross section radiography) of the head. Tohoku J. exp. Med. **56**, 311 (1952).

133. — — Rotatory crossgraphy (rotatory cross section radiography) of the neck. Tohoku J. exp. Med. **57**, 17 (1952).

134. — Theory of blurring of X-ray images and occurrence of obstructive shadows in rotatory cross section radiography. Tohoku J. exp. Med. **58**, 63 (1953).

135. —, and *T. Matsuda:* Clinical evaluation of rotatory cross section radiography (rotatory crossgraphy) applied to chest diseases. Tohoku J. exp. Med. **58**, 179 (1953).

136. —, and *T. Shinozaki:* Solidography of the heart. Acta radiol. (Stockh.) **41**, 435 (1954).

137. —, u. *T. Kitabatake:* Über einen Versuch zum ständigen Kontrollieren des Krankheitsherdes bei der Rotationsbestrahlung, mit Hilfe des Prinzips der transversalen Schichtaufnahme. Nagoya J. med. Sci. **17**, 461 (1954).

138. — High voltage macroradiography and high voltage rotation radiography. Recent Advanc. Tuberc. Res. (Tokyo) **15**, 44 (1956) [Japanese].

139. —, and *T. Matsuda:* Simultaneous multisection radiography by means of rotatory cross section radiography. Nippon Acta radiol. **18**, 191 (1958) [Japanese].

140. *Takahashi, S., and T. Matsuda:* Axial transverse laminagraphy applied to rotational therapy. Radiology **74**, 61 (1960).

141. — Axial transverse tomography and beam focus radiography applied to conformation radiotherapy. Jap. J. Cancer Clin. (Tokyo) **10**, 364 (1964) [Japanese].

142. *Takamatsu, I.,* and *Y. Imai:* Axial transverse tomogram of the mediastinal hernia. Hirosaki med. J. **3**, 349 (1952) [Japanese].

143. *Takeuchi, A.:* Experimental study on obstructive shadow formation in axial transverse tomography applied to chest. Nippon Acta radiol. **27**, 134 (1967) [Japanese].

144. — Obstructive shadow of ribs imaged on the axial transverse tomogram of the chest. Nagoya J. med. Sci. **31**, 509 (1969)

145. *Thomas, G.,* u. *A. Stecken:* Transversaltomographie normaler und pathologischer Befunde der Lungengefäße und der Aorta. Radiol. diagn. (Berl.) **2**, 375 (1961).

146. — Transversaltomographie normaler und pathologischer Befunde der Lungengefäße und der Aorta. II. Erweiterung der Diagnostik pathologischer Aortenbefunde durch das Schichtverfahren unter besonderer Berücksichtigung der Transversaltomographie. Radiol. diagn. (Berl.) **3**, 447 (1962).

147. *Vallebona, A.:* Nouvelle méthode roentgenstratigraphique. Radiol. clin. (Basel) **16**, 279 (1947).

148. — Vecchi e nuovi methodi stratigrafici. Radiol. med. (Torino) **33**, 601 (1947).

149. — L'esplorazione stratigrafica tridimensionale. Radiol. sperimentale **2**, 95 (1948).

150. — I nuovi orizzonti della stratigrafia nei verî campi della medicina. Inform. med. (Genova) **2** (4), 1—159 (1948).

151. — Prime ricerche su di un nuovo metodo radiografico: Stratigrafia assiale con radiazioni perpendicolari all'asse. Ann. Radiol. diagn. (Bologna) **20**, 57 (1948).

152. — Transversal Axial Stratography. Sci. med. ital. **1**, 152 (1950).

153. — Axial transverse laminagraphy. Radiology **55**, 271 (1950).

154. *Vallebona, A.:* La stratigrafia nelle sue origini e nei suoi attuali sviluppi. Minerva med. **2** (35), 1 (1950).

155. — Demonstration von transversalen Schichtbildern des Herzens. Fortschr. Röntgenstr. **76**, 508 (1952).

156. — Récents progrès dans le domaine de la stratigraphie. Seventh Internat. Congr. of Radiology (The invited papers). Acta radiol. (Stockh.), Suppl. **116**, 175—183 (1954).

157. — Three dimensional stratigraphic examination; axial transverse stratigraphy. I. Amer. J. Roentgenol. **74**, 769 (1955).

158. — Les récents développements de la stratigraphie et particulièrement de la stratigraphie axiale transversale. Gaz. Hôp. (Paris) **127**, 449 (1955).

159. — Methoden und Hilfsmittel zur Lokalisation tiefliegender Tumoren mit besonderer Berücksichtigung der Bewegungsbestrahlung. Strahlentherapie **97**, 489 (1955).

160. *Vallebona, D.:* La tomografia assiale trasversa nella preparazione del piano di trattamento dei tumori del polmone. Nunt. radiol. (Roma) **31**, 562 (1965).

161. *Vieten, H.:* Grundlagen und Möglichkeiten der Röntgendarstellung von Querschnitten (Transversalschichten) langgestreckter Körper mittels kreisförmiger Verwischung der nicht abzubildenden Objektteile. Fortschr. Röntgenstr. **73**, 226 (1950).

162. *Vignolini, R.:* Studio stratigrafico assiale dei seni costomediastinali. Radiol. med. (Torino) **36**, 36 (1950).

163. *Voigt, O.,* u. *M. Thümmler:* Zur Anwendung des transversalen Schichtverfahrens in der Lungenklinik unter Einsatz eines selbstkonstruierten Gerätes. Z. Tuberk. **118**, 274 (1962).

164. *Vulpian, P. de:* Tomographie transversale thoracique. J. Radiol. Électrol. **33**, 280 (1952).

165. *Wangermez, Ch., A. Rigaud, P. Bonjean* et *J. P. Meyruis:* La stratigraphie axiale transverse dans l'examen de la partie supérieure de l'abdomen. (Confrontations anatomo-radiologiques). J. Radiol. Électrol. **40**, 109 (1959).

166. *Watanabe, T., N. Ono,* and *K. Nagai:* Telecobaltradiation therapy which composed of rotatory cross section radiograph and rotatory conformation therapy unit. Nippon Acta radiol. **23**, 841 (1963) [Japanese].

167. *Watson, W.:* Differential radiography. Radiography **9** (1939).

168. *Wilk, S. P.:* Axial transverse tomography of the chest. Radiology **72**, 42 (1959).

2. Books on Axial Transverse Tomography

169. *Bonte, G., M. Brenot* et *G. Trinez:* La tomographie axiale transversale. Paris: Doin 1955.

170. *Farr, R. F., A. C. H. Scott, R. Ollerenshaw,* and *G. J. H. Everard:* Transverse axial tomography. Oxford: Blackwell Sci. Publ. 1964.

171. *Gebauer, A.,* u. *A. Schanen:* Das transversale Schichtverfahren. Stuttgart: Georg Thieme 1955.

172. —, *E. Muntean, E. Stutz* u. *H. Vieten:* Das Röntgenschichtbild. Stuttgart: Georg Thieme 1959.

173. *Takahashi, S.:* Tomography and axial transverse tomography. Tokyo: Igakushoin 1954 [Japanese].

174. *Takahashi, S.:* Rotation radiography Japan Society for the Promotion of Science. Tokyo: Maruzen 1957.

175. — Conformation radiotherapy. Rotation technique as applied to radiography and radiotherapy of cancer. Stockholm: Acta Radiologica Suppl. 242, 1965.

176. *Vallebona, A.* (by edited): La stratigrafia assiale trasversa. Genova: G. Sambolino e Figli 1947.

177. — Trattato di stratigrafia. Milano: Casa Editrice Dottore F. Vallardi 1952 [Excerpta Medica, Sect. 14, Vol. *7*, p. 97 (383), 1953].

3. Books on Anatomy of Axial Transverse Cross Section

178. *Doyen, E., J. P. Bouchon* et *R. Doyen:* Atlas d'anatomie topographique. Paris: A. Maloine 1911.

179. *Hovelacque, A., O. Monod* et *H. Evrard:* Treize coupes horizontales du thorax. Paris: Librairie Maloine 1938.

180. *Nishi, S., H. Oka, T. Sasa, K. Otsuki,* and *T. Hasegawa:* Clinical demonstration of axial transverse cross section of adult. Tokyo: Kanehara 1949.

181. *Nishi, S.* (by edited): Atlas of human anatomy. Tokyo: Kanehara 1956.

182. *Pernkopf, E.:* Topographische Anatomie des Menschen. München: Urban & Schwarzenberg 1943.

183. *Roy-Camille, R.:* Coupes horizontales du tronc. Paris: Masson & Cie. 1959.

184. *Eycleshymer, A. C.,* and *D. M. Schoemaker:* A cross-section anatomy. New York: D. Appleton-Century Co. 1938.

Author Index

The numbers in *italics* shown in paranteses are the numbers of the references in the bibliography.

Page numbers in *italics* refer to the bibliography.

Author Index

Subject Index

Normal type refers to figure numbers and *italics* refer to page numbers.

Promontorium 378, 381
Prostata 441, 446
Protuberantia occipitalis externa 87, 90
Protuberantia occipitalis interna 42, 72, 75,
 77, 80, 85, 87
Pulmo dexter 164, 169, 174, 179, 184, 189,
 194, 199, 204, 209, 214, 219, 224, 229, 234,
 239, 244, 249, 254, 259, 264, 269, 290
Pulmo dexter: Apex pulmonis 159, 162
Pulmo dexter: Lobus inferior 187, 192, 197,
 202, 207, 212, 217, 222, 227, 232, 237, 242,
 252, 257, 262, 267, 272
Pulmo dexter: Lobus medius 227, 232, 237,
 242, 252, 257, 262
Pulmo dexter: Lobus superior 167, 172, 177,
 182, 187, 192, 197, 202, 207, 212, 217, 222,
 227
Pulmo sinister 164, 169, 174, 179, 184, 189,
 194, 199, 204, 209, 214, 219, 224, 229, 234,
 239, 244, 249, 254, 259, 264, 269, 290
Pulmo sinister: Apex pulmonis 159, 162
Pulmo sinister: Lobus inferior 187, 192, 197,
 202, 207, 212, 217, 222, 227, 232, 237, 242,
 247, 252, 257, 262, 267, 272
Pulmo sinister: Lobus superior 167, 172, 177,
 182, 187, 192, 197, 202, 207, 212, 217, 222,
 227, 232, 237, 242, 252, 257, 262

Radius 477, 479, 481
Radix linguae 100, 105
R. profundus n. radialis 477
R. superficialis n. radialis 477
Rectum 398, 401, 403, 406, 408, 411, 416, 421,
 433, 436, 438, 441, 443, 446, 451, 459, 460
Ren dexter 312, 315, 317, 320, 322, 325, 327,
 330, 332, 335, 337, 340, 342, 345, 347, 350,
 352, 355
Ren sinister 302, 305, 307, 310, 312, 315, 317,
 320, 322, 325, 327, 330, 332, 335, 337, 340,
 342, 345, 347, 350
Retinaculum patellae laterale 492
Retinaculum patellae mediale 492
Rima pudendi 428, 431
Rotation center: Axial transverse tomograph
 8
Rotation center: Radiation therapy unit 574,
 301, 302
Rotation radiography 1

Sarcoidosis 532, 533, 534
Scapula 137, 140, 142, 145
Scapula: Acromion 147, 150

Scapula: Angulus inferior 229, 232
Scapula: Angulus superior 159, 162
Scapula: Facies costalis 172, 182, 202, 207,
 212, 217, 222, 227
Scapula: Fossa infraspinata 172, 202, 207,
 212, 217, 222, 227
Scapula: Margo lateralis 169, 174, 177, 179,
 182, 184, 187, 189, 192, 194, 197, 199, 202,
 204, 207, 209, 212, 214, 217, 219, 222, 224,
 227
Scapula: Margo medialis 147, 150, 169, 174,
 177, 179, 182, 184, 187, 189, 192, 194, 197,
 199, 202, 204, 207, 209, 212, 214, 217, 219,
 222, 224, 227
Scapula: Margo superior 150
Scapula: Spina scapulae 147, 150
Scrotum 453, 456
Septum nasi 70, 75, 77, 80
Simulator 303, 304
Sinus costomediastinalis 232, 237, 242, 247
Sinus frontalis 27, 30, 32, 35, 45, 47, 52, 55,
Sinus maxillaris 72, 75, 77, 80
Sinus occipitalis 85
Sinus petrosus superior 45
Sinus rectus 75
Sinus sagittalis inferior 50
Sinus sagittalis superior 10, 15, 20, 25, 30,
 35, 50, 55, 60, 65, 75
Sinus sigmoideus 75, 80, 85, 90
Sinus sphenoidalis 37, 40, 42, 45, 62, 65, 70,
 72, 75
Spatium retrooesophageum 140
Spatium retropharyngeum 90, 97, 100, 102,
 105, 107, 110, 112, 115, 117, 120, 122, 125,
 130
Spina scapulae 164, 167, 199, 202, 204, 207,
 209, 212
Sulcus lateralis 50
Sulcus parietooccipitalis 25
Suprarenal cyst 549, 550
Symphysis pubica 418, 421, 438, 441, 443,
 446

Talus 501
Tendo calcaneus (Achillis) 501
Tendo musculi bicipitis brachii 475, 477
Tentorium cerebelli 70, 80, 85
Thalamus 20, 30, 55, 60
Thickening of the periosteum 560, 561, 562,
 563
Thorotrast liver 551, 552
Tonsilla palatina 85, 90
Tonsilla pharyngea 102, 105